The Human Illnesses

The Human Illnesses

Neuropsychiatric Disorders and the Nature of the Human Brain

PETER C. WILLIAMSON, MD
Tanna Schulich Chair in Neuroscience and Mental Health
Schulich School of Medicine and Dentistry
University of Western Ontario
London, Ontario, Canada

JOHN M. ALLMAN, PhD
Frank P. Hixon Professor of Neurobiology
Division of Biology
California Institute of Technology
Pasadena, California

OXFORD
UNIVERSITY PRESS

2011

OXFORD
UNIVERSITY PRESS

Oxford University Press, Inc., publishes works that further
Oxford University's objective of excellence
in research, scholarship, and education.

Oxford New York
Auckland Cape Town Dar es Salaam Hong Kong Karachi
Kuala Lumpur Madrid Melbourne Mexico City Nairobi
New Delhi Shanghai Taipei Toronto

With offices in
Argentina Austria Brazil Chile Czech Republic France Greece
Guatemala Hungary Italy Japan Poland Portugal Singapore
South Korea Switzerland Thailand Turkey Ukraine Vietnam

Published by Oxford University Press, Inc.
198 Madison Avenue, New York, New York 10016

www.oup.com

Library of Congress Cataloging-in-Publication Data
Williamson, Peter, 1953-
The Human illnesses : neuropsychiatric disorders and the nature of the human brain /
Peter C. Williamson, John M. Allman.
p.; cm.
Other title: Neuropsychiatric disorders and the nature of the human brain
Includes bibliographical references and index.
ISBN 978-0-19-536856-7
1. Mental illness. 2. Nervous system--Diseases. 3. Neuropsychiatry. I. Allman,
John Morgan. II. Title. III. Title: Neuropsychiatric disorders and the nature
of the human brain.
[DNLM: 1. Mental Disorders--physiopathology.
2. Brain--physiopathology. WM 140 W732h 2011]
RC473.N48W55 2011
616.89—dc22

2010011751

1 3 5 7 9 8 6 4 2
Printed in the United States of America
on acid-free paper

This volume is dedicated to John Hughlings Jackson, Emil Kraepelin, Leo Kanner, and Arnold Pick—great clinicians who understood the nature of human illnesses.

Preface

The field of psychiatry has undergone profound changes over the past century. Beginning as an offshoot of neurology, it gradually became a psychological discipline with the popularity of psychoanalysis. In the past few decades, the swing has been almost as far in the opposite direction, to neuropsychopharmacology and molecular genetics. Many of these changes have been good for psychiatry: new treatments have emerged and much has been learned about genes associated with neuropsychiatric conditions. Although there are promising genetic correlates of some neuropsychiatric disorders such as frontotemporal dementia, no major genes have emerged to explain a substantial incidence of any of the major psychiatric disorders, and all too often treatments fall short of expectations. If we hope to better understand neuropsychiatric disorders, we are going to have to take a different approach.

One of the best clues about the nature of neuropsychiatric disorders has largely been ignored in recent years, and that clue is that these are human disorders. If we could understand more about what makes the human brain unique, then maybe we might understand how it breaks down, resulting in these conditions. The brain breaks down in discrete ways, and how it breaks down tells us something about how it was put together. What makes the human brain human is far from clear at this point, but we are beginning to understand some things about its nature.

We are also beginning to understand something about the neuronal pathways involved in major psychiatric disorders. Brain imaging allows us to look at brain structure, function, and chemistry as never before in these conditions. As we begin to understand these neuronal pathways, we could learn something about what makes us human. The pendulum is beginning to swing back, offering psychiatry another chance to regain a balance between neurobiological and psychological approaches to understanding neuropsychiatric conditions.

Our thesis is that the neuronal pathways that underlie neuropsychiatric conditions mirror unique human capabilities. Determining how these capabilities are represented in the human brain not only tells us about what makes the human brain human but also provides a framework for understanding neuropsychiatric disorders in a new way, much the same as the circulatory system provided a framework for understanding heart failure at the beginning of medicine 400 years ago.

The task of describing, let alone making sense of, such a diverse and complicated literature is a daunting one. We believed that the task required the cooperative effort of both a clinical neuropsychiatrist and an evolutionary biologist. In the process of working on this volume, we both learned a great deal, but we realized that it is impossible to be comprehensive in all fields, so we apologize in advance regarding shortcomings to specialists in the many fields on which we have touched. However, we hope we have captured a perspective that might be useful to clinicians and investigators working in these fields.

We would like to express our appreciation to the Schulich family for their generous support of the Tanna Schulich Chair in Neuroscience and Mental Health (P.W.) and to the Hixon family for the Frank P. Hixon Chair of Neurobiology (J.A.) and additional support from the James S. McDonnell Foundation, the Simons Foundation, the National Institutes of Mental Health, and the Canadian Institutes of Health Research. We would also like to thank Atiya Hakeem for the preparation of many of the illustrations and Sheri Bradshaw and Kathy Stuart for their assistance in preparing the manuscript.

Contents

The Human Illnesses

1

The Human Illnesses

Naturally occurring animal equivalents of some neuropsychiatric disorders such as depression, obsessive-compulsive disorder, and simple phobia can be found in many species. However, other more complex disorders, like schizophrenia, bipolar disorder, autism, and frontotemporal dementia, seem to be uniquely human illnesses. Like our vulnerability to disorders of the hip and knees—probably the consequence of our recently evolved bipedal stance—we believe our vulnerability to these neuropsychiatric illnesses is the consequence of our recently evolved capacity to live in complex social networks that persist in time but are continually changing in ways that often require rapid adaptation. Natural selection has endowed us with the molecular and neuronal systems to sustain both bipedal posture and the capacity to function in intricate social networks, but due to the recent and not yet stable nature of these adaptations and their enormous complexity, they carry with them the inherent vulnerability to dysfunction. Granted, it is possible to model some features of these disorders in animals with drugs and lesions during brain development. These models are helpful but always fall short of the actual conditions. Animals do not have language as we know it, nor do they likely experience a sense of self rooted in time and space as we do. They do seem to experience many of the same emotions that we do, but curiously they do not seem vulnerable to the exaggerated cycles of extreme elation and agitation followed by inactivity and sadness seen in many patients with bipolar disorder.

Descriptions of patients with disorders that resemble schizophrenia and bipolar disorder suggest that these disorders have been around since the beginning of civilization (Angst and Marneros, 2001; Jeste et al., 1985). It is likely that the same can said for autism and frontotemporal dementia, although it is difficult to separate them from other conditions on the basis of literary descriptions. While we sometimes think of these disorders as having been always present, there is actually a rich history of evolving concepts leading to our present classification system. One of the most important figures in this history is John Hughlings Jackson.

JOHN HUGHLINGS JACKSON (1835–1911)

John Hughlings Jackson worked in London at a time when many of the principal conditions in neurology were characterized. His influence was widespread, yet he was described as reclusive and notoriously difficult to engage in conversation. While most of his colleagues were preoccupied with clinical description, he developed a theoretical approach that still underpins our understanding of clinical neuroscience (Andermann, 1997; Swash, 2005).

Jackson was strongly influenced by Herbert Spencer's ideas on the evolution of the brain (Smith, 1982). Essentially, he saw three levels in which complex functions were superimposed on lower-level functions during evolution. Although the hierarchy was not strictly anatomical, the lowest level consisted mostly of the spinal cord and brainstem related to vegetative functions. The middle level

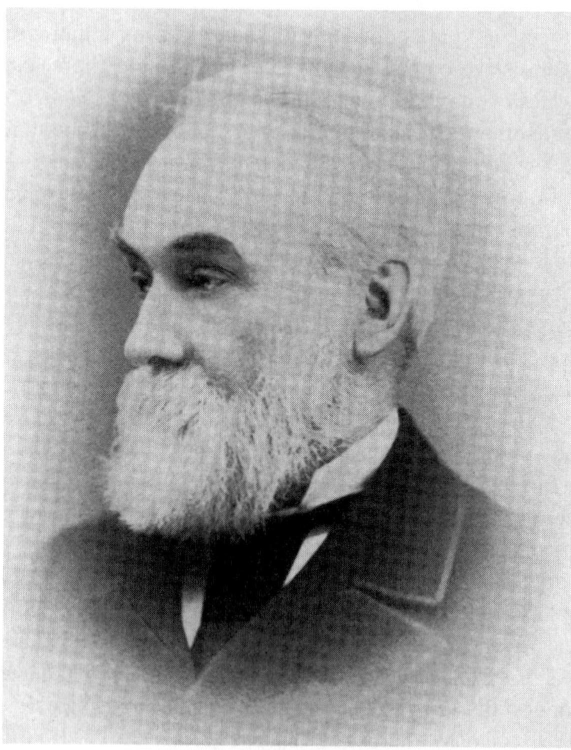

John Hughlings Jackson

included much of the basal ganglia, while the highest level, which was associated with higher cortical functions, included the prefrontal and occipital cortices. Complexity, specialization, integration, and interconnectedness were evident from the lowest to the highest level (Jackson, 1932a). Diseases of the nervous system were suggested to result from a "dissolution" or "reversal of evolution." In the case of aphasia, hemiplegia, and epilepsy, dissolution was proposed in lower cerebral centers, whereas insanity dissolution was seen as beginning in the "highest of all centres" (Jackson, 1932b).

In a paper on mental disorders published in *Medical Press and Circular* in 1882, Jackson (1932c, pp. 46-47) wrote:

> Disease is said to "cause" the symptoms of insanity. I submit that disease only produces negative mental symptoms answering to the dissolution, and that all elaborate positive mental symptoms (illusions, hallucinations, delusions, and extravagant conduct) are the outcome of activity of the nervous elements untouched by any pathological process; that they arise during activity on the lower level of evolution remaining. The principle may be illustrated in another way, without undue capitulation. Starting this time with health, the assertion is that each person's normal thought and conduct are, or signify survivals of the fittest states of what we may call the topmost "layer" of his highest centres: the normal highest level of evolution. Now, suppose that from disease the normal highest level of evolution (the topmost layer) is rendered functionless. This is the dissolution, to which answer the negative symptoms of the patient's insanity. I contend that his positive mental symptoms are still the survivals of his fittest states, are survivals on the lower, but then highest level of evolution. The most absurd mentation, and most extravagant actions in insane people are the survivals of their fittest states.

We see in Jackson's writing the suggestion that mental illness arises from the effects of deficit or *negative* symptoms in highest centers leading to *positive* or irritative symptoms in connected parts of the brain. The idea of negative and positive symptoms was widely applied in neurology and remains to this day as the positive and negative symptoms of schizophrenia. Jackson clearly saw mental disorders as human illnesses.

Jackson suggested that the type of insanity was related to the site of the deficit in higher cortical centers, anticipating current debates about hypofrontality and laterality anomalies in psychosis. He wrote (1932c, pp. 47–48):

> Disease may occur on any evolutionary level, on one side or both sides; it may affect sensory elements chiefly, or the motor elements chiefly. It must be particularly mentioned that there are local dissolutions of the highest centres. It will be granted that, in every case of insanity, the highest centres are morbidly affected. Since there are different kinds, as well as degrees, of insanity (for examples, general paralysis and melancholia), it follows of necessity that different divisions of the highest centres are morbidly affected in the two cases. Different kinds of insanity are different local dissolutions of the highest centres.

However, it was Emil Kraepelin who moved us toward our current classification system of psychotic disorders.

EMIL KRAEPELIN (1856–1926)

Emil Kraepelin worked for much of his career at Heidelberg with Franz Nissl, one of the pioneers of neurohistology, and Aloysius Alzheimer, who discovered the disease named after him in 1906. In 1899, in the sixth edition of his textbook on psychiatric disorders, Kraepelin separated a condition that he called *dementia praecox* from the *manic-depressive psychoses* on the basis of their symptomatology and clinical course. It was a brilliant deduction that eventually led to the current *Diagnostic and Statistical Manual of Mental Disorders, Fourth Edition, Text Revision* (DSM-IV-TR) classification system of psychiatric disorders. In fact, Shorter (1997) has suggested that it is "Kraepelin, not Freud, who is the central figure in the history of psychiatry."

Patients with dementia praecox were found to suffer both negative and positive symptoms, although he did not use those terms. Kraepelin's descriptions of

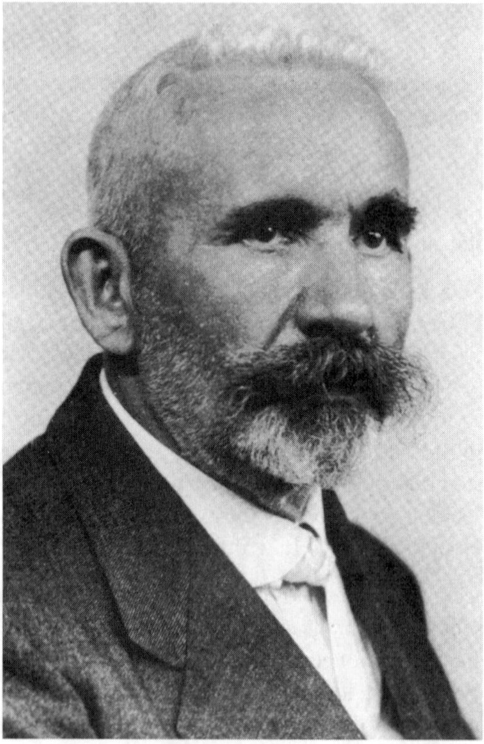

Emil Kraepelin. Photograph originally appeared in the *American Journal of Psychiatry* (Copyright 1927). Used with permission. American Psychiatric Association.

these conditions are truly remarkable. Negative symptoms included emotional dullness and a singular indifference toward others. To patients, "nothing matters" and "everything is the same." They had "no real joy in life and no human feelings." At the same time patients experienced positive symptoms such as hallucinations and delusions. Kraepelin had the following observations on hallucinations (1919, pp. 7–8):

> Sometimes it is only a whispering, "as if it concerned me" as a patient says, a secret language, "taunting the captive"; sometimes the voices are loud or suppressed, as from a ventriloquist, or the call of a telephone, "children's voices"; a patient heard "gnats speak." Sometimes they shout as a chorus or all confusedly; a patient spoke of "drumming in the ear"; another heard, "729,000 girls." Sometimes the voices appear to have a metallic sound, they are "resonant voices," "organ voices," or as of a tuning fork. At other times they do not appear to the patients as sense perceptions at all; they are "voices of conscience," "voices which do not speak with words," "voices of dead people," "false voices," "abortive voices." A patient said: "It appeared to me in spirit, as though they would find fault, without having heard it." There is an "inner feeling in the soul," an "inward voice in the thoughts"; "it is thought inwardly in me"; yet "sounded as if thought."

Delusions included the sense that "one's thoughts are being influenced" and sometimes the perception of knowing the thoughts of other people. His patients reported that they were frequently watched through the telephone or "connected up by wireless telegraphy or by Tesla currents," which seems now ironic with the advent of MR imagers that are quantified by Tesla units. Patients also suffered delusions of persecution and grandiose delusions (Kraepelin, 1919, p. 29):

> The patient is "something better," born to a higher place, the "glory of Israel," an inventor, a great singer, can do what he will. He is noble, of royal blood, an officer of dragoons, heir to the Throne of Bulgaria; Wilhelm Rex, the Kaiser's son, the greatest man in Germany, more than king or Kaiser. Or he is the chosen one, the prophet, influenced by the Holy Ghost, guardian angel, second Messiah, Saviour of the world, the little God who distributes grace and love, more than the Holy Ghost, the Almighty.

Kraepelin felt that memory was little affected, but he did observe that some patients had an "incoherence of the train of thought," resulting in marked disturbances in behavior and judgment (Kraepelin, 1919, p. 56):

> The most different ideas follow one another with most bewildering want of connection, even when the patients are quite quiet. A patient said, "Life is a dessert-spoon," another, "We are already standing in the spiral under a hammer," a third, "Death will be awakened by the golden dagger," a fourth, "The consecrated discourse cannot be over split in any movement."

In contrast to dementia praecox, manic-depressive illness was characterized (Kraepelin, 1921) by *manic states* and *melancholia* or *depressive states*. In some cases there was a mixture of both states. During mania, Kraepelin (1921, p. 63) observed:

> Mood is unrestrained, merry, exultant, occasionally visionary or pompous, but always subject to frequent variation, easily changing to irritability and irascibility or even lamentation and weeping.

During depressive periods, Kraepelin found a very different presentation (1921, p. 76):

> Mood is sometimes dominated by a profound inward dejection and gloomy hopelessness, sometimes more by indefinite anxiety and restlessness. The patient's heart is heavy, nothing can permanently rouse his interest, nothing gives him pleasure. He has no longer any humour or any religious feeling, he is unsatisfied with himself, has become indifferent to his relatives and to whatever he formerly liked best. Gloomy thoughts arise, his past and even his future appear to him in a uniformly dim light. He feels that he is worth nothing, neither physically nor mentally, he is no longer any use, appears to himself "like a murderer." His life has been a blunder, he is not suited for his calling, wants to take up a new occupation, should have arranged his life differently, should have pulled himself together more.

In addition to changes in mood, Kraepelin observed physical or vegetative symptoms. During depressive states, some patients had a "total absence of energy," while the opposite was often seen during mania. Sleep and appetite were affected in both states, with almost complete sleeplessness in some patients during mania. Delusions and hallucinations could also occur in some patients. Although they differed among patients, manic patients tended to develop grandiose delusions consistent with their mood. Depressed patients tended to develop ideas of persecution and hypochondriacal delusions (Kraepelin, 1921, p. 84):

> Ideas of persecution frequently exist in the closest connection with the delusion of sin. Disgrace and scorn await the patient everywhere; he is dishonourable, cannot let himself be seen anywhere any more. People look at him, put their heads together, clear their throats, spit in front of him. They disapprove of his presence, feel it as an insult, cannot tolerate him any longer among them; he is a thorn in the side to all. Speeches in the club have reference to him; there is secret talking of stories about females; he is a bully, should hang himself, because he has no character.

Dementia praecox was viewed, as the name implied, as a progressively deteriorating illness, but Kraepelin realized that the course of dementia praecox was extremely variable: some followed a malignant downward course, while others had periodic exacerbations with some degree of recovery in between. In the time before antipsychotic medication, the periods of improvement rarely lasted longer than 3 years. Manic-depressive illness was seen as a more benign illness. Attacks of mania could last a few days, several months, or longer. Depressive episodes tended to be longer, with variable periods of remission in between. Some features helped distinguish the two conditions (Kraepelin, 1921, p. 197):

> A well-marked manic or cyclothymic predisposition scarcely leads to dementia praecox; also the occurrence of mania or melancholia in parents or brothers and sisters will point in this direction, though certainly by no means absolutely. The question is more difficult to decide in individuals with depressive or irritable predisposition. It appears that here we must keep separate several, externally similar forms. Softness, sensitivity, dejection, lack of self-confidence are found to a greater extent in the previous history of manic-depressive insanity, shy, whimsical, repellent conduct in that of dementia praecox.

Kraepelin recognized that there were patients who suffered from depressive states that were not followed by manic episodes; however, he viewed these patients as having a variant of manic-depressive illness rather than a separate condition. This position was reconsidered by Leonhard, who suggested that some patients suffering only recurrent depressive episodes should be designated *monopolar* (later *unipolar*), while those with manic episodes should be referred to as *bipolar* (Leonhard, 1957). He noted that those patients with a history of mania had a higher incidence of mania in family members compared to those with recurrent depression; this was subsequently supported by more systematic family studies. Consequently, current classification systems distinguish between unipolar and bipolar mood disorders.

Eugen Bleuler broadened the concept of dementia praecox and coined the term *schizophrenia* in 1911 (Shorter, 1997), which eventually replaced the earlier term. Both dementia praecox and manic-depressive psychosis were suggested to begin in the second or third decade of life in the majority of cases. Bleuler recognized childhood cases, but it was not until 1943 that autistic disorders were recognized as being distinct from childhood schizophrenia (Kanner, 1965).

LEO KANNER (1894–1981)

Leo Kanner worked at Johns Hopkins Medical School in Baltimore for much of his career. In his memory, Leon Eisenberg (1981) wrote:

> As much as any one man can be so credited, he was the father of child psychiatry in the Americas. He was a man with a passion for social justice; a great teacher; a loving father, grandfather, and great-grandfather; and a scholar of great learning.
>
> Most astonishing of all was his capacity for entering the world of the child. Puffing away at his omnipresent cigar, he was a veritable Pied Piper whom no child could resist. He cared for children; they trusted him and told what they could reveal to no other.

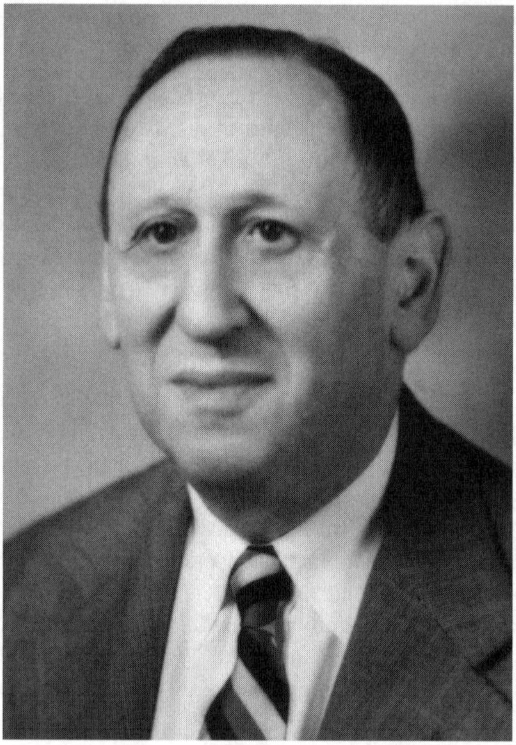

Leo Kanner

In 1943, Kanner published a careful clinical description of children with "autistic disturbances of affective contact," later known as "infantile autism." The group included 11 children, eight boys, and three girls, in keeping with an increased incidence in boys. A father of a 5-year-old boy observed (Kanner, 1943, p. 218):

> He seemed to be self-satisfied. He had no apparent affection when petted. He does not observe the fact that anyone comes or goes, and never seems glad to see father or mother or any playmate. He seems to draw into his shell and live within himself.

The mother of another child commented of her 6-year-old son (Kanner, 1943, p. 222):

> He doesn't care to play with the ordinary things that other children play with, anything with wheels on. He is afraid of mechanical things; he runs from them. He used to be afraid of my egg-beater, is perfectly petrified of my vacuum cleaner. Elevators are simply a terrifying experience for him. He is afraid of spinning tops.

Language development also seemed to be affected. The mother of a 3.5-year-old boy noted (Kanner, 1943, p. 233):

> Language developed slowly; he seemed to have no interest in it. He seldom tells experience. He still confuses pronouns. He never asks questions in the form of questions (with the appropriate inflection). Since he talked, there has been a tendency to repeat over and over one word or statement. He almost never says a sentence without repeating it. Yesterday, when looking at a picture, he said many times, "Some cows standing in the water." We counted fifty repetitions, then he stopped after several more and then began over and over.

At the same time, their rote memory was excellent, which often led the parents to "stuff them with more and more verses, zoologic and botanic names." Children frequently repeated what they had just heard (echolalia) and personal pronouns were repeated as heard without regard to *you* or *I*. Physically, the children were essentially normal, and all came from highly intelligent families (Kanner, 1943). Speaking of the preference of autistic children to static environments and inanimate objects, Kanner (1943, p. 246) observed:

> Objects that do not change their appearance and position, that retain sameness and never threaten to interfere with the child's aloneness, are readily accepted by the autistic child. He has a good relation to objects; he is interested in them, can play with them happily for hours. He can be very fond of them, or get angry at them if, for instance, he cannot fit them into a certain space. When with them, he has a gratifying sense of undisputed power and control.

Speaking of the relationship of autistic children to people, Kanner (1943, pp. 246–247) observed:

> The children's relation to people is altogether different. Every one of the children, upon entering the office, immediately went after blocks, toys, or other objects, without paying the least attention to the persons present. It would be wrong to say that they were not aware of the presence of persons. But the people, so long as they left the child alone, figured in about the same manner as did the desk, the bookshelf, or the filing cabinet.... Conversations going on in the room elicited no interest...he never looked into anyone's face. If an adult forcibly intruded himself by taking a block away or stepping on an object that the child needed, the child struggled and became angry with the hand or the food, which was dealt with per se and not as a part of the person. He never addressed a word or a look to the owner of the hand or foot.

Hans Asperger published a paper just one year after Kanner's classic paper on autism. It described four boys with impairments in social interaction. These patients resembled autistic patients in some ways but suffered from a milder disorder with no delay in cognitive development or language development.

Asperger (1944, p. 82) observed that another characteristic of autistic children is the absence of a sense of humor:

> They do not understand jokes, especially if the joke is on them. This is another reason for their often being the butt of teasing; if one can laugh at oneself, one can take the edge off of ridicule.

Unfortunately, Asperger's work was published in German and was not recognized outside of German-speaking countries for almost 50 years, when *Asperger's disorder* was included in the ICD-10 and DSM-IV classification systems (Neumärker, 2003).

ARNOLD PICK (1851–1924)

Behavioral disturbances are also common at the other end of the life cycle. Arnold Pick was a Czechoslovakian neurologist and psychiatrist who trained in Vienna in the same place as Carl Wernicke and worked for much of his career in Prague. He was known as an excellent clinician who held Hughlings Jackson

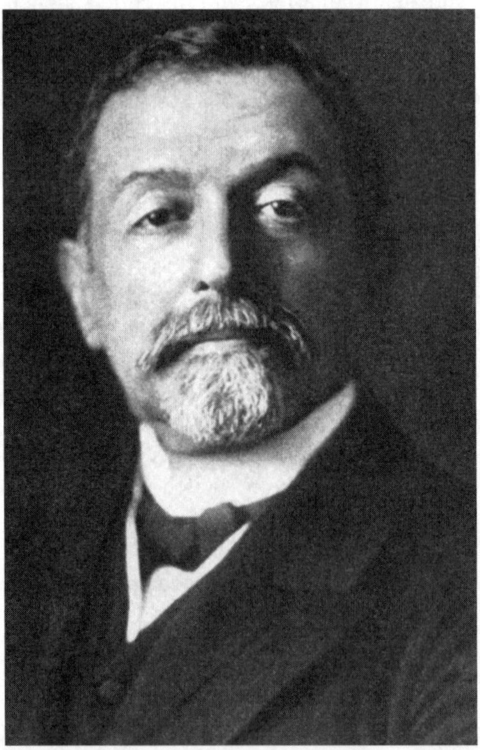

Arnold Pick. From Haymaker, W., and Schiller, F. (1970). *The Founders of Neurology.* Courtesy of Charles C. Thomas Publisher, Ltd., Springfield, Illinois.

in high esteem. In fact, he kept Jackson's portrait on his desk, and Jackson popularized Pick's work in England (Kertesz and Kalvach, 1996).

In a series of articles beginning in 1892, Pick described a patient with aphasic dementia and circumscribed lobar atrophy. Alzheimer later described inclusion bodies on postmortem examination that were associated with circumscribed atrophy; these were eventually known as Pick's bodies. Over time, frontal degeneration and personality changes were labeled as Pick's disease (Graff-Radford and Woodruff, 2007), although it became clear that patients with lobar atrophy did not often have Pick's bodies.

In the past few decades there has been increasing interest in slowly progressive aphasia without generalized dementia. Pick's disease is now generally considered to be a form of frontotemporal dementia. Frontotemporal dementias are divided into three clinical syndromes: frontotemporal dementia, progressive non-fluent aphasia, and semantic dementia. Frontotemporal dementia is a behavioral syndrome associated with progressive changes in social and personal conduct, disinhibition, and lack of insight. Progressive non-fluent aphasia is a type of aphasia with preservation of word meaning and other cognitive functions such as memory. Semantic dementia is a multimodal disorder of meaning (Mariani et al., 2006; Neary et al., 1998).

CURRENT DSM-IV-TR CLASSIFICATION

It is striking how closely the DSM-IV-TR classification system of psychiatric disorders (American Psychiatric Association, 2000) follows the categories and criteria described by Kraepelin more than a century before. However, schizophrenia is considered to be just one of several psychotic disorders, which include schizophreniform disorder, delusional disorder, brief psychotic disorder, shared psychotic disorder, psychotic disorder due to a general medical condition, substance-induced psychotic disorder, and psychotic disorder not otherwise specified. Kraepelin would likely have approved of these distinctions. He recognized milder forms of dementia praecox, which he referred to as the paraphrenias (Kraepelin, 1919). He also described a condition he called paranoia that is very similar to delusional disorder (Kraepelin, 1921). This system is under revision, but DSM-V is likely to retain the distinction between schizophrenia and bipolar disorders.

The DSM-IV-TR criteria for schizophrenia are shown in Box 1.1. The characteristic symptoms include both positive symptoms such as delusions, hallucinations, and disorganized speech and behavior and negative symptoms such as flat affect, alogia (poverty of speech), and avolition or an inability to initiate and persist in goal-directed activities. Only one of these symptoms is required if delusions are bizarre or hallucinations consist of a voice keeping up a running commentary on the person's behavior or thoughts or there are two or more voices conversing with each other. Consistent with Kraepelin's dementia praecox, schizophrenia is seen as a deteriorating disorder associated with disturbance in work, interpersonal relations, or self-care for at least a 6-month period.

Box 1.1 : DSM-IV-TR Diagnostic Criteria for Schizophrenia

A. *Characteristic symptoms*: Two (or more) of the following, each present for a significant portion of time during a 1-month period (or less if successfully treated):

(1) delusions
(2) hallucinations
(3) disorganized speech (e.g., frequent derailment or incoherence)
(4) grossly disorganized or catatonic behavior
(5) negative symptoms, i.e., affective flattening, alogia, or avolition

Note: Only one Criterion A symptom is required if delusions are bizarre or hallucinations consist of a voice keeping up a running commentary on the person's behavior or thoughts, or two more voices conversing with each other.

B. *Social/occupational dysfunction:* For a significant portion of the time since the onset of the disturbance, one or more major areas of functioning such as work, inter-personal relations, or self-care are markedly below the level achieved prior to the onset (or when the onset is in childhood or adolescence, failure to achieve expected level of interpersonal, academic, or occupational achievement).

C. *Duration:* Continuous signs of the disturbance persist for at least 6 months. This 6-month period must include at least 1 month of symptoms (or less if successfully treated) that meet Criterion A (i.e., active-phase symptoms) and may include periods of prodromal or residual symptoms. During these prodromal or residual periods, the signs of the disturbance may be manifested by only negative symptoms or two or more symptoms listed in Criterion A present in an attenuated form (e.g., odd beliefs, unusual perceptual experiences).

D. *Schizoaffective and Mood Disorder exclusion:* Schizoaffective Disorder and Mood Disorder With Psychotic Features have been ruled out because either (1) no Major Depressive, Manic, or Mixed Episodes have occurred concurrently with the active-phase symptoms; or (2) if mood episodes have occurred during active-phase symptoms, their total duration has been brief relative to the duration of the active and residual periods.

E. *Substance/general medical condition exclusion:* The disturbance is not due to the direct physiological effects of a substance (e.g., a drug of abuse, a medication), or a general medical condition.

F. *Relationship to a Pervasive Developmental Disorder:* If there is a history of Autistic Disorder or another Pervasive Developmental Disorder, the additional diagnosis of Schizophrenia is made only if prominent delusions or hallucinations are also present for at least a month (or less if successfully treated).

Mood disorders in DSM-IV-TR also follow the basic distinctions made by Kraepelin (Kraepelin, 1921). However, they are also influenced by Leonhard's ideas about monopolar (unipolar) and bipolar disorders. Thus, major depressive disorder stands alone and is distinguished from milder forms, including dysthymic disorder and depression not otherwise specified. Bipolar I disorder comes closest to Kraepelin's manic-depressive insanity and is characterized by one or more manic or mixed episodes, usually accompanied by major depressive episodes. Bipolar II disorder is characterized by one or more major depressive episodes accompanied by at least one hypomanic episode. Other mood disorders include the milder cyclothymic disorder and bipolar disorder not otherwise specified, as well as mood disorder due to a general medical condition and substance-induced mood disorder.

The DSM-IV-TR criteria for a major depressive episode are shown in Box 1.2. Key to the diagnosis is the presence of depressed mood or markedly diminished interest or pleasure most of the day, nearly every day for a 2-week period, associated with vegetative symptoms similar those described by Kraepelin, including sleep difficulty, fatigue, and weight changes, as well as poor concentration, feelings of worthlessness, and suicidal ideation.

The criteria for a manic episode are shown in Box 1.3. In this disorder, a period of abnormally elevated expansive or irritable mood lasting at least a week is accompanied by inflated self-esteem, decreased need for sleep, pressure of speech, flight of ideas, distractibility, increased activity, and excessive involvement in pleasurable activities to the point that there is marked impairment in social relations or occupational functioning. A hypomanic episode is characterized by mood change and the associated symptoms for at least 4 days and is not severe enough to lead to marked impairment or psychotic symptoms.

The comorbidity of schizophrenia and mood disorders in some patients is categorized as a schizoaffective disorder in DSM-IV-TR. In this disorder, there is a period of illness in which there is a major depressive episode, a manic episode, or a mixed episode concurrent with symptoms that meet Criterion A for schizophrenia. During this period of illness, there must be delusions or hallucinations for at least 2 weeks in the absence of mood symptoms. Symptoms cannot be due to the physiological effects of a substance or a general medical condition.

DSM-IV-TR distinguishes a number of pervasive developmental disorders, including autistic disorder, Rett's disorder, childhood disintegrative disorder, and Asperger's disorder. The criteria for autistic disorder are shown in Box 1.4. Essentially they are the same as those described by Kanner, falling into different aspects of social interaction impairment, communication impairment, and restricted repetitive and stereotyped patterns of behavior, interests, and activities prior to the age of 3. Rett's disorder is distinguished from autism by a higher incidence in girls, a characteristic pattern of head growth deceleration, loss of acquired hand skills, and the appearance of poorly coordinated gait or trunk movements. Childhood disintegrative disorder has a distinctive pattern of severe developmental regression in multiple areas of functioning following at least 2 years of normal development, in contrast to autistic disorder, where developmental abnormalities are usually noted in the first year of life. Asperger's disorder

Box 1.2 : DSM-IV-TR Diagnostic Criteria for Major Depressive Episode

A. Five (or more) of the following symptoms have been present during the same 2-week period and represent a change from previous functioning; at least one of the symptoms is either (1) depressed mood or (2) loss of interest or pleasure.

Note: Do not include symptoms that are clearly due to a general medical condition, or mood-incongruent delusions or hallucinations.

(1) depressed mood most of the day, nearly every day, as indicated by either subjective report (e.g., feels sad or empty) or observation made by others (e.g., appears tearful). **Note:** In children and adolescents, can be irritable mood.
(2) markedly diminished interest or pleasure in all, or almost all, activities most of the day, nearly every day (as indicated by either subjective account or observation made by others)
(3) significant weight loss when not dieting or weight gain (e.g., a change of more than 5% of body weight in a month), or decrease or increase in appetite nearly every day. **Note:** In children, consider failure to make expected weight gains.
(4) insomnia or hypersomnia nearly every day
(5) psychomotor agitation or retardation nearly every day (observable by others, not merely subjective feelings of restlessness or being slowed down)
(6) fatigue or loss of energy nearly every day
(7) feelings of worthlessness or excessive or inappropriate guilt (which may be delusional) nearly every day (not merely self-reproach or guilt about being sick)
(8) diminished ability to think or concentrate, or indecisiveness, nearly every day (either by subjective account or as observed by others)
(9) recurrent thoughts of death (not just fear of dying), recurrent suicidal ideation without a specific plan, or a suicide attempt or a specific plan for committing suicide.

B. The symptoms do not meet criteria for a Mixed Episode.
C. The symptoms cause clinically significant distress or impairment in social, occupational, or other important areas of functioning.
D. The symptoms are not due to the direct physiological effects of a substance (e.g., a drug of abuse, a medication) or a general medical condition (e.g., hypothyroidism).
E. The symptoms are not better accounted for by Bereavement, i.e., after the loss of a loved one, the symptoms persist for longer than 2 months or are characterized by marked functional impairment, morbid preoccupation with worthlessness, suicidal ideation, psychotic symptoms, or psychomotor retardation.

Box 1.3 : DSM-IV-TR Diagnostic Criteria for Manic Episode

A. A distinct period of abnormally and persistently elevated, expansive, or irritable mood, lasting at least 1 week (or any duration if hospitalization is necessary).
B. During the period of mood disturbance, three (or more) of the following symptoms have persisted (four if the mood is only irritable) and have been present to a significant degree:

   (1) inflated self-esteem or grandiosity
   (2) decreased need for sleep (e.g., feels rested after only 3 hours of sleep)
   (3) more talkative than usual or pressure to keep talking
   (4) flight of ideas or subjective experience that thoughts are racing
   (5) distractibility (i.e., attention too easily drawn to unimportant or irrelevant external stimuli)
   (6) increase in goal-directed activity (either socially, at work or school, or sexually) or psychomotor agitation
   (7) excessive involvement in pleasurable activities that have a high potential for painful consequences (e.g., engaging in unrestrained buying sprees, sexual indiscretions, or foolish business investments)

C. The symptoms do not meet criteria for a Mixed Episode.
D. The mood disturbance is sufficiently severe to cause marked impairment in occupational functioning or in usual social activities or relationships with others, or to necessitate hospitalization to prevent harm to self or others, or there are psychotic features.
E. The symptoms are not due to the direct physiological effects of a substance (e.g., a drug of abuse, a medication, or other treatment) or a general medical condition (e.g., hyperthyroidism).

   Note: Manic-like episodes that are clearly caused by somatic antidepressant treatment (e.g., medication, electroconvulsive therapy, light therapy) should not count toward a diagnosis of Bipolar I Disorder.

is not associated with the delay or deviance in early language development seen in autistic disorder.

DSM-IV-TR lists dementia due to Pick's disease. It is characterized by changes in personality early in the course, deterioration of social skills, emotional blunting, behavioral disinhibition, and prominent language abnormalities. Difficulties in memory, apraxia, and other features of dementia usually occur later in the course of illness. DSM-IV-TR acknowledges that Pick's disease often cannot be distinguished from atypical cases of Alzheimer's disease or from other dementias that affect the frontal lobes without postmortem examination. Dementia due to frontotemporal degeneration other than Pick's disease is diagnosed as dementia

Box 1.4 : DSM-IV-TR Diagnostic Criteria for Autistic Disorder

A. A total of six (or more) items from (1), (2), and (3), with at least two from (1), and one each from (2) and (3):

(1) qualitative impairment in social interaction, as manifested by at least two of the following:
(a) marked impairment in the use of multiple nonverbal behaviors such as eye-to-eye gaze, facial expression, body postures, and gestures to regulate social interaction
(b) failure to develop peer relationships appropriate to developmental level
(c) a lack of spontaneous seeking to share enjoyment, interests, or achievements with other people (e.g., by a lack of showing, bringing, or pointing out objects of interest)
(d) lack of social or emotional reciprocity

(2) qualitative impairments in communication as manifested by at least one of the following:
(a) delay in, or total lack of, the development of spoken language (not accompanied by an attempt to compensate through alternative modes of communication such as gesture or mime)
(b) in individuals with adequate speech, marked impairment in the ability to initiate or sustain a conversation with others
(c) stereotyped and repetitive use of language or idiosyncratic language
(d) lack of varied, spontaneous make-believe play or social imitative play appropriate to developmental level

(3) restricted repetitive and stereotyped patterns of behavior, interests, and activities, as manifested by at least one of the following:
(a) encompassing preoccupation with one or more stereotyped and restricted patterns of interest that is abnormal either in intensity or focus
(b) apparently inflexible adherence to specific, nonfunctional routines or rituals
(c) stereotyped and repetitive motor mannerisms (e.g., hand or finger flapping or twisting, or complex whole-body movements)
(d) persistent preoccupation with parts of objects

B. Delays or abnormal functioning in at least one of the following areas, with onset prior to age 3 years: (1) social interaction, (2) language as used in social communication, or (3) symbolic or imaginative play.

C. The disturbance is not better accounted for by Rett's Disorder or Childhood Disintegrative Disorder.

---

due to frontotemporal degeneration, one of the dementias due to other general medical conditions.

DEBATES ABOUT THE USEFULNESS OF CURRENT CLASSIFICATIONS

Bleuler's broader view of schizophrenia led to some confusion about schizophrenia for a time. While Europeans continued to have a narrow definition of schizophrenia, in North America the diagnosis of schizophrenia was assigned to many patients who in Europe would have been diagnosed with affective or personality disorders. However, current diagnostic systems have moved the disorder closer to that envisaged by Kraepelin. By and large, it is a reliable diagnosis with fairly good agreement between clinicians using standardized rating scales (Williams et al., 1977). Bipolar disorders can also be reliably diagnosed with standardized criteria (Williams et al., 1977). However, there has been considerable debate about the wisdom of putting all serious depressions into the unipolar category, whether they are recurrent or non-recurrent. Kraepelin put recurrent depressions together with manic-depressive disorder.

Unipolar depressive disorders are heterogeneous. Another problem is that about 1% of patients with unipolar depression convert to bipolar I disorder per year, while a further 0.5% convert to bipolar II per year (Angst et al., 2005). Despite this, early family studies suggested that bipolar patients were more likely to have a family history of affective disorder and a different clinical course and outcome (Perris, 1966; Winokur et al., 1967, 1993). Others argue that more recurrent unipolar patients resemble bipolar patients in that they have an earlier age of onset, a family history of mania, and a response to prophylactic lithium (Goodwin and Jamison, 2007).

There has been a trend to expand the concept of bipolar disorder. Bipolar II disorder was one of the first signs of this direction, but in recent years, bipolar disorder has grown to encompass cyclothymic and borderline personality disorders and even pediatric precursors of bipolar disorder (Akiskal, 1981; Faedda et al., 1995; Klerman, 1981). These conditions are suggested to be *bipolar spectrum* disorders, which share some phenotypic and familial overlap. Others consider this development as potentially misleading and issue "a plea for integrity of the bipolar concept" (Baldessarini, 2000). The issue is far from resolved, but the consensus appears to be moving closer to Kraepelin's position that at least highly recurrent depressive disorders are closely related to bipolar disorder.

The line between schizophrenia and bipolar disorders may not be a clean one. Although it was originally believed that there is not an excess of schizophrenic relatives in bipolar proband families or an excess of relatives with bipolar disorder in schizophrenic proband families, new evidence has shown that there may be some overlap (Lichtenstein et al., 2009). Other investigators have found higher-than-expected rates of psychotic mood disorder in the relatives of schizophrenic probands. This is also suggested by a Scottish family in which the chromosomal abnormality that disrupts DISC1 is linked to both schizophrenia and depression

(Chubb et al., 2008). Consequently, some susceptibility loci may be common to both nosological categories (Goodwin and Jamison, 2007). Some have pointed out that these and other genetic studies call into question the current approach to classification and diagnosis. A more dimensional approach looking at cognitive impairment, negative symptoms, positive symptoms, and mood symptoms determined by genetic variation and environmental influences has been offered (Craddock and Owen, 2010). While such an approach is reasonable, it fails to capture what clinicians have found to be useful for more than 100 years. Even Craddock and Owen (2010) acknowledge that there are non-shared genetic risk factors for schizophrenia and bipolar disorder and that the Kraepelinian dichotomy survives.

Pervasive developmental disorders also affect a heterogeneous group of patients. About 70% of patients with autistic disorder suffer from mental retardation and 30% suffer from seizures (Minshew and Williams, 2007). Many have questioned whether it is necessary to distinguish between autistic disorder and Asperger's disorder. Some have found no significant group differences in motor, visuospatial, or executive functions between patients with autistic disorder and Asperger's disorder, suggesting that Asperger's disorder may simply be *high-IQ autism* (Miller and Ozonoff, 2000). Others have argued that there is an *autistic continuum* and although there are similarities between autistic disorder and Asperger's disorder, there are enough differences in clinical presentation and outcome to justify the typology (Szatmari et al., 1989; Tantam, 1988; Wing, 1991). Despite these arguments, it is likely that DSM-V will abandon Asperger's disorder as a separate diagnosis and will include it in the autistic spectrum disorders.

The classification of frontotemporal dementia is very much a work in progress as our knowledge of specific genetic mutations progresses. It is likely that the syndrome may be linked to progressive supranuclear palsy and corticobasal degeneration in some cases (Neary et al., 2005). As with schizophrenia, bipolar disorder, and autism, no classification system is perfect. However, the current system generates reasonably consistent clinical presentations that are easily recognized by most clinicians.

COULD THE HUMAN BRAIN TELL US SOMETHING ABOUT THESE DISORDERS?

The fact that these conditions exist could tell us something about the unique features of the human brain. Conversely, the structure of the human brain may be a template for these conditions. If we can better understand those neuronal circuits related to self-awareness, affect regulation, and social behavior distinctive to the human brain, we may find some clues to the final common pathways of these disorders. We are at a very early stage of understanding these subtle functions in the normal brain and the brains of patients with these disorders, but we suggest that it is time to take stock of where we are and survey some possible directions for research.

OVERVIEW OF THE VOLUME

It is very difficult to appreciate the neural substrates of schizophrenia, bipolar disorder, autism, and frontotemporal dementia without some background regarding basic neuroanatomy, neurotransmitters, and neuronal circuits. We will give a brief overview of these topics, followed by an examination of what may make the human brain unique. Surprisingly, apart from size, there are no striking differences from other primates. However, some subtle differences are beginning to emerge with regard to brain structures involved in executive functions and language. There may also be some unique features with regard to cell types.

We will review what is known about schizophrenia, bipolar disorders, autism, and frontotemporal dementia from epidemiological, psychophysiological, neuropathological, genetic, structural and functional imaging, and pharmacological perspectives. These reviews will not be comprehensive but will highlight aspects of these conditions that might be relevant to a discussion of what makes the human brain vulnerable to them. We realize that there are other conditions that may be unique to humans, but it is beyond the scope of this volume to discuss all of the conditions. However, we believe that schizophrenia, bipolar disorders, autism, and frontotemporal dementia provide the most comprehensive group of disorders presenting with symptoms relating to human capabilities across the lifespan. In our discussion of autism, we have also included attention-deficit/hyperactivity disorder and anorexia nervosa because of the slightly different perspective that they offer on the capacity of humans to participate in complex long-term social networks. Although clearly different from autism, these conditions share some of the same deficits in self-awareness and self-control and possibly some of the same molecular and neuronal circuitry anomalies.

There are three aspects of human behavior that might be related to these conditions. The first is the ability to construct a *self* and understand another person's perspective or *theory of mind*. We will examine the brain circuits that might be involved in these capabilities from the perspective of the neuropsychiatric disorders that are associated with anomalies in this ability. The second unique capacity in humans is language. What is known about the circuits underlying this capacity will be reviewed. Anomalies in language development and brain asymmetry in neuropsychiatric disorders will be discussed. Finally, affective processing in humans will be reviewed with regard to the so-called *social brain*. It is proposed that some unique features of human and nonhuman primates may be related to this capacity. When they break down, neuropsychiatric disorders result.

Why do neuropsychiatric conditions occur? Do neuropsychiatric conditions tell us something about how the brain is constructed? What is the relationship between these disorders? Are there some features of the human brain that may make it vulnerable to these conditions? If so, what brain circuits might be involved? Are there unique human genes that lead to the development of these structures that are affected in these disorders? Some possibilities will be considered.

Studies of the concordance of most neuropsychiatric conditions in identical versus fraternal twins indicate that there are important genetic components contributing to the development of these disorders (Bailey et al., 1995; Barnett and Smoller, 2009; Bulik et al., 2007; Dworzyski et al., 2009; Faraone et al., 2005; Sullivan et al., 2003). Many genes have been found to be related to these disorders, and in several cases the same genes have been linked to multiple disorders; however, with the possible exception of frontotemporal dementia, no single gene is individually responsible for more than a tiny fraction of the incidence of these disorders (Chubb et al., 2008; Glessner et al., 2009; Guilmatre et al., 2009). These observations suggest that there may be many combinations of genes and environmental conditions that give rise to these disorders. These combinations probably work through specific neuronal and molecular circuits that constitute the final common pathways that are responsible for these disorders. The fact that they are human illnesses may be the most important clue of all, in that it implies that the defective circuits may reside in recently evolved features of the human brain.

2

Background on the Brain

This chapter describes some of the principal cell types and structures of the brain and their organization into functional units. We have learned much about the brain since conditions like schizophrenia and bipolar disorders were characterized. A basic understanding of some of these functional units is essential to the discussion of what makes the human brain vulnerable to these conditions.

The cells in the brain can be divided into two principal types: neurons and glial cells. There are well over 100 billion individual neurons in the human brain. Neurons form the signaling pathways in the brain by virtue of their ability to form synapses where chemicals called neurotransmitters are released to pass the message on to the next neuron. A number of neurotransmitters are involved in neuropsychiatric disorders. Some of those that are most likely to play a role include dopamine, norepinephrine, glutamate, serotonin, and gamma-aminobutyric acid (GABA). Within the neuron, there are several second-messenger pathways that interact with genes, leading to long-term changes in neuronal reactivity. Glial cells are the supporting cells of the brain, although they can also participate in signaling. The microglia participate in immune responses in the brain.

Functions such as language, memory, and attention depend upon complex interactions between cells and different parts of the brain. Specific functions can be specialized to one area, but the overall function depends upon the coordinated activity of several different brain areas. Affective responses interact with all of the functional networks. A single neuron can receive input from up to 150,000 other neurons (Kandel et al., 2000). However, this very large number of connections is true for a very specialized neuron type, the Purkinje cells of the cerebellum. Most of the neurons that make up the circuits described in this volume have much smaller sets of direct connection, probably numbering in the hundreds or low thousands. Input from these neurons develops in a systemic way through fetal development to adolescence and adulthood. Most of the structural changes are programmed by genes, but neuronal development is also heavily dependent on experience.

BRAIN DEVELOPMENT

Soon after conception, a neural plate folds onto itself to form the neural tube and eventually the brain. By 4 weeks three vesicles can be seen: the prosencephalon (forebrain), the mesencephalon (midbrain), and the rhombencephalon (hindbrain). The prosencephalon develops into the telencephalon and the diencephalon, while the telencephalon forms the cerebral cortex, the basal ganglia, the hippocampus, the amygdala, and the olfactory bulb. The diencephalon further differentiates into the thalamus, the hypothalamus, the retina, and the optic nerves. The mesencephalon and rhombencephalon develop into the brainstem, the cerebellum, and the spinal cord.

The cerebral cortex begins to form around the second trimester of pregnancy as six distinct cell layers migrate outwards from the subplate. These cortical neurons are highly topographically organized in that specific regions are responsible for particular types and locations of sensation and movement. Cortical specificity is highly dependent upon the neurons that arise from the thalamus and project up to the subplate (O'Leary et al., 1994). One of the earliest demonstrations of the role of thalamic projection neurons in cortical specificity was described in mice (Senft and Woolsey, 1991; Van der Loos and Woolsey, 1973). Rats have barrel fields in their somatosensory cortex that are very specific to sensation from a certain part of the rat's body (Schlaggar and O'Leary, 1993). The development of these barrel fields is not dependent on the somatosensory neurons themselves. Cells from the occipital cortex can be transplanted into the somatosensory cortex to form barrel fields, provided there are thalamocortical afferents. It is highly likely that thalamocortical neurons contribute to cortical specificity in other regions of the brain as well.

The brain develops in a highly predictable way dependent upon the activation of numerous genes and proteins. Cell migration related to the formation of cortical layers and cortical specificity occurs mostly in the second trimester of pregnancy. However, brain development does not stop at birth: myelinization of cortico-cortical pathways goes on well into adolescence and early adulthood (Benes et al., 1994). As a rough general principle, the phylogenetically newer brain regions appear to mature later than older ones (Flechsig, 1921; Gogtay et al., 2004). There is also an ongoing process of pruning to remove redundant connections throughout childhood to adulthood. About 60% of cortico-cortical connections involving associative regions such as the prefrontal and auditory cortices are lost in this way (Huttenlocher and Dabholkar, 1997). Thus, vulnerabilities due to anomalous early brain development can be uncovered by pruning at later stages of development.

RELEVANT BRAIN REGIONS

The brain takes in information about the environment through the five senses, filters and processes it, considers response options, and produces a behavioral response. These are complex processes that involve several brain regions. However, most brain regions have particular roles, and these seem to be consistent across species. For example, the occipital cortex processes visual information and the parietal cortex spatial information in all mammals. When we get to more complex behaviors involving the prefrontal and temporal lobes, things get a bit more complicated, so we will look at these brain regions and the structures they are connected to in a bit more detail. The principal brain regions are illustrated in Figure 2.1.

Prefrontal Region

The prefrontal cortex is one of the most important regions involved in complex behavior (Fuster, 1998; Stuss and Levine, 2002). Some have suggested that the prefrontal cortex orchestrates thought and action in accordance with internal goals through the active maintenance of patterns of activity that represent the goals and the means to achieve them. In effect, the prefrontal cortex biases signals to other brain structures, guiding the flow of activity along neural pathways that link inputs, internal states, and outputs needed to perform a task (Miller and Cohen, 2001).

The prefrontal cortex is divided into the dorsolateral region underlying the forehead and the orbital and medial regions, which lie above the eyes. The prevailing view has been that the ventrolateral and dorsal regions are involved in working memory and attention, whereas the orbital and medial regions are associated with behavioral inhibition (Fuster, 1989, Goldman-Rakic, 1987). Others have suggested that the dorsolateral region is responsible for the manipulation of information and the ventrolateral region is responsible for the retrieval of information from the posterior cortical areas (Owen et al., 1996; Petrides, 1996). More recently it has been suggested that the nature of the information being processed may lead to the apparent bias toward inhibition in the orbital and medial regions (Miller and Cohen, 2001)—that is, the medial and orbital regions process social and appetitive stimuli that elicit strong competing alternatives, leading to inhibition. In contrast, the information processed in the dorsal regions is more cognitive in nature, leading to less response competition and less need for inhibition.

The dorsolateral prefrontal cortex also plays an important role in the temporal flow of information. Constantinidis et al. (2002) used simultaneous single-cell recordings in primates to show that there are inhibitory interactions between neurons active at different time points relative to the cue presentation, delay interval, and response in a working memory task. This study suggests that the prefrontal cortex holds information on line in working memory and shapes the temporal sequence of response.

The orbitofrontal cortex is important in evaluating the reward value of stimuli (Rolls, 1999). Within the orbital and medial prefrontal cortex, there are

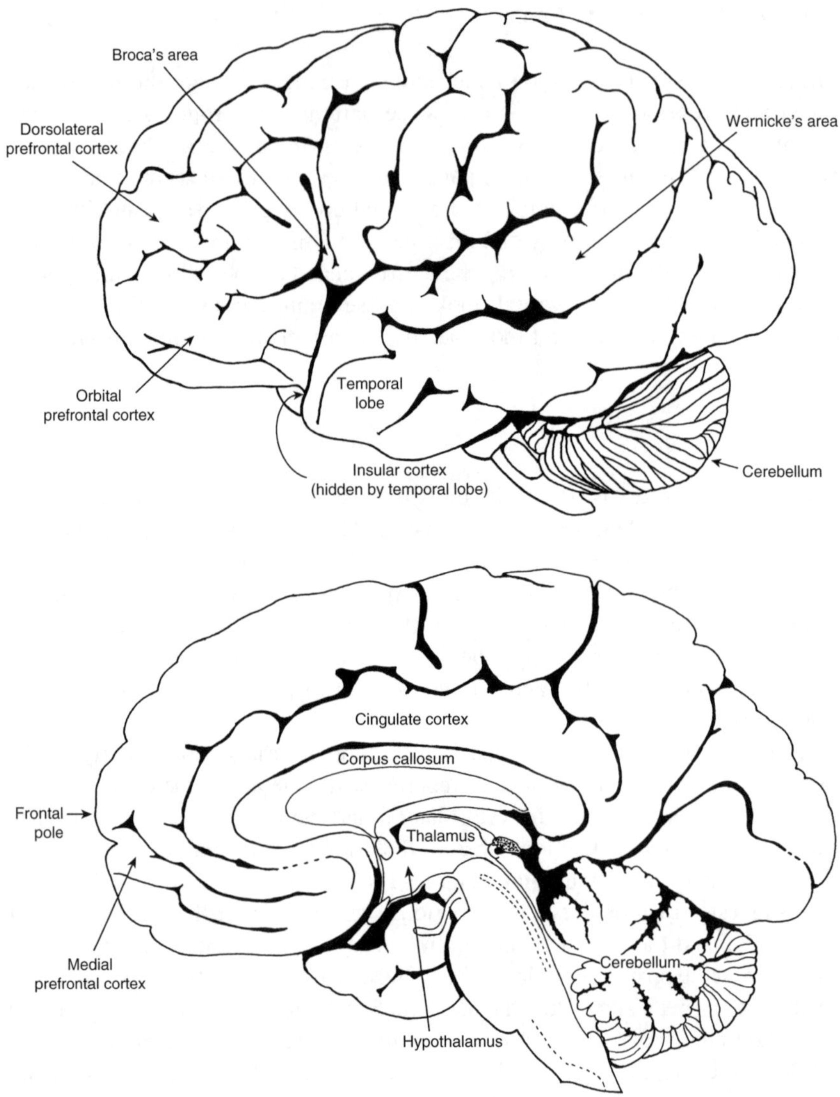

Figure 2.1 Principal brain regions. *Top*: Lateral view. *Bottom*: Medial view. Brain outline adapted with permission from DeArmond, S.J., and Fusco, M.M. *Structure of the Human Brain, a Photographic Atlas, 3rd ed.* New York, Oxford University Press. Copyright 1989.

two distinct networks. The orbital network receives sensory information from several modalities, including olfaction, taste, visceral afferents, somatic sensation, and vision. The medial network projects to visceromotor structures in the hypothalamus and brainstem (Ongur and Price, 2000). Thus, the orbital and medial prefrontal cortices guide reward-related behavior and the setting of mood, features that are important to social behaviors.

Damage to the orbitofrontal cortex can lead to impaired social behavior. One of the best-known examples is Phineas Gage, who was setting explosives with an iron bar while working on a railway more than a century ago. When the explosives prematurely ignited, the bar was hurled through his medial prefrontal cortex. Doctors at the time were surprised to find that his working memory was intact. In fact, he appeared to be more or less normal, apart from the appearance of socially inappropriate behaviors. He had been an upstanding and hard-working citizen before the accident; afterwards, he was no longer interested in work and took to alcohol and gambling. Thus, the learning of stimulus–reward associations is critical to appropriate social behavior.

Temporal Region

The temporal lobes contain a number of important structures that play a role in memory, emotion, and language. The hippocampus, which can be found on the inner aspect of the temporal lobe, is essential for long-term memory (Mesulam, 1990; Squire, 1992). The best demonstration of the role of these structures in memory comes from a case described by Brenda Milner at the Montreal Neurological Institute. H.M. had had neurosurgery to remove the medial temporal cortices on both sides, including the hippocampi, for intractable epilepsy. After the surgery, he had very good short-term memory and excellent recollection of events that had occurred long before the surgery. However, he could not transfer any short-term memories to long-term storage after the surgery. He could not recall having a meal less than an hour afterwards, and as time went on he could not recognize himself in a mirror because he did not recall aging (Kandel, 2006). This case showed that memories do not reside in the hippocampus because H.M. could recall his past. What the hippocampus seems to do is facilitate connections between different parts of the brain where memories are disturbed. The way this occurs is beyond the scope of this volume, but it has to do with the induction of genes by second messenger systems, leading to synaptic growth (Kandel, 2006).

Another structure in the temporal lobes that plays a role in memory is the amygdala, which is an almond-shaped structure at the end of the hippocampus (Aggleton, 1992). Damage to the amygdala in wild and fierce monkeys results in a marked change in behavior. Lesioned animals become tame and indifferent creatures, with changes in dietary and sexual behavior. Damage to the amygdala in this way was later termed Klüver-Bucy syndrome. What these studies showed was that the sight of humans was no longer coded as a threatening stimulus (LeDoux, 1996). The amygdala seems to be responsible for modulating fear, but it is also likely just as important for processing positive reward and reinforcement as it is for negative emotions (Murray, 2007).

The superior temporal gyrus is involved in language processing. Within the superior temporal gyrus is the Heschl gyrus, which is associated with auditory perception. Posterior to the Heschl gyrus is the planum temporale, which overlaps Wernicke's language association cortex and has close connections with the Heschl gyrus. Both the Heschl gyrus and planum temporale are critical to language processing. Not surprisingly, the planum temporale shows the most left–right asymmetry in the human brain (Mesulam, 2000).

Insular Cortex and Claustrum

The insular cortex, which lies between the frontal and temporal lobes and is buried in the lateral sulcus, is crucially involved in self-awareness and self-control (Craig, 2009). The insular cortex is important in speech articulation and pain perception and is often activated when subjects are asked to produce well-learned category-specific knowledge (Martin et al., 1996). Between the insular cortex and the striatum is a very thin structure called the claustrum (Latin for fence), which is unique to mammals. This structure has largely been ignored until recently. Francis Crick, the co-discoverer of the structure of DNA, and Christof Koch drew attention to this structure's possible role in consciousness because of its interconnections with all areas of the cortex (Crick and Koch, 2005).

Cingulate Cortices

The cingulate cortex is above the corpus callosum, which joins the left and right sides of the brain, and is closely connected with the amygdala, hippocampus, insula, and prefrontal cortex (Vogt, 2009a). The anterior cingulate is part of an attentional network involving the prefrontal, parietal, and temporal regions (Devinsky and Luciano, 1993). A large body of experimental work from monkeys and humans based on many different neural recording and imaging methods indicates that the superior part of the anterior cingulate participates in error detection and is often activated when subjects are asked to do an attention-demanding task involving a high degree of uncertainty (Allman et al., 2001; Botvinick et al., 2004). The activity of the superior parts of the anterior cingulate cortex increases with task difficulty (Paus et al., 1998). The inferior part of the anterior cingulate below the genu of the corpus callosum participates in processing emotion and tends to be suppressed when the dorsal anterior cingulate cortex is active (Bush et al., 2000).

Damage to the anterior cingulate often results in affective flatness and even mutism in severe cases. It is interesting that the anterior cingulate and medial prefrontal cortex are part of a primitive vocalization network in monkeys that is closely connected with the superior temporal gyrus and hippocampus (Barbas et al., 1999; Yukie and Shibata, 2009). The anterior cingulate is closely connected to the posterior cingulate, which may be part of a visual monitoring system for danger in animals (Raichle et al., 2001). Since visual sensory information is first processed in the cortical visual areas in the posterior part of the cortex, the flow of information in the cingulate cortex proceeds from these visual cortical areas through the posterior cingulate to the anterior cingulate cortex. This information is carried in large part through a large cable of fibers in the cingulum bundle that lies adjacent to the cingulate cortex. The retrosplenial cortex, which is inferior to the posterior corpus callosum, likely plays a role in consciousness and long-term memory (Vogt and Laureys, 2005). Curiously, there are two pathways from the dorsolateral prefrontal cortex to the hippocampus. One pathway goes directly to the hippocampus and the other goes indirectly through the retrosplenial cortex (Goldman-Rakic et al., 1984).

Thalamus

The thalamus, which lies deep in the brain, just above the brainstem, is the central switchboard of the brain. Neurons carrying information from all senses, except olfaction, synapse in the thalamus. Neurons from the thalamus project to the various sensory cortices. The occipital cortex directly receives visual information from the thalamus and sends it through different pathways to the parietal cortex and temporal lobes. Both project to the prefrontal cortex for further higher-level processing. Auditory information is processed in much the same way through the temporal lobe on its way to the prefrontal cortex. Olfaction follows a different pathway from the olfactory bulb to the orbitofrontal cortex. The thalamus also receives inputs from the dorsal and ventral striatum that project to the cortex.

Dorsal and Ventral Striatum

Immediately anterior and somewhat above the thalamus is the corpus striatum. The striatum consists of a dorsal tier, including the putamen, globus pallidus, and caudate nucleus, which is directly connected with the amygdala, and a ventral tier, which mostly includes the nucleus accumbens. The dorsal tier is connected with the prefrontal cortex and motor areas. The ventral tier is directly connected with the prefrontal cortex but receives input from the amygdala and hippocampus as well. The corpus striatum and subcortical structures such as the subthalamic nucleus and the substantia nigra make up the basal ganglia. Reinforcement and appetitive behaviors are associated with the ventral striatum, while the dorsolateral striatum is believed to mediate procedural or stimulus–response learning. Spatial learning is likely associated with both the dorsomedial striatum and ventral striatum (Voorn et al., 2004).

The nucleus accumbens in the ventral striatum merits further comment. This nucleus at the base of the brain is seen as the gateway between the limbic system and motor system (Mogenson et al., 1980). The core of the nucleus accumbens has much in common with the dorsal striatum, while the shell of this structure is likely a component of the extended amygdala. Converging input from prefrontal and limbic regions results in a synchronous discharge of cells that influences activity in the thalamus and prefrontal regions (Heimer, 2000; O'Donnell et al., 1999). Thus, the nucleus accumbens is a link between motivation and action.

Cerebellum

The cerebellum lies between the occipital cortex and the brainstem. It is a phylogenetically old part of the brain that was believed to be mostly involved in the coordination of motor movements. More recently, it has been recognized that it is involved in the performance of cognitive tasks and possibly self-awareness. We will discuss this further in subsequent chapters.

NEURONAL CIRCUITS RELATED TO LEARNING NEW BEHAVIORS

Basal ganglia-thalamocortical neuronal circuits are associated with learning new behaviors. The basal ganglia are considered to be part of the extrapyramidal motor system, which is associated with many skeletomotor, oculomotor, cognitive, and emotional processes. The basal ganglia have a unique position within the brain, which may explain the diversity of functions associated with them. They receive projections from the prefrontal cortex and project back to these same regions via the thalamus, allowing highly specific and coordinated control of neuronal activity. Five basal ganglia-thalamocortical neuronal circuits were characterized by Alexander and his colleagues (1990). There are likely more (Middleton and Strick, 2001), but most of the five circuits still hold up reasonably well, so they will be described in some detail.

The motor circuit projects via glutamatergic neurons from the supplementary motor area and motor cortex to the putamen, where it follows a direct and indirect GABA pathway to the thalamus. The indirect pathway passes through the subthalamic nucleus, allowing an extra synapse. Because GABA-ergic neurons are inhibitory, the indirect pathway has an opposite effect to the direct pathway. These pathways converge on the thalamus, which is reciprocally connected with the supplementary motor area and motor cortex, forming a loop circuit. Ocular movements are controlled by a similar pathway beginning in the frontal eye fields and supplementary eye fields. They project to the caudate by excitatory glutamatergic neurons and, like the motor circuit, they project directly and indirectly to the thalamus, where reciprocal connections are made with the sites of origin in the cortex.

Three basal ganglia-thalamocortical neuronal circuits were proposed to participate in cognition and emotion. Two of these follow very similar pathways and are referred to as the *prefrontal circuits*. One of these circuits originates in the dorsolateral prefrontal cortex and the other in the lateral orbital frontal cortex. Both the prefrontal circuits project via excitatory glutamatergic neurons to the caudate and directly and indirectly through the subthalamic nucleus via GABA-ergic neurons to the thalamus. The thalamic neurons are reciprocally connected with the sites of origin in the cortex.

The limbic basal ganglia-thalamocortical neuronal circuit follows a different route than the prefrontal circuits. This circuit begins in the anterior cingulate and medial orbitofrontal cortex and projects via glutamatergic neurons to the ventral striatum, including the nucleus accumbens. From the ventral striatum to the thalamus, there are direct and indirect GABA-ergic pathways similar to the other circuits. The thalamus is reciprocally connected with the anterior and medial orbitofrontal cortex. The limbic circuit receives substantial input from the amygdala and hippocampus.

The parallel arrangement of the direct and indirect pathways allows for opposing input back to the cortex, either inhibiting or stimulating certain pathways. Dopamine modulates these circuits by facilitating conduction through the direct pathway. This has an excitatory effect on the thalamus. Dopamine suppresses conduction through the indirect pathway, which has an inhibitory effect on the thalamus.

Regulation by Dopamine, Amygdala, and Hippocampus

Dopamine is released following the presentation of rewards (or stimuli that by learned association are connected to rewards) by the terminals of axons whose soma are located in the ventral tegmental area (VTA) and substantia nigra of the midbrain (Schultz, 2001). Recently it has been discovered that there are at least two types of dopamine neurons. One of these types is activated by reward and inhibited by aversive stimuli; the other is activated by both reward and aversive stimuli (Matsumoto and Hikosaka, 2009). This indicates that the dopamine system signals both reward and punishment. Excessive coupling or imbalances between reward and punishment may be important factors in the pathogenesis of neuropsychiatric illnesses. The location and connections of the VTA and substantia nigra and the responses of these neurons to rewarding and aversive stimuli are illustrated in Figure 2.2. Dopamine input to the nucleus accumbens can be modulated by the prefrontal cortex (Taber and Fibiger, 1995). It is likely that serotonin regulates dopamine input to the nucleus accumbens as well (Dewey et al., 1995; Kapur and Remington, 1996). In addition, glutamatergic inputs to the nucleus accumbens from the hippocampus and amygdala gate activity within these circuits. This feature allows behavior to be influenced by past experience through information made accessible by the hippocampus. Past emotional experience influences behavior via input from the amygdala. Input from the amygdala is able to override past experiential input from the hippocampus in certain circumstances (O'Donnell et al., 1999).

Role in Response Learning

There have been several theories about how changes in basal ganglia-thalamocortical neuronal circuits lead to response learning (Alexander et al., 1990; Graybiel, 1995). The prefrontal cortex seems to be necessary when new rules are required or older ones rejected. The basal ganglia seem to have a different role in potentiating previously learned rules based on the current context and reinforcement history. Wise et al. (1996) presented a model as to how this could come about. They suggested that direct-pathway neurons recognize the pattern of corticostriatal inputs promoting a rule through positive-feedback loops. Dopaminergic neuronal projections from the midbrain show increased activity during learning, leading to enhanced gene expression within the direct pathway. At the same time, neurons of the indirect pathway are suppressed. Dopamine potentiates direct-pathway activity through its effect on a subtype of dopamine receptors, the D_1 receptors, and suppresses the indirect pathway through another subtype of dopamine receptors, the D_2 receptors. Thus, dopamine activates context-dependent activity within behavioral modules on the basis of genetic changes associated with previous experience.

NEURONAL CIRCUITS RELATED TO EMOTIONAL REGULATION

In 1878, Broca described *le grande lobe limbique* as a broad band of brain tissue wrapped around the corpus callosum and including parts of the ventral forebrain.

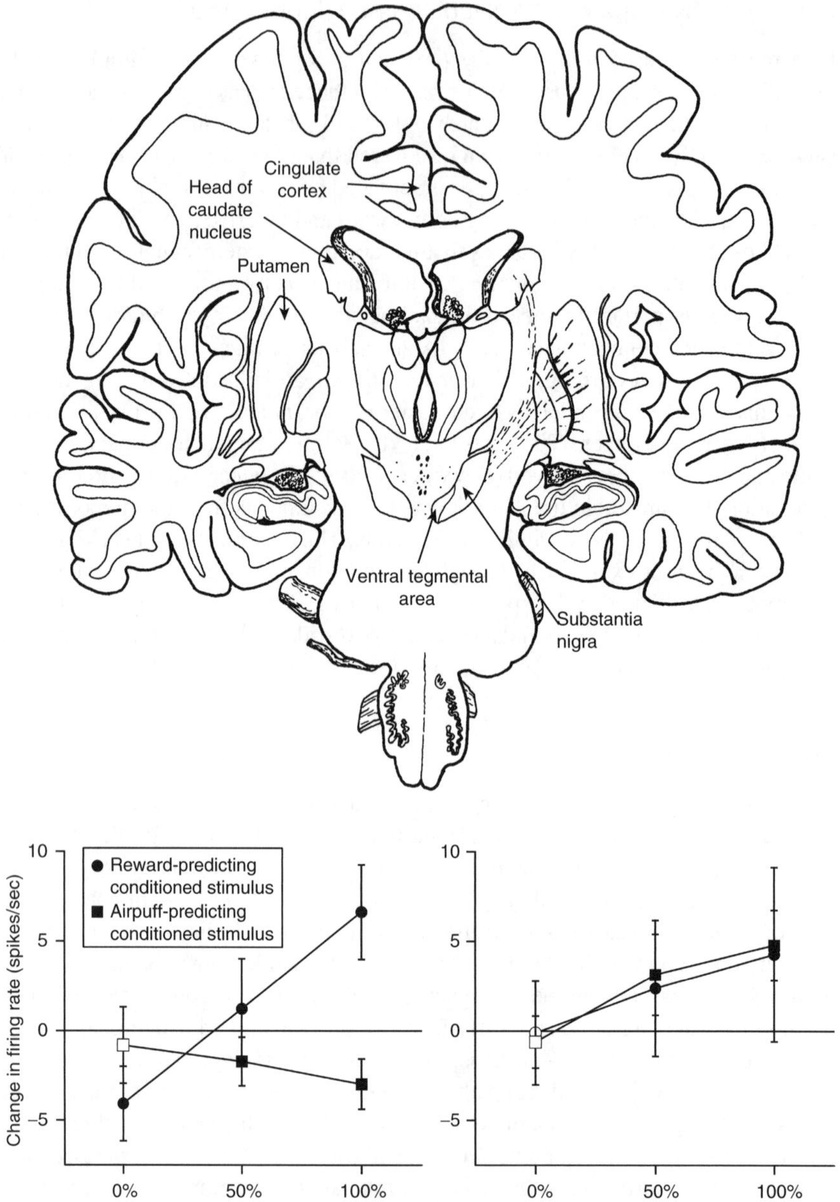

Figure 2.2 Dopamine pathways. *Upper panel*: The location of the major components of the dopaminergic system in a coronal section of the human brain. *Lower panel*: Graphs showing the responses of the two major types of dopaminergic neurons recorded from the ventral tegmental area and substantia nigra in macaque monkeys. The graphs show the firing rate of neurons as a function of responses to images predicting the probability of reward (juice) and punishment (air puff). The left graph shows one major type, which is

(Figure legend continues at top of next page)

(Continued from preceding page)

excited by reward and inhibited by punishment. The right graph shows the second major type, which is excited by both reward and punishment. Graphs adapted from Matsumoto, M., and Hikosaka, O. Two types of dopamine neuron distinctly convey positive and negative motivational signals. *Nature*, **459**, 837–841. Reprinted with permission from Macmillan Publishers Ltd., Copyright, 2009. Brain outline in the upper panel adapted with permission from DeArmond, S.J., and Fusco, M.M. *Structure of the Human Brain, a Photographic Atlas, 3rd ed.* New York: Oxford University Press, Copyright 1989.

This is the source of the modern term *limbic*, which is used to describe this collection of brain structures; it is derived from the Latin word *limbus*, which means border, but which also could be taken to mean an interface (Allman et al., 2001). Broca believed that the great limbic lobe was primarily involved in olfaction, but modern studies indicate that olfactory functions are restricted to only a small portion of the ventral part of the limbic lobe (Allman et al., 2001). The dorsal part of Broca's great limbic lobe is the cingulate cortex, so named because it forms a *cingulum* or collar around the corpus callosum. In 1937, Papez (Allman et al., 2001, p. 108) wrote:

> The cortex of the cingular gyrus may be looked on as the receptive organ for the experiencing of emotion as the result of impulses coming from the hypothalamic region, in the same way as the area striata is considered the receptive cortex for photic excitations from the retina.

Modern studies reviewed earlier in this chapter indicate that Papez's conclusion about the role of the cingulate cortex in emotion applies best to its most anterior and ventral parts, while it also has important roles in attention, effortful cognition, and the recognition of error. The limbic system also includes the parahippocampal gyri, the hippocampal formation, the amygdala, and the anterior nucleus of the thalamus (MacLean, 1978). The limbic system can be found in all mammals and was suggested to play a special role in the emotional aspects of behavior and memory.

Papez (1937) proposed that emotional experiences could be generated in two ways. The first was through the thalamus via the stream of feeling to the mammillary bodies, the anterior thalamus, and the cingulate cortex. The second way was through the stream of thought through the cerebral cortex, where memories about the stimulus are activated, leading to activity in the cingulate cortex. Thus, emotion could be activated at a cortical and subcortical level. It was a plausible idea that was consistent with Cannon's theory of emotion, but there has been considerable criticism of the involvement of the Papez circuit in emotion (LeDoux, 1996). Recent approaches to the study of emotional processing in the brain have been less influenced by the concept of the limbic system. However, many of the same brain structures, such as the cingulate cortex, dorsomedial and orbital ventromedial prefrontal cortex, nucleus accumbens, amygdala, and hypothalamus, are still viewed as key areas in emotional processing (Dalgleish, 2004). We will discuss some of these approaches further in Chapter 10.

Limitations of the Concept of the Limbic System

All of the disorders considered in this book involve some dysfunction of limbic system structures, and the concept of the limbic system has proved useful in understanding these disorders, but the concept does have serious limitations. Imbedded in the concept of limbic system is the notion that it is involved exclusively or primarily in emotions, yet there is a very large body of experimental work indicating that the dorsal anterior cingulate cortex is engaged in effortful cognition when the subject is doing hard mental work that requires focused attention and the discounting of distractions. The dorsal anterior cingulate and the anterior insular cortex appear to be crucial structures in error recognition and the initiation of error-correcting behaviors, which are the essential component of adaptive intelligence. These cognitive activities are the exact opposite of the popular conception of the functions of the limbic system; however, consistent with an enlarged conception of the limbic system are the major deficits in cognitive functioning that occur in all of the neuropsychiatric disorders considered in this book. In addition, the hippocampal formation is involved in all declarative memory, not just memories with a strong emotional content.

The structures that make up the limbic system are very heterogeneous in their anatomical microstructure. The hippocampi have a simple three-layered cortical structure, which is believed to be primitive. By contrast, the posterior cingulate cortex has six layers and is cytoarchitecturally very similar to the neocortex. The anterior cingulate cortex lacks layer 4, and this has been taken by some to be evidence that it is primitive; however, the adjacent neocortical motor cortex also lacks layer 4, and thus the lack of layer 4 is not a reliable indicator of primitive status. Some components are aggregations of neurons that do not have a laminar structure such as the hypothalamus, while the amygdala has parts that have a cortex-like structure and other parts that have an aggregrated-neuron architecture.

A similar heterogeneity is also present when one considers gene expression in limbic structures. There are genes and their protein products that are specifically localized in the limbic system, such as limbic system-associated membrane protein (LSAMP) (Horton and Levitt, 1988). However, the overwhelming majority of genes expressed in these structures do not follow a pattern of restricted co-expression throughout the limbic system. The evidence for this comes from the massive in situ gene expression studies done at the Allen Brain Institute for nearly 20,000 genes mapped throughout the entire brain in adult mice. By using the AGEA function at the Allen Brain Web site, one can select any site in the brain and observe the degree to which gene expression is correlated between that site and all other sites in the brain with a spatial resolution of 200 micra (http://mouse.brain-map.org/agea/all_coronal). For example, when one puts the cursor into the cingulate cortex one finds that gene expression is highly correlated with the rest of neocortex but is much lower for other brain sites. If one puts it into the nucleus accumbens, one finds that it is strongly correlated with the caudate-putamen but is much lower for other sites. If one puts it into the amygdala, one finds strong correlation with brainstem structures, and so on for all the components of the limbic system.

Thus, the functional imaging and electrophysiological recording data indicating a strong role for parts of the limbic system in focused attention, effortful cognition, error recognition, and adaptive intelligence require an enlarged concept of limbic system function. While there is strong connectivity among limbic system structures, there is great heterogeneity in micro-anatomy and gene expression among its components. Similarly, the limbic system, like other parts of the brain, comprises both phylogenetically ancient and recently evolved components.

SUMMARY

There are clearly a number of brain regions that might be relevant to neuropsychiatric disorders. The dorsolateral prefrontal cortex, anterior cingulate, and temporal lobes would be good places to look for abnormalities in patients with a thought disorder, flat affect, and auditory hallucinations. The dorsolateral prefrontal cortex, medial prefrontal cortex, anterior cingulate, and amygdala might be expected to be involved in patients with mood disorders. Similarly, the dorsolateral and medial prefrontal cortex and temporal lobes might be expected to be involved in patients with social deficits and repetitive behaviors such as those seen in autism and frontotemporal dementia.

With the possible exception of the dorsolateral prefrontal cortex, these brain structures can be found in most mammals, albeit in a modified form in some cases. These recently evolved features of the human brain provide clues pointing to the loci of vulnerability to neuropsychiatric illnesses in the human brain. The next chapter will take a closer look at some of the specializations that the human brain has undergone.

3

Unique Aspects of the Human Brain

Despite the obvious differences between humans and non-human primates, it has been difficult to establish what makes the human brain unique. In fact, the human brain looks a lot like a larger non-human primate brain, and these similarities extend to the microscopic structure as well. The differences are subtle. This chapter will review some of these differences with regard to brain size and morphology, unique cell types, and genetic investigations of genotype and gene expression in humans and non-human primates. We will then look at some of the unique aspects of human cognition compared to non-human primate cognition. Finally, we will offer some thoughts on whether human consciousness might be different from that of non-human primates.

THE EMERGENCE OF *HOMO SAPIENS*

About 6 million years ago the hominid lineage began to diverge from lineages leading to the modern African great apes. Each of these lineages contained many smaller branches. Within the hominids, two major lineages diverged: one characterized by heavy chewing muscles and very thick dental enamel, which eventually became extinct, and the other leading to *Homo habilis*, which inhabited east Africa about 2 million years ago. This species had a 600-gram brain and left evidence of the use of stone tools. *Homo erectus* first emerged 1.9 million years ago and moved beyond Africa to Europe and Asia. *Homo erectus* was close in body size to modern humans and had a brain weight of about 800 to 900 grams. With the larger brain, *Homo erectus* was able to make more sophisticated tools and control fire. About 500,000 years ago hominid brain size increased again, giving rise to the Neanderthals in Europe and western Asia and early *Homo sapiens* in Africa. Anatomically modern humans replaced the Neanderthals about 30,000 years ago. Contemporary humans have a brain size averaging around 1,300 grams (Allman, 1999; Killackey, 1995).

BRAIN SIZE AND MORPHOLOGY

Primates tend to have larger brains than other mammals. Within the primates there is considerable variation. Humans and chimpanzees are about the same body weight, but humans have brains that are three times larger. With a larger brain comes the capacity to adapt to an ever-changing environment. However, larger brains came with a cost: the relative energy consumed by the brain greatly increased, and the time required for the maturation of the brain extended to many years after birth. The large brain size co-evolved with the extended family and the intergenerational transfer of food and information, which supported a long post-natal period of dependency and development (Allman, 2000; Kaplan et al., 2009).

Mechanism of Increase

The cortex consists of a collection of narrow, vertical cell columns, the fundamental information-processing units of the brain. The columns are made up of pyramidal cells and interneurons that span the six layers described in Chapter 2. The predominant view is that evolution modifies brain structure by adding new columns, not changing the structure of the columns. Thus, the cortex grows more horizontally than vertically, leading to increased folding and the formation of gyri and sulci (Allman, 1990,1999). The enlargement of the cerebral cortex accounts for most of the difference in brain volume between humans and other primates. With the increase in the cortex, there is a marked increase in white matter connecting the neocortical sheet (Allman, 1998; Killackey, 1995; Preuss, 2000; Schoenemann et al., 2005). Some have argued that there is simply an increase in the number of these processing units and no new cortical areas in humans. While this may be the case, there are clearly some differences in the morphology of the human brain. We will look at some of these differences in more detail below.

Prefrontal Regions

The primate frontal cortex hyperscales relative to the rest of the cortex and the rest of the brain (Bush and Allman, 2004) in primates. The size of the frontal cortex expands at the 1.18 power relative to the rest of the cortex for primates. This differential expansion of the frontal cortex occurs not only in apes and humans but also in the more encephalized New World monkeys (capuchins and spider monkeys) and prosimians (aye-ayes). It appears to be a primate specialization because it does not occur in the taxonomic order Carnivores (Bush and

Allman, 2004). This expansion is partially the result of the differential enlargement within the frontal lobe of the prefrontal cortex, including area 10 in the frontal pole (Semendeferi et al., 2001).

Dorsolateral Region

Of particular interest is the dorsolateral prefrontal cortex (area 46) because of its role in mediating cross-temporal contingencies. There do seem to be some differences between human and monkey brains. Only a portion of area 46 has the same cytoarchitecture as area 46 in the human brain; the remaining part of area 46 in the monkey brain has the characteristics of the middle frontal gyrus in the human brain. This region has similar connections to other parts of the brain as area 46, with the exception that it does not receive input from the lateral parietal cortex (Petrides and Pandya, 1999). Some differences between the human and monkey brains can also be seen in ventrolateral prefrontal regions (Petrides and Pandya, 2001).

Frontal Polar Cortex

Another area of interest in the prefrontal region is frontal polar cortex (area 10). It has been suggested that area 10 has undergone some phylogenetic specializations in hominids. It is absolutely and relatively larger in humans but is also well developed in the great apes (Semendeferi et al., 2001). In a meta-analysis of over 100 imaging studies, Gilbert et al. (2006) found three subdivisions of the frontal polar cortex. The lateral part of the frontal polar cortex is involved in the retrieval of episodic memory and perhaps confers the ability to have autobiographical memory through the lifespan. The anterior medial part is related to multitasking. Just posterior to the multitasking region, activity on the medial aspect of the frontal pole extending into area 32 is related to *mentalizing*, or the conscious reflection on the thoughts and motivations of oneself and others. Mentalizing can be regarded as a special type of multitasking behavior since it typically involves comparisons between two different trains of thought. Related to the capacity for multitasking is prospective memory, the act of remembering to do something in the future, which also activates the anterior medial part of area 10 (Okuda et al., 1998). The capacity for prospective memory is necessary for the execution of plans for the future. These findings are consistent with the proposal that the anterior prefrontal cortex is involved when two or more separate cognitive operations must be integrated in pursuit of a higher behavioral goal (Ramnani and Owen, 2004). Some have referred to this region as a *gateway* between novel environmental stimuli and internal representations guiding behavior (Burgess et al., 2007).

Area 10 is activated in economic decision making (Knutson et al., 2003; Grether et al., 2007). The medial part of area 10 is selectively activated by the calculation of the costs and benefits of punishing cheaters (de Quervain et al., 2004). This area is also activated when making moral choices concerning the welfare of others (Greene et al., 2001). The differential expansion of the frontal polar cortex in humans may be related to evolution of the human extended family, with its unique capacity for the intergenerational transfer of food and knowledge and the complex cognitive functioning required to support this adaptation (Allman et al., 2002). Thus, the frontal polar cortex appears to help to endow humans with the ability to transcend the present into both the past and the future, to maintain more than one train of thought at a time, to consider the thoughts of others, and to make the kinds of resource allocation and moral decisions that are required to live in complex social networks that persist over long periods of time.

Anterior Cingulate Cortices

Although the anterior cingulate cortices are often associated with older limbic regions in the brain that are present in all mammals, they are larger and anatomically differentiated in primates, providing an interface between emotion and cognition (Vogt, 2009b). This interface has been suggested to allow self-control, focused problem solving, error recognition, and adaptive responses to changing conditions like those faced by early hominids. It is also the site of a highly specialized cell, the Von Economo neuron, which will we discuss further below (Allman et al., 2001).

Studies have failed to find conflict-related responses in the anterior cingulate in monkeys. This is curious because the anterior cingulate is clearly involved in conflict monitoring in humans. Methodological differences between the studies in humans and monkeys may account for this observation. However, it is also possible that humans have a unique region for monitoring conflict: area 32, which is just superior to area 24 (Cole et al., 2009). In any case, an argument can be made that the anterior cingulate cortices and the medial frontal cortex play a role in self-generated action and self-reflection in humans (Passingham et al., 2010).

Are Speech Areas Unique to Humans?

Wernicke's Area

Homologues of Wernicke's area and the inferior parietal cortex can be found in non-human primates. It is interesting that the anterior parietal cortex, ventral premotor area, somatic areas in the operculum and insula, and ventral prefrontal areas are interconnected in the macaque. Preuss and Goldman-Rakic (1989) suggested that they constitute a network of perisylvian areas representing the face and forelimb, all areas potentially important in communication. Non-human primates also have at least some of the asymmetries of speech areas seen in humans. The left sylvian fissure is usually longer on the left in Old World monkeys, apes, and humans. Some chimpanzees have planum temporale asymmetries similar to humans. Thus, the difference between humans and non-human primates is quantitative rather than qualitative in speech areas (Preuss, 2000).

Minicolumns in the left planum temporale may be organized differently in humans than in chimpanzees and rhesus monkeys. They are wider, perhaps because of an enlarged neuropil space that contains axons, dendrites, and synapses (Buxhoeveden and Casanova, 2002).

Broca's Area

Another area that is involved in motor aspects of speech is Broca's area, located in the frontal lobe just in front of the motor cortex. In monkeys, the region is involved in the guidance of motor acts. It is a region rich in mirror neurons, which respond when the subject observes a motor act performed by another individual (Rizzolattii and Sinigalia, 2008). Broca's area may be part of an older area for the observational guidance of movements and gestures that has been adapted for speech in humans. There is some evidence from surface impressions left by brains of *Homo habilis* that Broca's area has enlarged in early humans (Tobias, 1987). It is also an area that is particularly asymmetrical in humans.

Temporal Poles

It is likely that the temporal poles have undergone adaptational changes in humans to facilitate language processing. Lesion studies and functional imaging studies have demonstrated that they play a central role in word and concept retrieval (Damasio et al., 2004). These regions have also been suggested to be convergent regions that allow us to apply general knowledge about social situations to immediate situations (Frith, 2007). We will discuss this further in Chapter 10.

Thus, there are differences between the human and non-human brain in terms of size and morphology. Differences are most apparent in the association cortex but can be found in other functionally connected regions such as the anterior thalamic nuclei. The prefrontal cortex demonstrates the most specialization in humans, but this appears to be at the expense of some prefrontal motor regions. Regions associated with language also demonstrate some differences in human compared to non-human primates, but not as much as might be expected. Asymmetries in these regions can also be found in non-human primates, suggesting that language arose from regions used by non-human primates for gestural communication.

ARE THERE UNIQUE CELL TYPES?

Just as there are no uniquely human regions in the brain, there does not appear to be a unique cell type in humans. However, some specializations have occurred in several regions and cell lines. We will look at some of these changes in humans and higher primates.

Visual Area Differences

One of the regions that has undergone some changes in humans is the primary visual area, V1. Humans have only one band that stains for the metabolic enzyme cytochrome oxidase, whereas macaques and many Old World monkeys have two bands. Increased calbindin-immunoreactive cells in the primary visual region exist in humans compared to macaques; since these neurons are probably inhibitory, this finding suggests increased inhibitory regulation of these circuits (Preuss, 2000).

Pyramidal and Chandelier Cells

Humans and macaques differ in the characteristics of both pyramidal and chandelier cells. Humans have more pyramidal cells in the superficial cortical layers, which express nonphosphorylated neurofilament protein, than macaques. This observation suggests that the organization of upper cortical layers may be different in humans. It has been proposed that certain classes of cortico-cortical neurons are stronger in humans (Preuss, 2000). Chandelier cells, GABA-ergic neurons that exert a strong inhibitory influence on pyramidal cells, may also differ in their distribution and characteristics between humans and macaques, particularly in temporal regions (del Rio and DeFelipe, 1997).

Astrocyte Cell Differences

Human astrocytes or glial cells have a 3-fold larger diameter and show a 10-fold increase in primary processes compared to rodents. Unique to humans and primates are a population of layer 1 interlaminar astrocytes that extend long fibers and layer 5-6 polarized astrocytes that also have long processes. It has been proposed that human cortical evolution has been accompanied by increasing complexity of form and function of astrocytes, reflecting their roles in synaptic modulation and cortical circuitry (Oberheim et al., 2006).

Glial cells play a special role in signal transduction. Much of the energy in the cortex is related to glutamatergic signaling. Glial cells participate by converting glutamate to glutamine, which then diffuses back to the neuron, where it is made into glutamate for further signaling. Consequently, the local density of glia in the normal brain is a good indicator of metabolic demand from neighboring neurons. In the postnatal period in humans, there is tremendous growth of dendritic arbors and a four-fold increase in glial cell numbers. Studies across anthropoid primate species suggest that the human frontal cortex displays a higher glia-to-neuron ratio compared to other primates. However, the relative increase conforms to allometric scaling expectations, taking into account the larger human brain. Greater numbers of glia in the human brain seem to relate to the energy costs of supporting larger dendritic arbors and long-range projecting axons (Sherwood et al., 2006).

It has recently been shown that astrocytes must be present for synapses to form. They secrete a protein, thrombospondin, that triggers synapse formation (Christopherson et al., 2005). Cáceres et al. (2007) have shown that humans produce up to six times more thrombospondin messenger RNA in the forebrain and caudate than chimps or macaques.

Microglia

The microglia defend the brain against damage and infection and are thus crucial for survival. Since the brain is substantially isolated from the body's immune system by the blood–brain barrier, which restricts the passage of immune cells and proteins from the capillaries into the brain tissue, the brain has its own immune system, the microglia, which mount the defense against invading microorganisms and clear damaged tissue and metabolic waste. This is achieved through a process known as phagocytosis, in which the microglia detect and ingest these substances.

In a brilliant series of experiments, Nimmerjahn et al. (2005) directly observed the activity of microglia in the intact living brain through two-photo microscopy of mice that had been genetically engineered to express a marker restricted to microglia that emitted green fluorescence. Their experiments showed that the microglial cell bodies are relatively stationary but the fine processes of the microglia are in constant motion on a minute-to-minute basis and are much more active than other cell types in the brain. They observed that the microglia processes continually probe the brain and conduct a complete surveillance coverage of the brain tissue every few hours. When the microglial processes encounter damaged tissue, metabolic byproducts such as oxidized lipoproteins, or invading microorganisms, they expand and engulf these substances and transport them back to the microglial cell body, where they are stored for an indeterminate period of time. The microglial motility responds to the electrical activity of the nearby neurons. The microglia contact other types of glia and neurons as part of their constant surveillance, but when they encounter other microglia there is mutual repulsion of their processes. When neurons are damaged, the microglial processes can strip synapses away from their dendrites, suggesting that they may have a role in modifying neuronal connections in development and plasticity (Cullheim and Thams, 2007).

In conventional histological sections the static microglia can be seen in three phases (Kreutzberg, 1996). The first is the so-called *quiescent* stage characterized by thin, spider-like processes. In vivo brain imaging shows that these quiescent microglia are actually quite motile in their surveillance for damaged and foreign tissue. The microglia processes during the quiescent stage have many fine-caliber branches. The second stage is the *activated* microglia, in which the processes are much thicker. During the activated stage the microglia secrete a large number of cytokines such as interleukin-6 and toxins as part of their defense against invading organisms (Thomas et al., 2006). Thus, these necessary defenders can turn against their neighboring cells if inappropriately triggered, and this appears to happen in a number of pathologies such as Alzheimer's disease and autism, which we will discuss later in this volume. The third stage is the *phagocytic* stage, in which the processes and their engulfed contents are drawn back into the body of the microglial cell, causing it to expand as it becomes a garbage can filled with fragments of phagocytized cells, metabolic waste products, and foreign matter. The microglia originate outside the nervous system and are closely related to the macrophage cells, which originate in the bone marrow. They first appear in small numbers in the brain during embryogenesis but emerge mainly in the early postnatal period, when they enter the brain most likely from the bloodstream and form what has been called the *fountain of microglia*, in which they distribute along the course of the fibers of the corpus callosum to all parts of the brain (Imamoto and Leblond, 1978). There are subsequent invasions into the brain of macrophages, which transform in microglia (Schmid, et al., 2009).

A genetic defect in a subset of microglia is the cause of a remarkable neuropsychiatric disease that was first observed in Japan and Finland but has subsequently been found throughout the world. Nasu-Hakola disease is caused by a defect in the gene TREM2 or the closely linked gene DAP12. These defects impair the capacity of the microglia to phagocytose damaged tissue and increase the secretion of inflammatory cytokines, particularly in the frontal and cingulate cortices (Bianchin et al., 2004; Neumann and Takahashi, 2007). At around age 35, Bainchin et al. (2004, p. 3) report that in affected patients there are:

> Incipient personality changes that can only be noticed by relatives and close friends. The behavioral alterations then become progressively more evident during the next months. The patients start to present silly and facetious behavior, lack of insight, social inhibition, and other unrestrained behavior. They are easily distractible....Sometimes they seem to have a euphoric attitude, seemingly lacking adequate associated emotional components. As the disease progresses, the patients evolve to a state of profound dementia.

The breakdown in self-awareness, self-control, and social functioning in the early stages of Nasu-Hakola disease bears some resemblance to the early stages of the behavioral variant of frontotemporal dementia. As we will discuss elsewhere in this volume, inappropriate microglia triggering and functioning appears to be frequently associated with severe neurological disturbances that impair self-awareness and control.

Von Economo Neurons

A class of neurons found only in humans, great apes (bonobos, chimpanzees, gorillas, orangutans), elephants, and whales has been identified. Spindle or Von Economo neurons are characterized by a very long, gradually tapering, large soma that is symmetrical about its horizontal and vertical axes (Color Plate 3.1). In contrast to layer 5 pyramidal neurons, Von Economo neurons have less branched dendritic trees. Von Economo neurons are located in layer 5 in the anterior cingulate (see Color Plate 3.1) in both cognitive and affective processing regions and frontoinsular cortex (Allman et al., 2005; Nimchinsky et al., 1999; Watson et al., 2006).

The Von Economo neurons develop late in both phylogeny and ontogeny. Since they are present in all the great apes and humans, they probably arose about 15 million years ago in the common ancestor of this clade, around the same time as the appearance of the planum temporale, a structure later associated with language capabilities. The Von Economo neurons are probably related to a class of neurons found in the anterior cingulate and anterior insular cortex in all mammals that may be involved in the control of appetite (Allman et al., 2010). Von Economo neurons first appear in humans in small numbers around the 36th week of gestation. At birth, only 15% of the adult number is present. Von Economo neurons express serotonin 2_B-receptor and the dopamine D_3 receptor (Allman et al., 2005). They also express receptors for the cytokines interleukin 4, 6, and 8, which implicate them in the regulation of the immune system, which we will discuss later in this volume (Tetreault and Allman, unpublished data). The Von Economo neurons are more numerous in the fronto-insular and anterior cingulate cortex in the right hemisphere than in the left, which may relate to hemispheric specializations of these structures in sympathetic (right) and parasympathetic (left) responses, as will also be discussed later (Allman et al., 2005, 2010; Craig, 2005).

Von Economo neurons may convey to other parts of the brain the motivation to act based on the outcome of processing within the anterior cingulate and fronto-insular cortex. Of particular relevance to the capacity for self-control is the recognition of having committed an error because the anterior cingulate and fronto-insular cortex connect with areas storing information related to past experience in area 10 (Allman et al., 2010). This recognition allows the individual to initiate an adaptive response.

GENETIC STUDIES

There has been an intensive search for genes that might have undergone large sequence changes or acceleration in the rate of nucleotide changes in the human lineage. Some genes, such as a substantial proportion of those related to the olfactory receptor, have been deactivated in humans. Other genes appear to have undergone positive selection for amino-acid changes in humans (Carroll, 2003; Clark et al., 2003; Gagneux and Varki, 2001; Hacia, 2001; Preuss et al., 2004). The genetic basis of human evolution has been reviewed elsewhere, but we will comment on a few candidate genes that are relevant to this discussion (Vallender et al., 2008).

Genes Related to Cortical Size

Autosomal recessive primary microencephalopathy (MCPH) is a neurological disorder that has provided some powerful insights into the genetic mechanisms of cortical evolution. MCPH is characterized by greatly reduced cortical size with normal cytoarchitecture and mild to moderate mental retardation without other major neurological disorders (Woods et al., 2005). Figure 3.1 shows an MRI of a patient with microcephaly (left) compared to a normal patient (right).

The condition is most common in highly inbred populations resulting from cultural norms favoring consanguineous marriage, where the incidence can be as high as 1 in 10,000 (Woods et al., 2005). These mechanisms were anticipated in a proposal made by Pasko Rakic (1995) that the prime determinant of cortex size is the regulation of the type and number of cell division cycles in the cortical progenitor cells. Progenitor cell divisions can be symmetric, in which two daughter progenitor cells are made (early development); asymmetric, in which one progenitor cell and one neuron is made, which migrates into the cortex (midstage); or symmetric, in which two neurons are made, both of which migrate (late development) (Fig. 3.2).

MCPH is caused by genes located in at least seven distinct loci, and four specific genes have been described (Woods et al., 2005). One of these is the abnormal spindle-like microcephaly (ASPM) gene and the other is microcephalin. Both are involved in the control of cell cycle timing and DNA repair and have undergone substantial evolutionary change in apes and humans (Bond et al., 2002; Evans et al.,

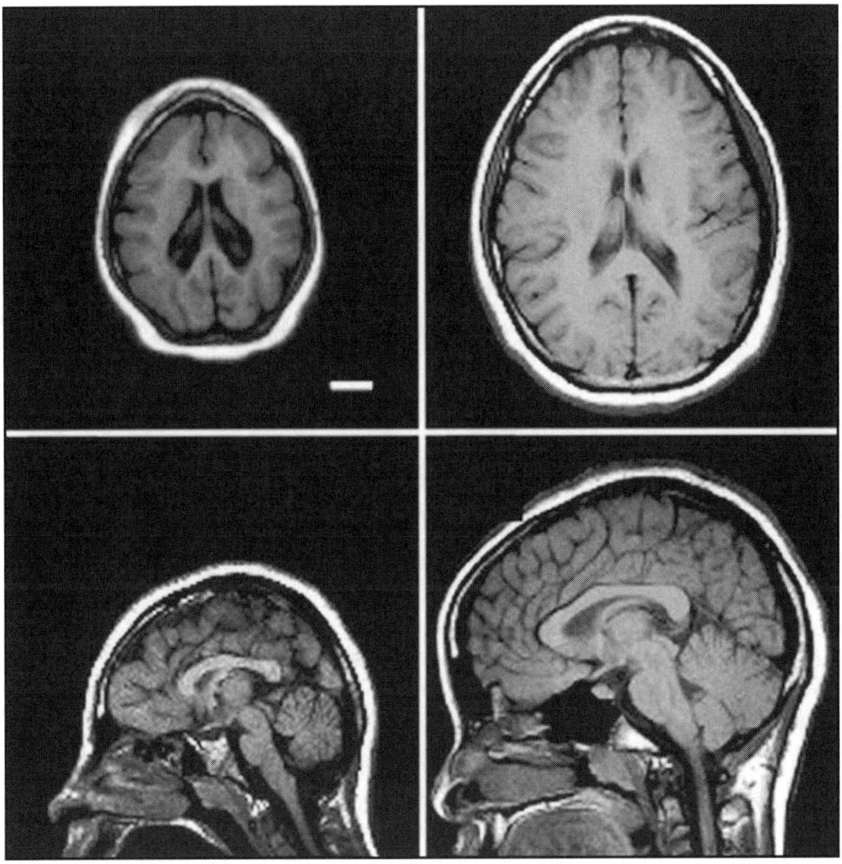

Figure 3.1 Magnetic resonance images of brains of individuals with an MCPH5 mutation. *Top left*: Axial T1-weighted image from a 13-year-old girl with an MCPH5 mutation, showing reduced size of cerebral cortex and some simplification of gyral pattern. *Top right*: Axial T1-weighted image from an unaffected 11-year-old female control. *Bottom left*: Sagittal T1-weighted image from a 13-year-old girl with an MCPH5 mutation, showing a striking reduction in the size of the cerebral cortex, prominent sloping of the forehead, and preserved midline structures. *Bottom right*: Sagittal T1-weighted image from an unaffected 11-year-old female control. Scale bar = 2 cm. Reprinted by permission from Macmillan Publishers Ltd: Bond, J., Roberts, E., Mochida, G.H., Hampshire, D.J., Scott, S., Askham, J.M., Springel, K., Mahadevan, M., Crow, Y.J., Markham, A.F., Walsh, C.A., and Woods, C.G. ASPM is a major determinant of cerebral cortical size. *Nature Genetics*, **32**, 316–320, Copyright 2002.

2005; Vallender et al., 2008; Woods et al., 2005). ASPM has also been implicated in cortical expansion in the highly encephalized spider and woolly New World monkeys (Ali and Meier, 2008). Mutations of ASPM are the most common cause of MCPH, and these account for about 40% of the cases; 57 such mutations have thus far been identified (Nicholas et al., 2009). APSM is the homologue of the *Drosophila* abnormal spindle gene (ASP), which is necessary for the formation of the mitotic spindles during cell division (Woods et al., 2005), and thus could regulate both cell

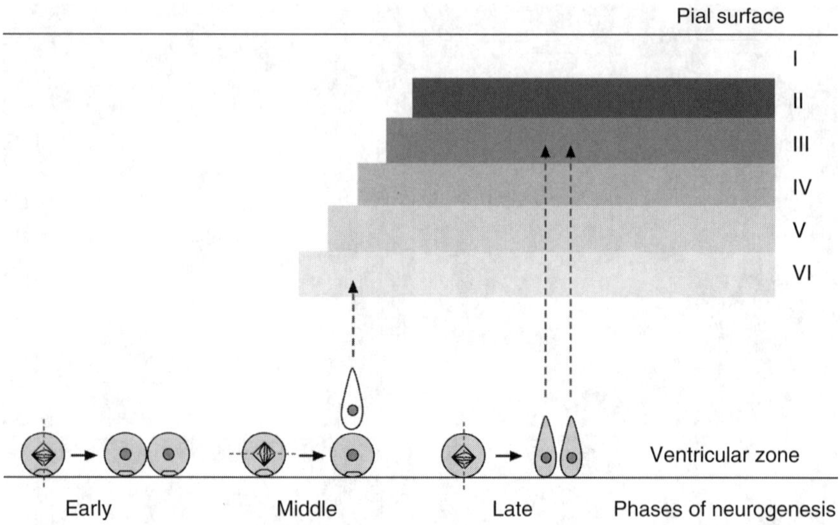

Figure 3.2 Development of the cerebral cortex. Neural progenitors (gray) proliferate in the ventricular zone adjacent to the ventricular lumen. As neurons are produced they migrate out of the ventricular zone (VZ) toward the pial surface. Later-born neurons migrate past earlier-born neurons to form six distinct cell layers (I–VI) in an inside-out fashion. Neural progenitors can divide in a symmetric or asymmetric fashion, producing daughter cells of identical or different fates, respectively. Two factors that determine the mode of cell division are the polarized localization of cell fate determinants (oval) along the apical-basal axis and mitotic spindle. Symmetric divisions are characterized by the equal partitioning of cell fate determinants between the two daughter cells, with the plane of cell division (*vertical dashed line*) perpendicular to the ventricular surface. Asymmetric divisions are characterized by unequal partitioning of cell fate determinants between two daughter cells, with the plane of division parallel to the ventricular surface (*horizontal dashed line*), resulting in one progenitor cell that remains in the VZ and one neuron that migrates toward the pial surface. Symmetric divisions producing two progenitor cells predominate during early stages of neurogenesis, expanding the progenitor pool. There is a subsequent shift toward more asymmetric divisions that maintain the progenitor pool and produce post-mitotic neurons. During late states of neurogenesis, there is a shift back to symmetric divisions, but progenitors divide to produce two neurons, depleting the progenitor pool while rapidly increasing neuronal production. Reprinted by permission from John Wiley & Sons: Chae, T.H., and Walsh, C.A. Genes that control the size of the cerebral cortex. Novartis Foundation Symposium, 288, 79–90, Copyright 2007.

cycle type and number of cycles in cortical neurogenesis in a manner directly relevant to the model proposed by Rakic (1995) and presented in Figure 3.2. Finally, there is recent evidence that some of the genes that cause microcephaly regulate the sizes of particular regions of the cortex (Rimol et al., 2010).

HAR1F: A Gene Related to Cortical Development

David Haussler and his colleagues screened the chimpanzee and human genomes for regions that showed strong evidence for recent evolutionary change in humans

(Pollard et al., 2006). The region (HAR1) showing the highest number of coding changes in this analysis is located in the gene HAR1F, and these coding changes are specific to the human lineage, but probably are more than 1 million years old. HAR1F appears to have a role in regulating cortical development. In the fetal human brain, HAR1F is very selectively expressed in the Cajal-Retzius cells from gestational weeks 7 through 19, during the period in which the laminar structure of the cortex is established. Co-expressed in the same Cajal-Retzius cells at these stages is the gene RELN, which produces the protein reelin, which plays a key role in the formation of the cortical layers. As shown in Figure 3.2, the precursors of the cortical pyramidal neurons are born in the ventricular zone and migrate along radial glia to the reach the cortex. Reelin serves as a stop signal indicating that migrating neurons have arrived at their appropriate laminar destination (Chai et al., 2009). Thus, the recent evolutionary change in HAR1F may be modulating the laminar structure in the human cortex. HAR1F is also expressed in the frontal cortex and the hippocampus in the adult human brain, although its functional role in adults is unknown at present.

Variations in the Promoter Region of the Serotonin Transporter

Within the clade comprising monkeys, apes, and humans there is a variation in the length of the promoter region of the gene that encodes the serotonin transporter (5-HTT), which regulates the amount of serotonin at synapses (Lesch et al., 1997). The short form has been associated with an increased risk of the development of alcoholism and depression in highly stressed individuals (Jedema et al., 2010). However, short-form subjects have improved performance relative to long-form subjects on tasks involving visual episodic memory, set shifting, and probabilistic reward learning (Jedema et al., 2010). Both humans and macaque monkeys who have the short form of the serotonin transporter gene have reduced volumes in the subgenual anterior cingulate cortex and prefrontal cortex and increased volume in the pulvinar complex of the thalamus (Jedema et al., 2010). The pulvinar mediates selective attention and may compensate for the reductions in cingulate and frontal cortex. The short-form monkeys also had superior performance in reversal learning tasks and were able to adapt their behavior more rapidly when reward contingencies changed. The performance of the short-form monkeys on this task and related probabilistic reward tasks showed a strong parallel with the human short-form subjects (Jedema et al., 2010). Thus, the short form of the serotonin transporter appears to endow both humans and monkeys with superior cognitive capacities in some changing environments, but this capacity appears to come at the cost of greater vulnerability to depression when stressed. When Jedema et al. (2010) compared the activity of the serotonin transporter in monkey using positron emission tomography (PET), they found no difference between the short- and long-form monkeys, suggesting that the differences in their performance may have been due to structural differences in the brains of these subjects. Serotonin influences brain development, and it is possible that the structural and behavioral differences arise from this developmental role.

FOXP2 Gene

Another gene that has received considerable attention is the forkhead box P2 (FOXP2) gene. FOXP2 has been identified as the gene underlying a human developmental language abnormality. Individuals with a FOXP2 mutation exhibit prominent deficiencies in orofacial movements but perform other movements normally. They are impaired on tests of verbal fluency and language comprehension and production. Interestingly, songbirds express similar genes, suggesting that these genes are related to vocal control (Lai et al., 2001; Teramitsu et al., 2004). Complementary DNAs that encode for the FOXP2 protein were sequenced in the human, chimpanzee, gorilla, orangutan, rhesus, macaque, and mouse. Changes in human FOXP2 amino-acid coding and pattern of nucleotide polymorphism suggested that this gene has been the target of selection during recent human evolution (Enard et al., 2002; Konopka et al., 2010).

Glutamate Dehydrogenase 2

Glutamate dehydrogenase is an enzyme that metabolizes the neurotransmitter glutamate, which has been implicated in schizophrenia (see Chapter 4). It has been suggested that a retrotranspositional event occurred in the ape lineage after divergence from Old World monkeys that resulted in a new form of the enzyme that supported the higher level of neurotransmitter turnover seen in the human brain (Burki and Kaessmann, 2004).

Monoamine Oxidase A

The monoamine amine oxidase A gene encodes the enzyme in the mitochondria that breaks down neurotransmitters, including dopamine, serotonin, and norepinephrine. There may have been a non-synonymous change in this gene in the human lineage after the human–chimpanzee divergence (Andrés et al., 2004). These neurotransmitters are implicated in mood disorders (see Chapter 5).

Gene Expression

An area that has borne some fruit is the investigation of the temporal and spatial patterns of gene expression in the human brain (Cáceres et al., 2003; Enard et al., 2002). Cáceres et al. (2003) identified 169 genes that exhibited expression differences between human and chimpanzee cortex. Ninety percent of these genes were upregulated or more highly expressed in humans. Between humans and chimpanzees, about 10% of genes differ in their expression in at least one region of the brain (Khaitovich et al., 2004). Both chimpanzees and humans showed particular differences from gorillas in the gene expression related to aerobic energy metabolism in the anterior cingulate region (Uddin et al., 2004).

While these differences in the human genome make some sense in view of specializations of the human brain, they are likely only a tiny fraction of the actual genetic differences that characterize the human brain. A recent comparison of 7,645 human and chimpanzee gene sequences identified several hundred genes that had probably undergone positive selection for amino-acid changes in humans (Clark et al., 2003).

Copy Number Variation

There is very little molecular difference between humans and great apes. The proteins across these species are almost identical. However, there are some striking differences between gorillas, chimpanzees, and humans in segmental duplication of genes, which might lead to similar proteins but very different phenotypes. Copy number mutations seem to be more evident in gorillas and chimpanzees than humans, but there appears to be a burst in genomic duplication activity during human evolution. Many of the genes affected are involved in signal transduction (Marques-Bonet et al., 2009). As we will see in later chapters, copy number variation anomalies can also be found in many neuropsychiatric conditions. In many cases, the genes duplicated are associated with signal transduction and forming neuronal networks.

HUMAN COGNITION COMPARED TO NON-HUMAN COGNITION

What makes human cognition different from non-human primates is slowly beginning to emerge (Premack and Premack, 2003). As cognitive studies have become more sophisticated, it has become apparent that animals are capable of many abilities once thought unique to humans. However, Premack (2007) has presented an argument that even though there are similarities between animal and human abilities, they are much smaller than the dissimilarities. Eight cognitive abilities were considered: teaching, short-term memory, causal reasoning, planning, deception, transitive interference, theory of mind, and language. We will briefly comment on Premack's observations in each of these areas.

Many animals teach their young to stalk or gather food, but a single target is in mind. Human teaching, on the other hand, is not domain-specific and has many targets. Chimpanzees are able to remember about five to seven items, the same as humans. However, humans are able to count past the number of items stored in their short-term memory owing to their ability for both recursive numbers and language. When events are temporally and spatially contiguous, human adults believe that the first event caused the second event. The difference between animals and humans is illustrated by the example that animal may recognize that a large rock is more likely to break a branch than a small one, but an animal will not infer that a large rock lying by a crushed plant actually crushed the plant.

Similar arguments are offered for differences between humans and other species in planning. Some birds store food for future use, but planning is much more complex in humans, sometimes involving more than one individual with several steps. Deception is an area suggested to be uniquely human, but other species are capable of "fooling" others; a plover leads intruders away from a nest, for example. Yet even in deception differences can be pointed out. In the human, deception occurs across domains to serve many goals. Transitive interference is another area where some animals demonstrate competence. Fish will prefer to swim with fish that they have observed losing fights with size-matched rivals. It is suggested that this may be a hard-wired process, not based on reasoning. Chimpanzees, for example, do not spontaneously place dolls in order the way human children do.

The two cognitive functions that are most closely identified with humans are theory of mind and language. Human mothers do know what their children are capable of and respond appropriately. This ability to infer the mental condition of another individual, or so-called *theory of mind*, provides enormous advantages to survival in social groups, a topic we will return to in Chapters 8 and 10. Chimpanzees lack voluntary control of their voice and are not capable of language. However, chimpanzees are able to learn a symbolic language to some degree when it is presented in a visual format. We will examine human language capabilities in more detail in Chapter 9.

CONSCIOUSNESS

We are at a very early stage of understanding the brain circuits that mediate consciousness (Chalmers, 1996; Damasio, 1999; Metzinger, 2000). A basic subjective awareness of surroundings is likely maintained via brainstem nuclei, hypothalamus, and somatosensory cortex. Self-awareness may require the involvement of other brain structures such as the medioprefrontal cortex, cingulate and insular cortex, thalamus, and superior colliculus. There is little doubt that mammals have a basic subjective awareness of their internal body states and their surroundings. However, there is still a great deal of debate as to whether they are self-aware in the sense of being distinct from other individuals within their social group. Inherent in this concept of self-awareness is the capacity to be aware of the subjective states of other individuals. We will discuss this further in Chapter 8, but at this point it may be helpful to consider some more general aspects of conscious experience.

40-Hz Oscillations

Specific aspects of conscious experience correlate with changes in activity in brain regions in association with specific stimuli or memories, but conscious experience as a whole involves the activation or deactivation of widespread brain regions. Subjects who are comatose or in slow-wave sleep demonstrate markedly reduced activity in the cerebral cortex and thalamus. On the other hand, mental activity is associated with temporal binding of 40-Hz oscillations, reflecting synchronous activity of re-entrant corticothalamic loops (Llinás and Pare, 1991; Tononi and Edelman, 1998a, 1998b). Activity within the loops is focused by an attentional network involving the dorsolateral prefrontal cortex, right inferior parietal lobe, anterior cingulate, and some temporal lobe structures. Comparison of ongoing experience with past experiences and its emotional valence is enabled by input from the hippocampus and amygdala, respectively.

The Binding Problem

How does a complex collection of sights, sounds, smells, and physical sensations become integrated into a unitary experience with a subjective and objective sense of self in an external, ever-changing world? The question is referred to as the *binding problem*. There have been several theories about how consciousness becomes a unitary experience (Cleeremans, 2003; Crick, 1984; Gray, 1995, 2004; Jones, 2001; Laberge, 1995; Llinás and Pare, 1991; Llinás et al., 1994; Newman 1997a, 1997b; Newman and Grace, 1999; Posner, 1994; Tononi and Edelman, 1998a, 1998b). All of these theories recognize the importance of thalamocortical connections and the 40-Hz activity generated by these connections simultaneously at multiple cortical locations in the maintenance of consciousness. There is also a consensus that attention involves many brain regions, such as the prefrontal cortex, anterior cingulate, and parietal cortex. Nevertheless, there are differing mechanisms suggested for how attention is shifted and how current experience is compared to past experience.

Gray (1995) proposed that a hippocampal *comparator* is responsible for the contents of consciousness—that is, the current state of an organism's perceptual world is compared with a predicted state. However, patients with damage to the hippocampus have full consciousness, albeit in a somewhat chaotic and altered form, which would not be predicted by the model (Gray, 2004). Newman and Grace (1999) proposed that the comparative function was mediated by hippocampal inputs to the nucleus accumbens, which in turn influenced the nucleus reticularis, a thin shell covering the thalamus. This model integrates the role of the reticular activating system, which is involved in sleep/wake cycles. It also accounts for gating from the hippocampus, which is important in providing context, and it is consistent with the role of thalamocortical loops synchronized by fast activity. Unfortunately, it is very difficult to test these models in humans. It is also not clear what aspects of the proposed circuitry might be unique to humans.

Craig (2009) has suggested that monkeys and especially humans are endowed with a more fine-grained awareness of internal body states; this awareness proceeds through specialized circuits involving highly differentiated circuits arising from the spinal cord and through the posterior part of the ventral medial nucleus of the thalamus and the insular cortex. We will discuss these findings in detail in Chapter 10.

SUMMARY

Although the human brain is constructed from the same building blocks as the brains of non-human primates, there are some clear differences. Beyond differences in size, there are regional differences in structures that support capabilities such as theory of mind and language. The difference can be seen at all levels. At a genetic level, there appear to be a number of differences in gene expression, although almost all of these have yet to be characterized. At a cellular level, we see differences in metabolic rates, synaptic proliferation, and perhaps cell lines.

More interestingly, we see a striking difference in connectivity, suggesting that unique cognitive functions in humans are related to different parts of the brain acting together. We are just beginning to understand some of these differences in connectivity. Human experience is very complex and not easily reduced to this level. However, it is possible that understanding what happens when these circuits break down in mental illness may shed some light on the nature of the circuitry itself. We will begin with schizophrenia.

4

Schizophrenia

Much has been learned about schizophrenia since the condition was first described by Kraepelin (Williamson, 2006). This chapter will review what we know about the epidemiology and natural course of the disorder. We will then look at some of the psychophysiological and neuropathological findings. Although no major genes have emerged, there are some intriguing findings that may point toward anomalies in brain development. Other aspects of schizophrenia, such as which neurotransmitters might be involved and in vivo structural and functional brain imaging studies, offer some clues about circuitry. No discussion of this type can hope to be complete, but we hope to highlight the findings that may be relevant to a discussion of what makes the human brain more vulnerable to this condition.

EPIDEMIOLOGY AND NATURAL COURSE

Incidence and Prevalence

Schizophrenia tends to have its onset just as the prefrontal cortex is completing its development. The diagnosis is usually made in the third decade of life, but a prodromal phase precedes the first admission by an average of 6 years, with women presenting about 3 to 4 years later than men (Häfner and an der Heiden, 1997). Although there was some heterogeneity among studies, pooled 1-year and lifetime prevalence was 0.34 per 100 and 0.55 per 100, while 1 year incidence rates were 11.1 per 100,000. More recent epidemiological studies have found higher male than female incidence rates (Goldner et al., 2002), although almost all prevalence studies have shown similar gender rates. A possible explanation may be that the duration of illness is shorter in males due to a higher mortality rate.

Environmental Factors

Epidemiological studies have implicated a number of environmental factors that could affect early brain development. On the whole, schizophrenic patients have more labor and delivery complications. Up to a nine-fold increase in risk for schizophrenia has been reported with pre-eclampsia, possibly due to fetal hypoxia. An increased risk of schizophrenia has also been associated with exposure to influenza and nutritional deficiencies (Jones and Cannon, 1998). The role of cytokines potentially related to maternal influenza and other infections has been examined by Brown et al. (2004) in a large cohort of pregnancies followed in the Kaiser Foundation Health Plan in Alameda, California. Fifty-nine of the individuals born to the mothers in this study eventually developed schizophrenia spectrum disorders, and they were compared with 105 matched individuals born in the study who did not suffer from schizophrenia or affective disorders. Brown et al. (2004) measured the levels of the cytokines interleukin (IL)-6, IL-8, IL-1B, and tumor necrosis factor (TNF)-alpha in serum samples taken from the mothers during the second trimester of their pregnancies and found a strong relationship between the levels of IL-8 and the later development of schizophrenia spectrum disorders in their mature offspring. They found no relationship with the other cytokines or any other maternal attribute, such as age, smoking status, ethnicity, or education.

Course of Illness

Many patients with schizophrenia show no signs before developing the illness, but others have a variety of nonspecific findings, such as minor differences in head circumference at birth or dermatoglyphic (fingerprint) anomalies. The dermatoglyphic abnormalities are interesting because viral infections in the first 6 months of pregnancy can affect their development (McGrath and Murray, 1995). Other anomalies include soft neurological signs such as disorders of equilibrium, tremor, and adiadochokinesia, many of which were described by Kraepelin long before the introduction of neuroleptics (Kraepelin, 1919). However, none of these findings are specific to schizophrenia.

Although Kraepelin observed that dementia praecox was a progressively deteriorating condition in many cases, other patients had a less malignant course, with periodic exacerbations and some degree of recovery in between. Before antipsychotic medications, recovery rarely lasted longer than 3 years. Follow-up studies since the introduction of antipsychotic medication have shown a significant improvement in outcome (Ciompi, 1980; Hogarty et al., 1974; Huber et al., 1980; May et al., 1981). However, antipsychotic medications control positive symptoms such as hallucinations and delusions much better than they control negative symptoms such as lack of motivation and flattened affect. Schizophrenic patients have difficulty coping with critical comments from family members and often break down under stress (Norman and Malla, 1993). The overwhelming majority are not employed at their expected occupational level, married, or raising a family. In fact, the World Health Organization placed schizophrenia on the list of the 10 most disabling medical illnesses (Murray and Lopez, 1996).

NEUROPSYCHOLOGICAL FINDINGS

Social and intellectual deficits are often seen in childhood in individuals who later develop schizophrenia. Scholastic test scores are nonsignificantly below average in primary grades but drop significantly between the ages of 13 and 16, perhaps marking cognitive impairment associated with the illness (Fuller et al., 2002). Even home movies of children who later develop schizophrenia show some differences from other children. In one well-known study, raters were able to fairly accurately determine which patients would develop schizophrenia on the basis of atypical emotion expressions and movements (Walker and Lewine, 1990). All of this suggests that schizophrenia actually begins long before the development of hallucinations and delusions, but what is the nature of the psychological impairment?

Prefrontal Psychological Deficits

Perhaps not surprisingly, schizophrenic patients demonstrate fairly consistent deficits in prefrontal functions. As discussed in Chapter 2, the prefrontal cortex plays a role in language production, working memory, and executive functions. With something as simple as producing as many words starting with a certain letter as you can, schizophrenic patients fail to come up with as many words as comparable controls (Gruzelier et al., 1988; Kolb and Whishaw, 1983). The question always arises as to whether such deficits reflect widespread effects, but the fact that schizophrenic patients can do many visuospatial tests, which involve posterior regions of the brain, quite well suggests that deficits may affect frontal regions more than other parts of the brain (Morrison-Stewart et al., 1992). This deficit also appears to be independent of intellectual functioning (Crawford et al., 1993).

More sophisticated tests of executive reasoning ability, such as the Wisconsin Card Sorting Test (WCST), are difficult for schizophrenic patients. Generally, they complete fewer categories and show tendencies to perseverate on the same category, similar to neurological patients who have had a frontal lobe injury (Van der Does and Van den Bosch, 1992). Comparable deficits can be seen in schizophrenic patients on other executive function tasks, such as the Tower of Hanoi task (Goldberg et al., 1990). These tests also rely on working memory to some extent.

Memory

Working memory enables information to be held after sensory input so that a course of action can be planned. Working memory deficits have been demonstrated in schizophrenic patients with a number of tasks, including the Letter-Number

Sequencing Test, the N-Back, Delayed Response, and Delayed Match to Sample tasks (Carter et al., 1998; Gold et al., 1997; Keefe, 2000). Such on-line storage may be related to many of the cognitive performance deficits seen in schizophrenic patients (Silver et al., 2003). A deficit on working memory tasks can also be seen in the relatives of schizophrenic patients (Park et al., 1995).

Most patients with schizophrenia are well oriented and can recall a few words after a few minutes when asked to do so. However, schizophrenic patients generally perform poorly on both short-term and long-term memory tasks in standard test batteries, with an effect size in the moderate to large range (Aleman et al., 1999; Heinrichs and Zakzanis, 1998). Prospective memory tasks that may be linked to frontal area 10 deficits are particularly difficult for patients (Wang et al., 2009). Some have suggested that schizophrenic patients have an impaired ability to process contextual information (Bazin et al., 2000; Hemsley, 1987; Rizzo et al., 1996; Servan-Schreiber et al., 1996). This deficit seems to be largely in the binding together of different contextual information to form a memory representation (Danion et al., 1999; Waters et al., 2004). It is likely that the brain regions for content and context of memory may be different (Nyberg et al., 1996), but the processes that bind different elements into a unified memory representation are just beginning to be understood (Chalfonte and Johnson, 1996).

Attention

It has been suggested that schizophrenic patients complain of being bombarded by stimuli that they are unable to filter out, leading to an inability to distinguish self from other (McGhie and Chapman, 1961). This suggestion has been borne out to some degree by the performance of schizophrenic patients on attentional tasks such as the Continuous Performance Test (CPT). About 40% of chronic schizophrenic patients have markedly impaired performance on this test (Orzack and Kornetsky, 1966). Based on well over 40 CPT studies in schizophrenic patients, Cornblatt and Keilp (1994) argue that impaired attention is evident in schizophrenic patients independent of clinical state and even before the onset of illness, suggesting that it is not a medication effect. However, the CPT task involves a number of functions and it is not entirely clear whether impaired performance on this task may be due to early perceptual processing abnormalities dependent on working memory or attentional difficulties (Neuchterlein et al., 1994).

Deficits in Early Visual Processing

Early clinical observations of schizophrenia, such as those of Bleuler (1950), noted that patients often complained of altered sensory experience, but these were attributed to deficits in association and emotion (Javitt, 2009). Sensory processing was considered one of the intact functions in schizophrenia, but a large body of recent work indicates that there are significant deficits in some of the functions performed in the lower cortical visual area in schizophrenia. These deficits include contrast sensitivity (Kéri et al., 2009), Vernier acuity (Kéri et al., 2004), the discrimination of object shape and spatial location (Tek et al., 2002), the capacity to track moving objects (Kelemen et al., 2007), and the abnormal perception of common visual illusions, such as the Muller-Lyer test (Kantrowitz et al., 2009). Also compromised in schizophrenia is the capacity to discriminate the emotional content in facial expressions, which probably arises from these low-level deficits; this impairs social functioning in schizophrenics (Butler et al., 2009). Corresponding to these psychophysical deficits are abnormalities in early visual processing indicated in electrophysiological, imaging, and neuroanatomical studies (reviewed later in this chapter). These deficits in early vision are to some extent consistent with the overall hypothesis of this book, which is that neuropsychiatric illnesses are often related to novel behavioral capacities brought about by recent evolutionary change. One of the major innovations in the evolution of the visual system in anthropoid primates was the enhanced capacity to discriminate individual faces and the facial expression of emotions (Allman, 1982, 2000).

Is There a Core Deficit on Neuropsychological Tests?

Schizophrenic patients have widespread impairments on neuropsychological tests involving both hemispheres. In keeping with unique specializations in the human brain, the frontal and temporal regions seem to be more affected. However, not all patients have deficits. The effect size for most of the findings is on the order of 1.0, indicating that only about 25% of patients would have scores outside the normal range if the data were normally distributed (Heinrichs and Zakzanis, 1998). When anomalies are found, they usually involve working memory in some way (Goldman-Rakic, 1994; Silver et al., 2003). However, more recent work directly implicates early visual processing in schizophrenia. Several investigators have also commented on the difficulties with encoding of information in schizophrenic patients (Carter and Neufeld, 1999). Difficulties at his stage depend on working memory capacity, but not exclusively. What seems to be missing with many patients is the ability to efficiently link the current stimulus with a cognitive set necessary for the task at hand.

It is possible that traditional neuropsychological tests cannot detect the core deficit in schizophrenia. Frith (1995) suggested that it was more useful to think about two main deficits: a *poverty of will*, which accounts for negative symptoms and difficulties on word fluency tasks, and a *failure of self-monitoring*, leading to positive symptoms like thought insertion (failure to recognize your own thoughts) and auditory hallucinations (attribution of internal speech to someone else). We will discuss this possibility further in Chapter 8.

ELECTROPHYSIOLOGICAL FINDINGS

Electroencephalographic (EEG) Studies

Hans Berger, a psychiatrist, was the first to show that an EEG could be recorded from the human head, reflecting mostly thalamocortical activity (Berger, 1929). Some of the original surface EEG reports in schizophrenic patients described little alpha activity, with disorganized, very fast random frequency described as *choppy*. Other findings included a high incidence of sharp waves suggestive of epilepsy, reduced reactivity to external stimuli, and frontal slowing. A few EEG studies have been done with implanted electrodes in patients with chronic schizophrenia (Hanley et al., 1972; Heath, 1954). Spike activity was recorded from the septal area, which likely included the head of the caudate, lateral septal nuclei, nucleus accumbens, and olfactory tubercle. While these patients did not have epilepsy, the spikes could suggest partial denervation from other structures (Stevens, 1973).

More recently, there has been an increased interest in EEG studies in schizophrenia, with the suggestion that the ability to perceive different sensory modalities as a unified experience, or *binding*, occurs in association with localized gamma synchronization at cortical and thalamic levels (Cleeremens, 2003; Llinás and Pare, 1991; Tononi and Edelman, 1998a, 1998b). Some have suggested that there are abnormalities in gamma synchronization in schizophrenia (Spencer et al., 2004), while others have suggested that abnormalities may not be limited to this frequency band (van der Stelt et al., 2004). It is likely that gamma synchrony depends on GABA-ergic chandelier cells (Lewis et al., 2005), which are abundant throughout the prefrontal cortex and may differ in their biochemistry in humans (del Rio and DeFelipe, 1997).

Event-related Potential (ERP) Findings

With ERP recordings, it is possible to look at the response of the brain to various sensory stimuli in a very short time. Very-low-voltage changes within the first 400 milliseconds (ms) following a stimulus can be measured with this technique by averaging hundreds of responses to a stimulus. Early components (<250 ms) depend on the physical properties of the stimulus, while later components (particularly P300) reflect cognitive processes associated with the stimulus. Abnormalities in early ERP components have been described, suggesting impaired reticular filtering or subcortical monitoring (Holzman, 1987). In other cases, there was a reversal of normal lateral asymmetry in early ERP components (Gruzelier, 1999). However, findings were not specific to schizophrenia in that they could be seen in a number of other conditions, such as depression (Friedman and Squires-Wheeler, 1994).

One of the more consistent ERP findings in schizophrenia is called *prepulse inhibition*. Essentially, it is normal inhibition of the stimulus response caused by an earlier warning stimulus (Braff and Geyer, 1990). Prepulse inhibition deficits can be found in a number of other conditions, such as obsessive-compulsive disorder, Huntington's disease, attention-deficit disorder, and Tourette syndrome (Swerdlow and Geyer, 1998). Later ERP components are studied with an oddball paradigm in which a repeated tone is interspersed with a less frequent event to which the subject must respond in some way. The majority of these investigations have found a reduction in the amplitude of the P300 in schizophrenia. ERP abnormalities are present in a number of other conditions, such as dementia, alcoholism, and major depression (Friedman and Squires-Wheeler, 1994). Although ERP findings are not specific to schizophrenia, they suggest that schizophrenic patients have difficulty attending to relevant stimuli and suppressing irrelevant stimuli, consistent with some of the neuropsychological findings.

NEUROTRANSMITTER ABNORMALITIES

Dopamine

Dopamine is clearly involved in schizophrenia. Dopamine agonists lead to hallucinations and delusions that look a lot like schizophrenia, while the effectiveness of antipsychotic medications is correlated with the ability to block D_2 receptors (Carlsson, 1988; Seeman, 1987)—with the exception of clozapine, which has a low dopamine receptor occupancy. This would suggest an increase in dopamine activity in schizophrenia. However, it is likely that there is a decreased level of dopamine in the prefrontal region on the basis of a neurodevelopmental abnormality combined with a subcortical increase in dopamine activity (Weinberger, 1987). The decreased levels in the prefrontal cortex may be associated with negative symptoms, while increased subcortical levels may be associated with positive symptoms (Davis et al., 1991; Swerdlow and Koop, 1987; Weinberger 1987). More recently, Grace (1993) suggested that low dopamine levels could lead to excessive phasic or burst firing of dopaminergic neurons, resulting in positive symptoms.

Stress increases the release and turnover of dopamine, which may explain why schizophrenic patients often relapse under stress (Deutch, 1993; Moghaddam 2002). Some of the difficulties that schizophrenic patients have with cognitive tasks may also be related to dopamine regulation (Servan-Shreiber et al., 1998). Dopamine-releasing drugs such as amphetamines or dopamine receptor-stimulating drugs such as apomorphine lead to some schizophrenic-like behaviors in animals when given chronically (Robinson and Becker, 1986). Even a single exposure to amphetamines can be associated with lasting changes in behavior and sensitization (Vanderschuren et al., 1999). Prepulse inhibition changes similar to those seen in many schizophrenic patients are also seen in these animals (Swerdlow et al., 2000; Tenn et al., 2003). These effects can be reversed by antipsychotic drugs.

Glutamate

Drugs that block *N*-methyl-D-aspartate (NMDA) glutamate receptors such as phencyclidine (PCP) cause both positive symptoms such as paranoia and thought disorder and negative symptoms such as amotivation and blunted affect when given to normal volunteers and schizophrenic patients (Krystal et al., 1994; Lahti et al., 1995b). NMDA receptor antagonists are capable of inducing the many cognitive deficits found in some schizophrenic patients. For example, healthy volunteers show deficits similar to schizophrenic patients on the CPT when given ketamine, an NMDA blocker (Umbricht et al., 2000). Single-dose PCP has also been shown to disrupt prepulse inhibition in rats, similar to the startle-gating deficits seen in schizophrenic patients (Jentsch and Roth, 1999).

When higher doses of PCP are given to mature (but not immature) rats, a neuron-necrotizing reaction can be seen that spreads to other parts of the limbic system, including the anterior cingulate; parietal, temporal, piriform, and entorhinal cortices; hippocampus; amygdala; and taenia tecta (Olney and Farber, 1995). This kind of reaction can be understood by the fact that glutamatergic neurons maintain tonic inhibitory control over several pathways that converge on the posterior cingulate by their stimulation of inhibitory GABA-ergic neurons. With the blockage of this stimulation, there is a paradoxical increase in activity in excitatory pathways, leading to the neuronal damage (Olney and Farber, 1995). Acute administration of NMDA antagonists increases forebrain dopamine transmission, which might explain why some antipsychotic drugs can attenuate the effects of PCP on rats (Jentsch and Roth, 1999). Subchronic treatment with PCP leads to increased responsivity in the mesolimbic dopamine pathway to *d*-amphetamine or mild stress, much like the positron emission tomography (PET) findings in schizophrenic patients (Jentsch et al., 1998). Thus, glutamatergic activity may be closely linked with dopamine transmission.

There is now some evidence that glutamatergic drugs can be helpful in the treatment of schizophrenia. Sarcosine, which enhances NDMA function through glycine transporter 1, improved both positive and negative symptoms when added to risperidone in acutely ill patients (Lane et al., 2005). Similarly, LY404039, a selective agonist for metabotropic glutamate 2/3 receptors known to reverse PCP effects in animal models, has recently been shown to be effective in the treatment of both positive and negative symptoms in schizophrenic patients (Patil et al., 2007).

Other Neurotransmitters

Several other neurotransmitters have been implicated in schizophrenia, but the case for their involvement is not so strong. It has been suggested that serotonin is implicated by the effects of atypical neuroleptics on serotonin 5-TH_{2A} receptors. Serotonin also modulates dopamine neurotransmission in several regions relevant to schizophrenia: the prefrontal cortex, the striatum, including the nucleus accumbens, and the ventral tegmentum (Kapur and Remington, 1996). There has been increasing interest in the role of gamma-aminobutyric acid (GABA) in schizophrenia (Wassef et al., 2003). Glutamatergic neurons synapse on subcortical GABA-ergic neurons, which in turn synapse on neurons in the thalamus projecting back to the cortex. A deficit in these GABA-ergic neurons could result in a similar pattern of overactivity in limbic regions to the effects of NMDA antagonists because glutamatergic release at NMDA receptors potentiates activity in GABA-ergic neurons (Olney and Farber, 1995). If NMDA receptors are blocked, GABA-ergic neurons are less active, much like a deficit in GABA-ergic neurons. Consequently, there is reason to believe that all these neurotransmitters interact with one another. Anomalies in one neurotransmitter system often lead to dysfunction in another.

NEUROPATHOLOGICAL STUDIES

Early Findings

Often described as the graveyard of neuropathology, interest increased when studies of the hippocampus and entorhinal cortex suggested cytoarchitectural differences consistent with early neurodevelopmental abnormalities (Falkai and Bogerts, 1993). Generalized atrophy, neuronal loss, reduced neuronal size, and pyramidal cell disarray have been reported in the hippocampus (Benes et al., 1991b; Bogerts et al., 1985; Falkai and Bogerts, 1986; Kovelman and Scheibel, 1984), while a loss of normal clustering has been found in the entorhinal cortex (Jacob and Beckmann, 1986). A reduction in the number and volume of neurons has also been reported in the mediodorsal thalamus and nucleus accumbens, but these changes could have occurred after the onset of the illness (Pakkenberg, 1990, 1992; Stevens, 1982; Young et al., 2000).

Cell Migration Anomalies

There have been a number of reports of abnormalities in cell migration early in brain development (Falkai and Bogerts, 1993). Cortical cell migration is dependent upon the subplate, which receives projections from the thalamus. Akbarian et al. (1993a, 1993b) found that neurons involved in subplate migration were more deeply distributed in frontal and temporal cortex white matter in schizophrenic patients than controls. This could indicate difficulties with the formation of connections at the subplate, which are critical for the development of basal ganglia-thalamocortical neuronal circuits and cortical specificity. Other neuropathological findings support cell migration anomalies. Selemon et al. (1995, 1998) found elevated neuronal density in the dorsolateral prefrontal cortex in schizophrenic patients using stereological methods, suggesting reduced neuropil. Decreased neuropil could be consistent with anomalies in the pruning of cortical–cortical connections during adolescence, which some have thought to be involved in the pathophysiology of schizophrenia (Feinberg, 1982/1983).

Dopamine

The majority of postmortem investigations have demonstrated striatal increases in D_2 receptors in chronic patients (Soares and Innis, 1999). However, the issue of effects of medication invariably arises, as treatment with neuroleptic medication is usually associated with a compensatory increase in the number of receptors. Investigations of the serotonergic receptor in schizophrenia have been inconclusive (Soares and Innis, 1999).

Glutamate

Postmortem investigations of glutamate receptors in schizophrenia have produced seemingly contradictory findings (Krystal et al., 2000). Studies of the prefrontal region in schizophrenia have shown some evidence of an excess of glutamatergic receptors and uptake sites (Deakin et al., 1989; Ishimaru et al., 1994; Toru et al., 1988). Increased glutamate-immunoreactive axons have been found in the cingulate cortex of schizophrenic patients (Benes et al., 1992). However, a decrease in aspartate and glutamate and an increase in *N*-acetylaspartateglutamate, a neuropeptide concentrated in glutamatergic neurons, has also been reported (Tsai et al., 1995). A more consistent pattern emerges in temporal regions. Several studies have shown that the expression of some glutamate receptor subtypes is decreased in the hippocampus (Meador-Woodruff and Healy, 2000). Similar decreases can also be seen in the hippocampus in kainate receptor expression (Meador-Woodruff and Healey, 2000). Overall, the postmortem studies suggest increases in glutamatergic receptors in the anterior cingulate and prefrontal/orbitofrontal regions and deficits in hippocampal and temporal regions. This pattern argues against a generalized loss of glutamatergic synapses but could be in keeping with abnormal glutamatergic activity and/or a loss of synapses in specific neuronal circuits.

GABA

GABA-ergic abnormalities have also been reported. Benes et al. (1991a) reported a deficit in small interneurons, which are GABA-ergic, in the prefrontal and cingulate cortices of schizophrenic patients. Indicators of the activity of the synthesizing enzyme for GABA, glutamate decarboxylase (GAD), have been assessed in a number of postmortem studies in schizophrenic patients. Messenger RNA expression of GAD was found to be decreased in the prefrontal region in two studies (Akbarian et al., 1995; Volk et al., 2000). Contradicting these findings, another study found increased prefrontal GAD activity using a different methodology (Gluck et al., 2002). Another study has found complex changes in GABA-ergic terminals in both schizophrenia and bipolar patients (Benes et al., 2000). However, it is likely that one or more populations of GABA neurons are altered in schizophrenia (Lewis and González-Burgos, 2008). One of these populations is the chandelier neuron. It has been suggested that layer 3 pyramidal neurons, certain types of local circuit GABA neurons, and dopamine afferents are synaptically linked and undergo considerable maturational changes during adolescence (Lewis, 1997). These observations arise largely from studies in monkeys, but there is reason to believe that these structures may be the neural substrate for delayed response tasks, on which schizophrenic patients perform poorly (Lewis et al., 2002).

Lewis and Gonzalez-Burgos (2006) proposed a link between reduced activity of chandelier neurons, dopamine, and glutamatergic activity. They suggested that NMDA hypofunction in the dorsolateral prefrontal cortex leads to decreased excitatory input to the dopamine neurons in the brainstem from the dorsolateral prefrontal cortex. As these excitatory projections synapse on GABA-ergic neurons before reaching the dopaminergic neurons, which project to the striatum from the brainstem, dopaminergic activity is increased in the striatum. The excitatory projections from the dorsolateral prefrontal cortex to the brainstem dopaminergic projections back to the prefrontal cortex do not go through GABA-ergic neurons, so the dopaminergic activity in the prefrontal cortex is reduced. Reduced dopamine levels in the prefrontal cortex lead to altered D_1-mediated signaling and reduced chandelier neuron activity.

Primary Visual Cortex

A well-documented recent finding comes from a study of primary visual cortex (Brodmann's area 17) in schizophrenics versus controls (Dorph-Petersen et al., 2007). These authors used robust stereological methods to estimate the total volume and neuron numbers in area 17 in postmortem brains from 10 subjects with schizophrenia and 10 matched normal comparison subjects. They found a significant reduction in total neuron numbers (25%) and volumes (22%) in area 17 in the schizophrenia group relative to the normal subjects. Using the same stereological procedures, they subsequently found that there was no difference in neuron numbers or volume between schizophrenics and controls in the lateral geniculate nucleus of the thalamus, which relays the visual input from the retina to area 17 (Dorph-Petersen et al., 2009). These results suggest that the loss of neurons in area 17 in schizophrenia is independent of the thalamic input and thus specific to cortex. The authors of this study argue persuasively that the reduction in the volume and neuron counts in area 17 in schizophrenia is probably a developmental abnormality in which the size of area 17 is reduced relative to other cortical areas (Dorph-Petersen et al., 2007). Schizophrenics and controls do not differ in cortical thickness or neuronal density in area 17, and thus the reduction is limited to the size of area 17. There are also consistent reports of the reduction in the size and neuron counts in the pulvinar, a major thalamic structure involved in visual attention, with strong connections with both area 17 and extrastriate cortical visual areas (Byne et al., 2009). As reviewed early in this chapter, there are many observations of deficits in early visual processing in schizophrenic subjects, as well as abnormalities in visual evoked potentials (Foxe et al., 2005; Yeap et al., 2008) and reduced activity in primary visual cortex (Desco et al., 2003). Since many of these studies controlled for potential effects of medication and length of illness, these studies appear to indicate that early visual processing deficits are essential features of schizophrenia.

Asymmetry and Gliosis

In a large structural magnetic resonance imaging (MRI) study, Makris et al. (2006) found that the anterior insula, particularly on the left side, was reduced in volume in schizophrenic subjects. Eight previous studies also found evidence of reduced insular volume in schizophrenia, with some additional evidence of a greater involvement on the left side. The anterior insula is particularly involved in self-awareness and self-control (Craig, 2009), which is consistent with the difficulty schizophrenic patients have in discriminating hallucinations from reality. Some evidence of decreased or even reversed asymmetry has been found on postmortem examination. Probably the most interesting finding was reversed asymmetry of pyramidal cell density in the dorsolateral prefrontal cortex in schizophrenic patients (Cullen et al., 2006). However, asymmetrical findings in other regions such as the planum temporale have been found to be inconclusive (Holinger et al., 2000; Shapleske et al., 1999).

Postmortem studies have failed to observe gliosis, which has been taken as evidence that schizophrenia must be a neurodevelopmental disorder since other degenerative conditions such as Alzheimer's disease are associated with evidence of active inflammation and/or repair reflected in gliosis. But, as reviewed later, there is some evidence for increased expression of genes related to inflammation in the brains of schizophrenics. Moreover, gliosis is not always demonstrable after neural injury, nor is it associated with apoptosis, a type of cell breakdown that may occur in schizophrenia (Harrison, 1999). There are also limited forms of apoptosis that lead to synaptic loss but not cell death that may be evident in the early stages of schizophrenia (Jarskog, et al., 2005).

Few postmortem findings have been reliably replicated, for reasons mostly related to the nature of postmortem work. Often, older, medicated patients with comorbid conditions are studied. There are also many limitations related to the method of collection of specimens and the small numbers of patients studied. In vivo brain imaging overcomes some of these difficulties.

GENETIC INVESTIGATIONS

The heritability of schizophrenia has been estimated to be in the range of 60% to 90%, based on overwhelming evidence from family, twin, and adoption studies (Cardno and Gottesman, 2000; Ingraham and Kety, 2000; Kendler et al., 1993). With advances in molecular genetic techniques, it has been possible to examine linkage of a particular marker with schizophrenia within families or the association of a candidate gene with the disorder in individuals from different families. It is clear from these studies that no major gene is associated with schizophrenia; it is much more likely that a large number of genes interact with a number of environmental factors (Jones and Cannon, 1998).

Genome Scans

There are now at least 20 genome scan studies that have examined schizophrenic patients and their families. Many of these have insufficient power, and most have not accounted for heterogeneity (Waterworth et al., 2002). Nevertheless, there appears to be a consensus that there are modest linkages with a number of genes (DeLisi, 2000; Kato et al., 2002; Lewis et al., 2003; Owen et al., 2004, 2007; Rapoport et al., 2005; Riley and Kendler, 2006; Ross et al., 2006). Not surprisingly, some of these genes are involved in dopaminergic signal transduction, such as catechol-O-methyltransferase (COMT), an enzyme that inactivates dopamine (Egan et al., 2001). Other genes are involved in glutamatergic signal transduction, such as neuregulin, which regulates the expression of glutamate receptor subunits (Stefansson et al., 2002; Tosato et al., 2005); RGS4 proteins, which inhibit metabotropic receptor signaling (Chowdari et al., 2002); dysbindin, which affects NMDA receptor activity (Straub et al., 2002); and a calcineurin subunit gene that could be involved in NMDA-mediated plasticity (Gerber et al., 2003). There is also linkage to a nicotinic receptor involved in gating deficits seen in many schizophrenic patients (Leonard et al., 2002). A recent genome-wide survey of copy number variations has found multiple rare structural variants, both genome-wide and at specific loci, that have been implicated in other studies (International Schizophrenia Consortium, 2008). Copy number variants are essentially deletions and duplications of genes.

Candidate Genes

Abnormalities in genes involved in neurodevelopment are beginning to emerge in some studies, but none seems to account for a large amount of the variance, nor are they likely specific to schizophrenia (Harrison and Owen, 2003; Harrison and Weinberger, 2005; Perlman et al., 2004). However, one of these genes, Disrupted in Schizophrenia (DISC1), is particularly interesting because of its role in neuronal migration, neurite outgrowth, and neuronal maturation as well as synaptic transmission and plasticity in adults (Ross et al., 2006). Another neurodevelopmental gene variant of neuregulin-1 has been associated with lateral ventricular volume increases in schizophrenic patients (Mata et al., 2009). It is also likely that many of the genes affecting glutamatergic signal transduction also affect brain development (Rapoport et al., 2005, Harrison and Weinberger, 2005).

DISC1 is a gene that was discovered in a large Scottish family with a very high incidence of mental disorders (Chubb et al., 2008). It is a gene located on chromosome 1 that in many family members was disrupted by the translocation of part of the gene to chromosome 11. Of the 29 family members carrying the disrupted gene, 7 had schizophrenia, 1 had bipolar disorder, and 10 had recurrent major depression. Thus, 18 of the 29 carriers of the disrupted gene were diagnosed with a major mental illness, whereas none of the 38 family members with the non-disrupted gene were found to be so affected (Chubb et al., 2008). Apart from the major disruption of the gene found in the Scottish family, small sequence variations of the DISC1 gene have been linked to schizophrenia, schizoaffective disorder, bipolar disorder, and major depression in other populations in Scotland, as well as in Iceland, Finland, North America, Taiwan, China, and Japan (Chubb et al., 2008). Small sequence variations in DISC1 have also been linked to autism spectrum disorders in Finland (Kilpinen et al., 2008). Although such evidence comes from many populations from throughout the world, such variations in DISC1 account for a very small portion of the prevalence of these disorders. Through the comparison of the sequences, Crespi et al. (2007) showed that DISC1 has undergone considerable recent evolution: several parts of the DISC1 gene have undergone substantial positive selective changes since the divergence of apes from monkeys and also since the divergence of humans from apes. These changes were caused by alterations in the amino acids in the DISC1 protein and thus potentially modified its functions. The site of the largest evolutionary divergence maps to exons 1 and 2 in the part of the DISC1 gene that binds to MAP1a (microtubule associated protein 1a), which is involved in the control of activity-dependent dendritic branching (Szebenyi et al., 2005). This is consistent with the localization of the DISC1 protein in dendritic shafts and spines in human cortical neurons (Kirkpatrick et al., 2006). Duan et al. (2007) blocked the expression of DISC1 in postnatally generated neurons in the dentate gyrus of the mouse hippocampus through the use of selective interference of DISC1 RNA. When DISC1 expression is blocked in these neurons, there is considerably more branching of the secondary and tertiary dendrites than when DISC1 expression is normal. Thus, DISC1 reduces secondary and tertiary dendritic branching in these neurons and may have a similar function regulating dendritic branching in the human brain.

Since DISC1 is strongly and preferentially expressed on the apical and basal dendrites in the Von Economo neurons described in Chapter 3, it could be part of the genetic circuitry responsible for the relative absence of higher-order branching in the Von Economo neurons (Allman et al., 2010). A single nucleotide variation in another part of the DISC1 gene is linked to increased risks of major depression and schizophrenia, and this variation was also linked to reduced volume of anterior cingulate cortex and reduced connectivity in frontal polar cortex in an MRI and diffusion tensor imaging study involving a large population of Japanese subjects (Hashimoto et al., 2006). Variations in the DISC1 gene have been frequently associated with changes in cognitive functioning, particularly with respect to tasks that involve maintaining and shifting attention (Chubb et al., 2008).

Thus, DISC1 has undergone considerable recent evolution and may be related to enhanced cognition in apes and humans. The recent evolutionary changes in DISC1 may carry increased vulnerabilities to dysfunction, which may manifest in multiple neuropsychiatric disorders.

NRXN1 (neurexin-1) is a gene with a similar set of findings with respect to schizophrenia. The connection was discovered in a Bulgarian family in which two siblings, both schizophrenic, were found to have a small deletion (Kirov et al., 2009), but no such deletion was found in a large number of control subjects. Shortly thereafter, a pair of identical twins, both schizophrenic, were also found to have a deletion in NRXN1 (Walsh et al., 2008). Subsequently, NRXN1 deletions were found in schizophrenic subjects in several additional studies in European countries, America, and Japan (Kirov et al., 2009), and these deletions were much more common in schizophrenic subjects than in controls (Kirov et al., 2009). Abnormalities in the NRXN1 gene have also been reported in seven studies of autistic subjects; the functional properties of this gene will be discussed in more detail in Chapter 6.

BRAIN IMAGING STUDIES

MRI

Although lateral and third ventricular enlargement and asymmetry anomalies were found in schizophrenic patients with computed tomography (Shelton and Weinberger, 1986), it was not until the MRI studies that the extent of structural abnormalities became known in the disorder. With MRI, it became possible to examine all brain structures in living patients with close to the same precision as gross postmortem samples.

One of the questions that can be addressed with this technique is whether schizophrenic patients have a smaller brain size, which could be associated with perinatal and/or neurodevelopmental abnormalities. There may be a small reduction in brain and intracranial size in schizophrenia, but there is no evidence of a reduction of extracranial size (Shenton et al., 2001; Ward et al., 1996). The evidence for increased cerebrospinal fluid in schizophrenic patients is more convincing, suggesting an abnormality of brain growth or neuronal degeneration

(Narr et al., 2003; Woods, 1998; Woods and Yurgelin-Todd, 1991; Woods et al., 1996). Although the lateral ventricles were found to be enlarged, particularly the temporal horns on the left side, in the majority of studies, the increases were modest (Shenton et al., 2001, Wright et al., 2000).

Gray Matter Losses

Widespread gray matter reductions have been reported in schizophrenic patients, their unaffected siblings, and patients at risk for schizophrenia (Cannon et al., 1998; Gur et al., 1999; Lawrie et al., 1999; Zipursky et al., 1992, 1998). However, more specific volumetric losses have been found. A classic study of 15 monozygotic twin pairs discordant for schizophrenia found that 14 of the 15 affected twins had smaller left and 13 of the 15 had smaller right hippocampi than their normal twin (Suddath et al., 1990). Other temporal lobe structures, such as the superior temporal gyrus, have also been found to be smaller in schizophrenic patients in the majority of investigations (Shenton et al., 2001). In some cases, superior temporal losses precede the onset of psychosis in at-risk patients (Takahashi et al., 2009). Hippocampal and superior temporal gyrus volume reductions may be related to memory-processing abnormalities in schizophrenic patients (Goldberg et al., 1994; Nestor et al., 1993). A correlation between smaller hippocampi and pregnancy and/or birth complications has also been reported in schizophrenic patients (McNeil et al., 2000; Stefanis et al., 1999).

Modest volume deficits have been found in a number of other brain regions, including the prefrontal, parietal, thalamic, and cerebellar regions and corpus callosum (Shenton et al., 2001). Some meta-analyses of prefrontal and thalamic regions have found very small effect sizes (Davidson and Heinrichs, 2002; Konick and Friedman, 2001). However, more recent meta-analyses support a reduction in the median dorsal nucleus and pulvinar of the thalamus (Byne et al., 2009). In the temporal regions, several meta-analyses of MRI findings in this region have suggested that the effect sizes are smaller than those in neuropsychological and neurophysiological studies (Lawrie and Abukmeil, 1998; Nelson et al., 1998; Wright et al., 2000; Zakzanis et al., 2000), on the order of 0.40, with an overlap of as much as 90% between schizophrenic and control groups on many volumetric measures. These inconsistencies may be due to methodological issues. This methodological issue is highlighted by the robust reduction in area 17 (primary visual cortex) found in schizophrenic brains based on the histological study of postmortem brains (Dorph-Petersen et al., 2009).

Progressive Changes

Volumetric deficits seem to be present at the first episode, in keeping with a neurodevelopmental abnormality (Vita et al., 2006). Ventricular enlargement is not usually seen in first-episode patients, suggesting that it might be a consequence of cortical change (DeLisi, 2008). Later in the illness, there is progressive enlargement of the left lateral ventricle and reduction of many cortical, subcortical, and cerebellar structures in many patients (Color Plate 4.1). In fact, all but 3

(Garver et al., 2000; James et al., 2002; Keshavan et al., 1998) of more than 19 longitudinal studies have found progressive changes. However, the pattern of changes has varied, with some finding ventricular enlargement (Cahn et al., 2002; Delisi et al., 1995; Lieberman et al., 2001; Mathalon et al., 2001; Nair et al. 1997; Rapaport et al., 1997; Sporn et al. 2003) and others whole brain (Cahn et al., 2002; Sporn et al., 2003; Wood et al., 2001), prefrontal (Ho et al., 2003; Mathalon et al., 2001; Nakamura et al., 2007; Pantelis et al., 2003; Thompson et al., 2001; Vidal et al., 2006), temporal (Ho et al., 2003; Jacobsen et al., 1998; Kasai et al., 2003; Mathalon et al., 2001; Nakamura et al., 2007; Pantelis et al., 2003; Salisbury et al., 2007; Takahashi et al., 2009; Thompson et al., 2001; Vidal et al., 2006), parietal (Sporn et al., 2003), cingulate (Pantelis et al., 2003; Vidal et al., 2006), cerebellar (Pantelis et al., 2003), and thalamic (Rapaport et al., 1997) gray matter losses. Another study found primarily white matter losses (Gur et al., 1998). Progressive brain volume losses have been found in both members of sets of twins in which only one twin had schizophrenia, suggesting that genetic factors are involved (Brans et al., 2008). Progressive brain volume changes, particularly in gray matter in the first year, correlate with clinical and functional outcome at 5 years (Cahn et al., 2006).

Clinical Correlations

There have been many attempts to look at the correlates of negative symptoms with MRI in recent years. Most have found an association between prefrontal deficits and negative symptoms (Anderson et al., 2002; Paillère-Martinot et al., 2001; Roth et al., 2004; Sigmundsson et al., 2001; Wible et al., 2001). Positive symptoms have correlated with many structural deficits, but the most-replicated finding has been a correlation between left superior temporal gyrus volume and auditory hallucinations, which is not surprising in view of the role of this structure in speech (Barta et al., 1990; Flaum et al., 1995; Levitan et al., 1999).

Diffusion Tensor Imaging

Within white matter, water molecules tend to diffuse more freely along myelinated tracts. This directional dependence is referred to as *anisotropy*. Generally, low anisotropy would imply tissue with low connectivity. Lower levels of anisotropy have been found in schizophrenic patients in widespread regions extending from frontal to occipital regions, whether or not there is a deficit in white matter volumes (Buchsbaum et al., 1998; Davis et al., 2003; Lim and Helpern, 2002). However, more recent studies have found mostly altered white matter integrity in tracts connecting the frontal cortex with the temporal and parietal cortices (Burns et al., 2003; Shergill et al., 2007). Like gray matter deficits, fractional anisotropy deficits are much more striking in chronic schizophrenic than first-episode patients (Friedman et al., 2008). Interestingly, anisotropy was actually *increased* in frontotemporal tracts associated with speech in those patients prone to auditory hallucinations (Shergill et al., 2007). Reduced fractional anisotropy in the anterior cingulum (Wang et al., 2004) has been found to correlate with performance deficits on the WCST (Kubicki et al., 2003). Other investigators have found reduced posterior cingulate anisotropy in patients prone to positive symptoms (Fujiwara et al., 2007). Although there are different patterns in individual patients, there seem to be fairly consistent anomalies in the white matter connections between the prefrontal and temporal regions (Ellison-Wright and Bullmore, 2009).

In Vivo Brain Chemistry

^{1}H-Magnetic Resonance Spectroscopy (MRS)

N-acetylaspartate (NAA), a marker of neuronal integrity, glutamate, and its precursor/metabolite, glutamine, can be quantified in living patients with ^{1}H-MRS. Normal NAA levels have been found in three of four first-episode, never-treated patients in the anterior cingulate and prefrontal regions (Bartha et al., 1997; Cecil et al., 1999; Stanley et al., 1996; Théberge et al., 2002), while decreased levels were found in two of three studies in the temporal region (Bartha et al., 1999; Cecil et al.,1999; Fannon et al., 2003). Just over half of the investigations of the temporal region in medicated and unmedicated chronic patients have shown decreased NAA levels (Bertolino et al., 1996; Buckley et al., 1994; Deicken et al., 1998; Delamilliere et al., 2002; Fukuzako et al., 1995; Heimberg et al., 1998; Kegeles et al., 2000b; Maier et al., 1995; Nasrallah et al., 1994; Yurgelun-Todd et al., 1996). NAA levels have correlated negatively with length of illness in the anterior cingulate and thalamus (Ende et al., 2001; Théberge et al., 2003), but no correlation has been found in the hippocampus or prefrontal regions (Deicken et al., 1999; Stanley et al., 1996). NAA levels have been correlated with both negative and disorganized symptoms (Callicott et al., 2000; Delamillieure et al., 2000; Fukuzako et al., 1999b), activation of working memory cortical networks (Bertolino et al., 2000b), and evoked release of striatal dopamine (Bertolino et al., 2000a).

Increased glutamine levels have been reported in first-episode never-treated patients in the anterior cingulate and medial prefrontal (Bartha et al., 1997; Théberge et al., 2002) and thalamic regions (Théberge et al., 2002), but not in dorsolateral or temporal regions (Bartha et al., 1999; Stanley et al., 1996). Increased glutamine in these first-episode patients likely indicated increased physiologically active glutamate, as 80% of glutamate released at the receptor is made from glutamine. Most of the glutamate measured by this technique is found throughout the cell and not physiologically active. Interestingly, chronic patients had decreased levels of both glutamate and glutamine in the anterior cingulate, which could indicate a loss of neurons and/or neuropil (Théberge et al., 2003). A longitudinal study of first-episode, never-treated patients suggested that glutamine levels fall in the first few years of illness. This decrease in glutamine is strongly correlated with gray matter losses in the superior temporal gyrus (Théberge et al., 2007).

^{31}P MRS Studies

Investigations of first-episode, never-treated schizophrenic patients have been fairly consistent in their findings of decreased membrane precursors or phosphomonoesters (PME) and increased membrane breakdown products or phosphodiesters (PDE) in prefrontal (Pettegrew et al., 1991; Stanley et al., 1995) and temporal (Fukuzako et al., 1999a) regions. Findings in chronic patients have been less consistent but suggest a trend toward decreased membrane metabolite levels in chronic patients in prefrontal and temporal regions (Calabrese et al., 1992; Deicken et al., 1994; Fujimoto et al., 1992; Kato et al., 1995; O'Callaghan et al., 1991; Shiori et al., 1994; Williamson et al., 1991; Volz et al., 1997, 1998b, 2000a, 2000b; Yacubian et al., 2002). The finding of increased membrane breakdown products at the beginning of the illness could suggest glutamatergic excitotoxicity, in keeping with the increase in glutamine followed by a loss of gray matter found in some first-episode patients, but it could also reflect a downregulation or neurodevelopmental anomalies in these regions.

Functional Brain Imaging Studies

Dopamine In Vivo Imaging

Two meta-analyses of earlier postmortem and brain imaging studies found evidence of increased D_2 density in the striatum, but there was considerable overlap with healthy controls (Laruelle, 1998; Zakzanis and Hansen, 1998). More recent PET studies have examined presynaptic dopamine activity. As ^{18}F fluorodopa is taken up in presynaptic monoaminergic neurons and metabolized to dopamine, increased uptake suggests increased dopaminergic activity. Six of eight studies have found increased ^{18}F fluorodopa uptake in the ventral striatum in medicated chronic schizophrenic patients (Dao-Castellana et al., 1997; Elkashef et al., 2000; Hietala et al., 1995, 1999; Lindström et al., 1999; McGowan et al., 2004; Meyer-Lindenberg et al., 2002; Reith et al., 1994). One of these studies found a strong correlation between striatal dopamine uptake and performance on the WCST in schizophrenic patients (Meyer-Lindenberg et al., 2002).

Similar investigations with dopamine transporter ligands have not revealed overall differences in the striatum but have found a lack of asymmetry in schizophrenic patients (Hsiao et al., 2003; Laasko et al., 2000). Surprisingly, second-generation PET cameras, which can examine prefrontal dopaminergic activity, have not found the predicted decrease (McGowan et al., 2004). However, the occupancy of striatal dopamine receptors in schizophrenic patients was twice the level of normal subjects with pharmacological stimulation (Abi-Dargham et al., 1998; Breier et al., 1997; Laruelle et al., 1996). These studies point to a problem of dopamine regulation in schizophrenia rather than a deficiency or excess.

Resting Blood Flow Studies

Since Ingvar and Franzen's classic xenon cerebral blood flow study (Ingvar and Franzen, 1974), the majority of investigators have found some evidence of resting hypofrontality in schizophrenia, but the effect size is modest (Buchsbaum and Hazlett, 1998; Davidson and Heinrichs, 2003; Hill et al., 2004). As in the Ingvar and Franzen (1974) study, hypofrontality tends to be more characteristic of chronic patients and cannot be explained by medication (Hill et al., 2004).

Cognitive Activation Studies

Weinberger et al. (1986) showed that schizophrenic patients are not able to activate their dorsolateral prefrontal cortex during the WCST. Interestingly, affected monozygotic twins also have hypofrontality during the WCST, and the degree of hypofrontality during the WCST was related to the volume loss in the left hippocampus (Berman et al., 1992). These studies were done with xenon cerebral blood flow techniques but have been largely borne out by more precise PET and single photon emission computed tomography (SPECT) studies. A meta-analysis of 41 functional neuroimaging studies has confirmed deficits in the dorsolateral prefrontal cortex, anterior cingulate cortex, and mediodorsal nucleus of the thalamus in schizophrenic patients during the performance of executive function tasks, although schizophrenic patients tended to activate a similar network to healthy controls (Minzenberg et al., 2009). More recent studies have also demonstrated fairly consistent prefrontal and temporal deficits during various memory tasks, although there is considerable overlap between patients and controls (Davidson and Heinrichs, 2003).

Clinical Correlations

Most PET and SPECT studies have found that negative and deficit symptoms tend to be associated with lower prefrontal metabolism or prefrontal activation deficits (Andreasen et al., 1992; Heckers et al., 1999; Kawasaki et al., 1993; Lahti et al., 2001, 2006; Liddle et al., 1992; Molina Rodriguez et al., 1997; Sabri et al., 1997; Schröder et al., 1996; Tamminga et al., 1992; Wolkin et al., 1992). A number of PET investigations of patients experiencing auditory hallucinations during the scan have implicated a wide network of activity throughout the limbic system, including the thalamus, hippocampus, cingulate gyri, and orbitofrontal cortex, as well as auditory processing regions (Copolov et al., 2003; Sabri et al., 1997; Silbersweig et al., 1995).

Patients who are prone to hallucinations but not necessarily experiencing them during the scan tend to have increased anterior cingulate and decreased hippocampal activity (Lahti et al., 2006). A pattern of activation in mesotemporal and ventral striatal regions has been described in patients experiencing paranoid delusions (Epstein et al., 1999). Schizophrenic patients with passivity phenomena (the delusion of being controlled by an outside force) showed hyperactivation of the parietal and cingulate cortices (Spence et al., 1997). Patients showing high levels of thought disorder tend to have high levels of activity in Broca's and temporoparietal language areas, which may extend into the anterior insula (Horn et al., 2009; Lahti et al., 2006).

SCHIZOPHRENIA, INCREASED APOLIPOPROTEIN L-1, AND RESISTANCE TO TRYPANOSOME BRAIN INFECTION

The gene for apolipoprotein L-1 (APOL-1) has significantly increased expression in the prefrontal cortex of postmortem schizophrenic brains relative to controls (Mimmack et al., 2002). APOL-1 confers resistance to infections by the trypanosomes, a family of protozoan parasites that contain the agent that causes the encephalitis known as sleeping sickness and is transmitted by the tsetse fly in Africa (Vanhollebeke et al., 2007). APOL-1 brings about the destruction of trypanosomes by several different mechanisms that cause them to lyse (Vanhollebeke et al., 2007). In situ hybridization studies indicate that APOL-1 is selectively expressed in neurons in human prefrontal cortex (Mimmack et al., 2002). The increased expression of APOL-1 may influence the activity of these neurons and play a role in their abnormal functioning in schizophrenia; however, this increased expression may have conferred resistance to cerebral trypanosome infections in the African hominid past. There are also two studies indicating the significant upregulation of immune and inflammation-related genes in the prefrontal cortex of schizophrenics (Arion et al., 2007; Saetre et al., 2007).

OVERVIEW

Schizophrenia affects many of the brain regions and functions unique to humans. Patients sometimes feel that an outside force is controlling their actions. They hear their thoughts aloud or hear voices that no one else can hear. Although findings are widespread in schizophrenia, most involve regions that have undergone adaptations in the human brain, particularly the frontal and temporal regions. The involvement of the prefrontal cortex is evidenced by poor performance on neuropsychological tests and an inability to activate this region on brain imaging during these tasks. Other difficulties with encoding and putting information in context also point to this region. Attentional deficits in schizophrenic patients point to other regions, such as the anterior cingulate and parietal cortex, which form the attentional network.

The subtle affective and cognitive deficits during childhood in many schizophrenic patients suggest anomalies in early brain development. Many structural findings, such as lateral ventricular increases and gray matter losses, do not seem to be prominent early in the illness. The illness does seem to progress with the onset of florid symptoms. Gray matter losses are particularly evident in temporal regions involving language and memory. Gray matter loss in language regions correlates highly with ratings of auditory hallucinations. These regions, along with other parts of the limbic system, are usually found to be activated when patients are experiencing hallucinations. Negative symptoms tend to correlate with structural and functional deficits in the prefrontal region.

We know that positive symptoms are relieved by dopamine-blocking agents. This is interesting because dopamine projects to the anterior cingulate and prefrontal cortex. We also know that types of glutamatergic receptor antagonists involving the NMDA receptor can cause both positive and negative symptoms in normal subjects and schizophrenic patients. There is now some evidence that glutamatergic activity is increased early in the illness in the anterior cingulate and thalamus. Later in the illness, losses of glutamatergic metabolites are seen that correlate highly with gray matter losses in temporal regions. These observations suggest there may be both a neurodevelopmental and a neurodegenerative process in schizophrenia.

The heterogeneity of clinical findings and genetic linkages suggest that there is likely no major factor but a combination of genetic and environmental factors resulting in dysfunction in multiple neuronal circuits as the brain matures. Damage to any part of these circuits could lead the whole circuit to fail, which might explain some of the heterogeneity. If this is the case, then we might be able to understand some of the fundamental architecture of the human brain by piecing together the anomalies in disorders like schizophrenia that seem to involve abnormalities of self and language. However, we first have to examine how the findings in other psychiatric conditions differ. In the next chapter, we will contrast the findings in schizophrenia with those in bipolar disorders.

5

Bipolar Disorders

This chapter will review what we know about the epidemiology and natural course of bipolar disorder. We will then look at some of the psychophysiological and neuropathological findings in the disorder. As with schizophrenia, no major genes have emerged, but there are several genes associated with the disorder that may offer some insight into its pathophysiology. Other aspects of bipolar disorder, such as which neurotransmitters might be involved and in vivo structural and functional brain imaging studies, offer further clues about neuronal circuitry. Our purpose here, as in the previous chapter, is to highlight the findings that may be relevant to a discussion of what makes the human brain more vulnerable to this condition and to discuss how findings differ from schizophrenia.

EPIDEMIOLOGY AND NATURAL COURSE

Incidence and Prevalence

The incidence of bipolar I and II disorders falls into roughly the same range as schizophrenia. The incidence is usually around 9.0 per 100,000 for men and 9.6 per 100,000 for women (Bebbington and Ramana, 1995). In a recent face-to-face household survey of 9,282 respondents, 12-month prevalence was 2.6% and the lifetime prevalence was 3.9% (Kessler et al., 2005a, 2005b). In the 12-month cases, 82.9% were judged to be severe as defined by a serious suicide attempt, work disability, psychotic symptoms, substance dependence, or repeated serious violence (Kessler et al., 2005b). The median age of onset is about 25 for bipolar I and II disorders (Kessler et al., 2005a). There is a high rate of both anxiety and substance use comorbidity in bipolar patients (Bauer et al., 2005; Kessler et al., 2005b).

Course of Illness

Kraepelin was right to some degree about the course of bipolar disorders. There is a consensus that the long-term outcome in bipolar disorder is better than in schizophrenia (Tsuang et al., 1979). However, in a recent study, 28% of patients remained symptomatic, only 43% of patients achieved functional recovery, and more than half of the patients had a new illness episode within 2 to 4 years of the first hospitalization for mania (Tohen et al., 2003). Many suggest that the psychosocial impairment associated with mania and depression is associated with all areas of functioning and persists for years (Coryell et al., 1993; Goldberg et al., 1995). Psychotic features are associated with greater symptom severity and higher morbidity in the long term (Coryell et al., 2001). Men and women hospitalized for affective disorders also have elevated mortality rates from suicide and circulatory disorders (Angst et al., 2002).

Environmental Factors

There have been few investigations of either obstetrical complications or exposure to viruses before birth in patients who develop bipolar disorders. However, there is some evidence that prenatal and perinatal complications are more frequent (Buka and Fan, 1999).The relationship between prenatal exposure to viral infections and the development of mood disorders is controversial, but there is some evidence that the rate of major affective disorder may be increased to those exposed to the 1957 influenza epidemic in the second trimester (Machón et al., 1997). There is also some evidence that patients with bipolar disorder are indistinguishable from schizophrenic patients in terms of neurological soft signs at the presentation of illness (Whitty et al., 2006). Thus, a case for a neurodevelopmental origin for bipolar disorder can be made, although it is not as strong as in schizophrenia.

NEUROPSYCHOLOGICAL FINDINGS

Kraepelin suggested that there was substantial cognitive decline with schizophrenia but not bipolar disorder. While general intellectual function is preserved in bipolar disorder, there is now evidence that bipolar disorder is associated with significant cognitive impairment (Bearden et al., 2001; Malhi et al., 2004; Olley et al., 2005; Quraishi and Frangou, 2002).

Nature of Impairment

There is consistent evidence of impaired sustained attention in both mania and depression that persists into the euthymic state (Clark and Goodwin, 2004).

Verbal memory is impaired in both acute and euthymic states, but visuospatial memory deficits are variable (Quraishi and Frangou, 2002). All aspects of executive functioning, including planning, abstract concept formation, and set shifting, are impaired in symptomatic patients. Some have suggested that executive function may be normal in recovered patients (Quraishi and Frangou, 2002), while others suggest ongoing deficits (Arts et al., 2008; Torres et al., 2007). The effect sizes for executive function deficits fall into the large range ($d \geq 0.8$), while effect sizes for immediate and delayed verbal memory, abstraction, and set-shifting fall into the medium effect range ($0.5 \leq d \leq 0.8$) (Arts et al., 2008; Robinson et al., 2006; Torres et al., 2007).

Specificity

Bipolar patients usually score higher than schizophrenic patients on measures of intellectual functioning even if they are acutely ill. On measures of sustained attention, verbal memory, and executive functioning, there are few differences between acutely ill bipolar patients and schizophrenic patients. However, unlike schizophrenic patients, these deficits improve or remit with clinical improvement in bipolar patients (Quraishi and Frangou, 2002). On the whole, bipolar patients suffer cognitive deficits that are milder but qualitatively similar those seen in schizophrenia (Schretlen et al., 2007).

PSYCHOPHYSIOLOGICAL FINDINGS

Electroencephalographic (EEG) Studies

Although initial studies of bipolar patients suggested that there were a number of nonspecific abnormalities, such as excessive fast or slow activity, subsequent studies have failed to reliably discriminate bipolar patients from healthy controls (Shagass, 1975). Similarly, early studies of EEG coherence showed laterality abnormalities, with engagement of the nondominant hemisphere during verbal tasks in mania and activation of the dominant hemisphere during spatial processing in depression and mania. However, these suggestions did not hold up under critical analysis (French and Beaumont, 1984).

Event-related Potential (ERP) Findings

There are few ERP studies of bipolar disorder, but it has been suggested that first-episode bipolar patients do not have the reduced P300 amplitude observed in schizophrenic patients (Salisbury et al., 1998). However, this study may have been confounded by drug and alcohol abuse, as a subsequent study controlling for these factors found reduced P300 amplitude and prolonged P300 latency in both schizophrenia and bipolar disorder (O'Donnell et al., 2004). Twin investigations have also found strong genetic correlations with both P300 and P50 abnormalities in bipolar patients (Hall et al., 2007). P300 abnormalities can be seen in the relatives of bipolar patients as well (Pierson et al., 2000). Thus, ERP abnormalities consistent with impaired attentional processing can be seen in both schizophrenia and symptomatic bipolar disorder.

Circadian Rhythm Disturbances

Mood tends to correlate with circadian phase in normal subjects (Boivin et al., 1997). In both depressed and manic patients these fluctuations tend to be amplified, in that most patients experience depressive symptoms in the morning and improvement in mood later in the day (Bouhuys, 1991). A number of disturbances of sleep architecture have been found in both major depression and mania, such as insomnia or hypersomnia, early morning awakenings, and reduced sleep efficiency and rapid eye movement (REM) sleep latency (Hudson et al., 1992). Increased levels of cortisol and corticotrophin-releasing hormone are consistently observed during the night in depressed patients, consistent with a decreased response to dexamethasone seen in many of these patients during the day. There may also be a phase advance in the diurnal rhythm of melatonin secretion in bipolar disorder (Boivin, 2000).

Many of these findings suggest an abnormal phase advance of the endogenous circadian pacemaker, but most studies are confounded by the effect of activity and light exposure (Boivin, 2000). In fact, seasonal variations in mood are often observed (Rosenthal et al., 1984) and relapses of mania tend to increase in the spring (Hunt et al., 1992). Nevertheless, other evidence could point to circadian rhythm disturbances in mood disorders. One of the more interesting observations is that approximately 50% to 60% of depressed patients respond at least temporarily to sleep deprivation (Wu and Bunney, 1990). In some cases, sleep deprivation can also precipitate a manic episode (Wehr, 1992). Consequently, there is now considerable evidence to suggest that mood disorders are associated with circadian rhythm disturbances.

NEUROTRANSMITTER ABNORMALITIES

Norepinephrine

One of the first clues to the pathophysiology of bipolar disorder arose from the observation that patients given reserpine often developed symptoms indistinguishable from major depression. As reserpine depletes norepinephrine, catecholamines were implicated in depression (Bunney and Davis, 1965). What followed was an intensive search for catecholamine abnormalities in cerebrospinal fluid, plasma, and urine; generally increased levels were found in both unipolar and bipolar depression. However, more convincing evidence comes from the effects of different classes of antidepressant drugs, all of which desensitize beta-adrenergic receptors with chronic administration. Curiously, lithium, a mood stabilizer, facilitates the release of norepinephrine and reduces the beta-adrenergic-stimulated adenylyl cyclase response. Other mood stabilizers also have noradrenergic system effects, providing a strong case for the involvement of norepinephrine in bipolar disorders (Goodwin and Jamison, 2007).

Serotonin

Lower concentrations of serotonin metabolites have been consistently reported in the cerebrospinal fluid of bipolar depressed patients (Mahmood and Silverstone, 2001; Shiah and Yatham, 2000). Serotonin stimulates the release of pituitary hormones such as prolactin, growth hormone, and adrenocorticotropic hormone. Neuroendocrine responses to serotonin have generally been found to be reduced in bipolar depressed and bipolar euthymic patients (Mahmood and Silverstone, 2001). Selective serotonin reuptake inhibitors (SSRIs) are the mainstay of antidepressant treatment. In some cases, they can precipitate mania. Mood stabilizers such as lithium and valproate enhance serotonergic transmission (Shiah and Yatham, 2000). Thus, serotonin is clearly involved in the pathophysiology of bipolar disorders.

Other Neurotransmitters

Not surprisingly, dopamine, which is known to mediate reward and motor activity, has been indirectly implicated in bipolar disorders. It has long been known that depression is common in Parkinson's disease. L-dopa also produces hypomania in bipolar patients. Some antidepressants increase intrasynaptic dopamine, and electroconvulsive therapy consistently enhances dopamine function (Goodwin and Jamison, 2007). However, other neurotransmitters such as acetylcholine, GABA, and glutamate may be implicated in the pathophysiology of bipolar disorders. In the case of acetylcholine, effects are likely mediated by the modulation of affective behavior by the cholinergic–adrenergic balance. Evidence for the involvement of glutamate comes mostly from the effects of lithium, valproate, and carbamazepine on glutamatergic function, while evidence for the involvement of GABA comes mostly from postmortem studies (Goodwin and Jamison, 2007).

Signal Transduction Pathways

There has been an explosion of information about what happens in the neuron after the neurotransmitter binds to an ion channel or receptor. Although a detailed discussion of this topic is beyond the scope of this volume, there are several intracellular signal transduction pathways that might be relevant to bipolar disorders and the effects of mood-stabilizing drugs. These include guanine nucleotide-binding proteins, adenylyl cyclases, and protein kinase A and C isoenzymes (Bezchlibnyk and Young, 2002; Manji and Lenox, 2000). Changes in these pathways can be linked to a maladaptive stress response consistent with the hypothalamus–pituitary–adrenal axis abnormalities seen in many patients (Quiroz, et al., 2004).

NEUROPATHOLOGICAL STUDIES

Postmortem studies of major depressive disorder and bipolar disorder have demonstrated specific neuronal and glial histopathology, such as cell loss in the subgenual prefrontal cortex, cell atrophy in the dorsolateral and orbital cortex, and increased numbers of cells in the hypothalamus and dorsal raphe nucleus. Many of these findings could be associated with stress-mediated toxicity, which is partially reversed by antidepressant and mood-stabilizing medication (Rajkowska, 2000). Postmortem anomalies more directly implicating stress response systems have been reported in mood disorders. In a large and carefully controlled stereological study, Manaye et al. (2005) found a selective loss of neurons in the paraventricular nucleus of the hypothalamus in patients who had major depression and bipolar disorder compared with normal and schizophrenic subjects. The paraventricular nucleus is an important site for the production of corticotrophin-releasing hormone and other neuropeptides.

There is also some postmortem evidence of neurotransmitter abnormalities in bipolar disorders. Young et al. (1994) found elevated frontal, temporal, and occipital norepinephrine turnover in bipolar patients at postmortem examination. In contrast, serotonin turnover in the temporal cortex and dopamine turnover in the occipital cortex was found to be decreased. The density of GABA synthetic enzyme terminals was decreased in the anterior cingulate and prefrontal regions. Other investigators have reported postmortem abnormalities in the function of 5-HT_{1A} receptors (Bowen et al., 1989).

GENETIC INVESTIGATIONS

The risk of developing a bipolar disorder is increased by a factor of 10 and the risk of developing a major depression is more than doubled in relatives of patients who suffer from a bipolar disorder. Concordance rates for monozygotic twins are in the order of 63% to 77%, compared with 13% to 23% for dizygotic twins (Goodwin and Jamison, 2007). Meta-analyses of linkage studies have shown strong evidence for linkage to bipolar disorder on chromosomes 6q, 8q, 13q, and 22q. However, these regions were also associated with an increased risk for schizophrenia (Badner and Gershon, 2002; McQueen et al., 2005).

There are several promising candidate genes, the most studied of which has been the serotonin transporter gene. A variation in DNA in the promoter region of the serotonin transporter gene has been found to be associated with the illness (Lasky-Su et al., 2005; Serretti and Mandelli, 2008). Several other candidate genes have been associated with bipolar disorder, including those associated with monoamine oxidase A, an enzyme that degrades dopamine, norepinephrine, and serotonin; catechol-O-methyltransferase, an enzyme involved in the degradation of dopamine and norepinephrine; brain-derived neurotrophic factor (BDNF); and the disrupted in schizophrenia gene (DISC1). However, the number of studies finding a positive association with these candidate genes was generally much smaller than those finding a negative association (Goodwin and Jamison, 2007).

As with schizophrenia, no clear answers have emerged from genetic studies. There are several weak linkages, many of which overlap with schizophrenia, and a few candidate genes that make sense, such as the serotonin transporter gene.

Borna Virus

Borna virus causes a disease in horses and other mammals that is characterized by depression and agitation; it sometimes progresses to death but is more commonly a chronic condition (Ludwig and Bode, 2000). The virus resides and replicates in the nuclei of neurons and other cells, particularly in the limbic system. Borna virus also infects humans, and in a small trial the symptoms of mania were reduced by treatment with the antiviral drug amantadine in bipolar patients who were seropositive for this virus (Olhmeier et al., 2008). There is also evidence that some Borna virus genes have become incorporated directly into the human genome and even express proteins (Horie et al., 2010). These observations raise the possibility that Borna virus infections or Borna genes incorporated into the human genome may play a role in bipolar disorder in humans.

Epigenetic Changes Linking Childhood Abuse to Suicide

In a very carefully controlled study of suicide victims who had suffered childhood abuse versus matched controls who did not, McGowan et al. (2009) found evidence for epigenetic changes in the neuron-specific glucocorticoid receptor gene (NR3C1). These epigenetic changes result from the methylation of cytosine bases in the DNA in the 1F exon of this gene, which reduces the gene's expression. DNA methylation is a stable, long-lasting event. The reduction in the expression of glucocorticoid receptor in the hippocampus causes an increase in the activation of the hypothalamic–pituitary–adrenal axis response to stress, which is a characteristic feature of depressed patients. Thus, early childhood events can have a long-lasting epigenetic influence on gene expression and influence a person's vulnerability to neuropsychiatric illnesses later in life. It would be very interesting to determine whether these DNA-methylation changes that increase the stress response might be related to loss of neurons found in the paraventricular nucleus of the hypothalamus reported by Manaye et al. (2005), which also might increase the stress response in depressed and bipolar subjects.

BRAIN IMAGING STUDIES

Magnetic Resonance Imaging

Although there are robust changes in brain volume in bipolar subjects compared to healthy volunteers, none are diagnostically specific (Arnone et al., 2009). Widespread loss of gray matter has not generally been found in mood disorders, in contrast to schizophrenia (Sheline, 2003). However, subgenual prefrontal cortical reductions have been found in some but not all studies of patients with major depression and bipolar disorder (Drevets et al., 1997; Haldane and Frangou, 2004; Soares, 2003). The amygdala has been found to be fairly consistently enlarged in most studies of bipolar patients (Haldane and Frangou, 2004; Soares, 2003). White matter hyperintensities, particularly in frontal regions, have been described in mood-disordered patients by many investigators (Stoll et al., 2000).

Although somewhat less enlarged than in schizophrenic patients, lateral ventricles have been found to be larger in patients with major depression and bipolar disorder, particularly in patients with multiple episodes (Elkis et al., 1995; Kempton et al., 2008; Strakowski et al., 2002). Regions showing changes in bipolar disorder in the later stages of illness also include the cerebellar vermis, lateral ventricles, and left inferior prefrontal regions (Strakowski et al., 2005). Hippocampal reductions are generally not found in bipolar patients but have been reported in depressed patients, particularly those with multiple episodes (Campbell et al., 2004; MacQueen et al., 2003), suggesting that glutamatergic neurotoxicity related to glucocorticoids could play a role in the volume losses in this region (Sapolsky, 2000). A similar maladaptive response to stress has been hypothesized in bipolar disorders (Manji et al., 2001).

In contrast to schizophrenic patients, there are few studies of brain volumes in mood-disordered patients that examine the same patients over time. However, a recent 3-year longitudinal study of brain morphology demonstrated a decline in the gray matter density of the hippocampus, anterior cingulum, left amygdala, and right dorsomedial prefrontal cortex in patients with major depression (Frodl et al., 2008). Many of these regions have been shown to be associated with a loss of neuropil in response to stress. It is also interesting that progressive volumetric changes seem to preferentially affect regions involved in processing affect.

Diffusion Tensor Imaging

Decreased fractional anisotropy has been reported in the frontal white matter tracts of bipolar patients (Alder et al., 2004; Haznedar et al., 2005; Sexton et al., 2009). More sophisticated tractography approaches have demonstrated a significantly increased number of reconstructed fibers between the left subgenual cingulate and the amygdalo-hippocampal complex (Houenou et al., 2007). This is very interesting in view of the enlargement of the amygdala in many structural studies. Some lateralized differences from controls have been found as well. Elevated left and reduced right orbitomedial prefrontal fractional anisotropy has been reported in a large group of bipolar patients (Versace et al., 2008).

In Vivo Brain Chemistry

[1]H-Magnetic Resonance Spectroscopy (MRS)

Decreased levels of N-acetylaspartate (NAA) have been reported in just over half of studies in depressed patients in the prefrontal region (Yildiz-Yesiloglu and Ankerst, 2006a). Temporal and hippocampal regions have not been found to have decreased NAA levels in most studies. Findings are inconsistent in the thalamus, anterior cingulate, basal ganglia, and amygdala. A recent comprehensive review of findings in bipolar disorders suggested a pattern of decreased NAA levels in the frontal lobes and hippocampus and higher choline ratios in the basal ganglia (Yildiz-Yesiloglu and Ankerst, 2006b).

Myo-inositol levels, which may be correlated with glial cell function, can also be estimated with ^{1}H MRS. Although some studies have found decreased levels in major depression and bipolar disorder, no consistent patterns have emerged. Levels of glutamate/glutamine and GABA have been found to be decreased in prefrontal regions in depressed patients (Hasler et al., 2007). Lithium has been associated with an increase in NAA, while valproate seems to have little effect (Yildiz-Yesiloglu and Ankerst, 2006a).

^{31}P MRS Studies

Patients with major depression have been found to have increased levels of phosphomonoesters (PME) and reduced levels of adenosine triphosphate (ATP) in the frontal lobe (Volz et al., 1998b). A meta-analysis (Yildiz et al., 2001) of eight ^{31}P MRS frontal and temporal lobe studies in bipolar patients found that PME levels of euthymic patients were lower than healthy controls. Depressed bipolar patients had higher PME levels compared with euthymic bipolar patients. No differences were seen between the phosphodiester (PDE) levels of bipolar patients and controls. Overall, PME has been generally increased in the depressed state and decreased in the euthymic state. Although lithium has generally been found not to affect PME levels, a recent proton-decoupled study showed an increase in PME levels with lithium treatment (Yildiz et al., 2001).

Functional Brain Imaging Studies

Resting Studies

The most replicated functional imaging resting state abnormality in depression is the inverse relationship between prefrontal activity and depression severity, which may explain some of the cognitive difficulties in these patients (Mayberg, 2003). Activity in the dorsolateral prefrontal cortex on PET has been found to be decreased most often, but subgenual prefrontal cortex activity (Color Plate 5.1) has also been found to be decreased in depressed patients (Drevets, 2000; Videbech, 2000). When loss of gray matter is accounted for in the subgenual prefrontal cortex, there may actually be an increase in subgenual prefrontal activity (Drevets, 1999). Increases in activity are consistently found in the amygdala as well, in both unipolar and bipolar depressed groups (Drevets, 2003). Left amygdala metabolism was found to have a positive correlation with plasma cortisol levels, implicating emotional and stress-response systems that include the amygdala (Drevets et al., 2002). Decreased basal ganglia activity has been reported in some studies (Videbech, 2000).

The findings in manic patients are limited by the difficulties of studying these patients. Consequently, the findings are not often contradictory. Nevertheless, increased activity has been found in many patients in the orbital prefrontal cortex, left dorsal anterior cingulate, and left caudate regions (Blumberg et al., 1999, 2000). Most of the findings in both depressed and manic patients appear to be state dependent. The possible exception may be elevated amygdala activity, which has been found in euthymic bipolar patients not taking mood-stabilizing medications (Drevets et al., 2002). Improvement in depressive symptoms with pharmacological treatment correlates with increases in prefrontal activity and decreases in amygdala and subgenual cingulate activity (Drevets, 1999; Mayberg, 2003).

Activation Tasks

Depressed patients may have decreased activation during affective processing tasks. George et al. (1997) found that depressed patients had an attenuated temporal and right insular response to faces with varied emotions compared to controls. In a functional MRI study, decreased dorsolateral prefrontal and increased amygdala response to fearful faces was seen in bipolar patients, many of whom were mood elevated (Yurgulen-Todd et al., 2000). More recently, functional connectivity has been found to be decreased between the perigenual anterior cingulate and amygdala in bipolar patients during the emotional processing of face stimuli. Anomalies on diffusion tensor imaging in these patients suggested that the decreased connectivity was associated with aberrant white matter connections between these structures (Wang et al., 2009).

L-Tryptophan Depletion

Patients with major depression who were L-tryptophan (serotonin precursor) depleted had decreased brain metabolism on PET in the dorsolateral prefrontal cortex, thalamus, and orbitofrontal cortex if they had a depressive relapse. Decreased brain metabolism in these regions correlated with increased depressive symptoms (Bremner et al., 1997).

Receptor Binding Studies

An early *N*-methylspiperone PET study found that unmedicated psychotic bipolar disorder patients had elevated D_2 dopamine receptor levels similar to schizophrenic patients (Pearlson et al., 1995). However, a more recent study of never-treated manic patients failed to find an increase in [^{18}F] 6-fluoro-L-dopa uptake in the striatum compared to healthy volunteers (Yatham et al., 2002).

In keeping with postmortem anomalies, reduced 5-HT_{1A} binding has been reported in midbrain, limbic, occipital, and parietal regions in recurrent, familial mood disorders (Drevets et al., 2000; Sargent et al., 2000). Chronic antidepressant treatment does not seem to affect 5-HT_{1A} receptor density (Moses-Kolko et al., 2007). Brain serotonin transporter binding can also be assessed using PET. Unfortunately, results have been conflicting, with both decreased and increased levels reported in limbic and neocortical regions (Cannon et al., 2007; Oquendo et al., 2007). Attempts to link serotonin transporter binding in vivo to genetic polymorphisms of the serotonin transporter gene promoter were unsuccessful in one study (Oquendo et al., 2007). Another study found that brain serotonin turnover, measured by direct jugular venous sampling rather than brain imaging, was elevated two-fold in unmedicated patients with major depressive disorder carrying the s allele compared to the l allele of the serotonin transporter gene. A marked reduction in serotonin turnover after successful treatment with SSRIs suggested that brain serotonin turnover may be a biological substrate for major depressive disorder (Barton et al., 2008).

There have been few studies looking at other in vivo transmitters in bipolar patients. However, a preliminary study using a newly developed type 2 muscarinic (M_2) receptor label found decreased M_2 binding in the anterior cingulate in bipolar depressed patients compared to healthy controls and patients with major depression (Cannon et al., 2006). This study provided the first direct evidence that altered M_2 receptor function contributes to mood dysregulation in bipolar disorder.

DEPRESSION AND INFLAMMATION

Benjamin Hart (1988) proposed that "the behavior of a sick individual is not a maladaptive and undesirable effect of illness but rather a highly organized behavioral strategy that is at times critical to the survival of an individual if it were living in the wild state." He further suggested that the cytokines were responsible for depression and social withdrawal as the animal devotes its limited resources to mounting energetically costly defenses, such as fever, against infection. A large body of experimental work in rodents supports this hypothesis and particularly implicates interleukin 1 (IL-1-alpha and beta), interleukin 6 (IL-6), and tumor necrosis factor in inducing sickness behavior and symptoms of depression (Dantzer et al., 2007). Interferon-alpha stimulates the production of these inflammatory cytokines, and when this drug is used to treat infections and cancer, nearly half of the human patients undergoing this therapy develop clinical depression (Raison et al., 2006). High serum levels of IL-6 have also been found to be strongly associated with major depression in the elderly (Bremmer et al., 2008). Serum levels of IL-6 are also correlated with poor-quality social relationships and poor sleep quality in elderly women (Friedman et al., 2005).

Harrison et al. (2009a) investigated the role of IL-6 in a double-blind study involving 16 healthy male volunteers who received either a typhoid vaccination or placebo. The subjects who received the typhoid vaccination (but not the placebo) experienced a substantial reduction in mood after 3 hours, and their negative change in mood was strongly related to the amount of increased signal recorded from their subgenual anterior cingulate cortices when the subjects observed emotional faces (Color Plate 5.2). The subgenual anterior cingulate cortices have often been implicated in depression, and the activated site in Color Plate 5.2 (Harrison et al., 2009a) is very close to the site where deep brain stimulation relieves the symptoms of depression in severely depressed patients (Mayberg et al., 2005).

The serum levels of IL-6 in the vaccinated subjects were related to reduced connectivity between the subgenual anterior cingulate cortices and other mood-related brain structures, including the amygdala, nucleus accumbens, and parts of the prefrontal cortex. In a second paper based on the same experiments, Harrison et al. (2009b) found that measures of fatigue and mental confusion were related to increased activity in the dorsal anterior cingulate cortices when the subjects performed the Stroop task, which requires subjects to discount distracting information. The Stroop task is very effective in driving the dorsal anterior cingulate cortices in normal subjects (Bush et al., 2000), and the increased activity probably reflects the increased cognitive effort required to focus on this task when fatigued and confused. The activity of the dorsal anterior cingulate cortices is related to task difficulty in physical and mental exertion (Critchley et al., 2000; Paus et al., 1998).

In an MRI study of 18 women who had recently experienced the loss of a mother or sister and were presented with a photograph of their lost loved one, the activity of the subgenual anterior cingulate cortex was strongly related to the production of IL-1-beta in their saliva (O'Connor et al., 2009). Thus, there is evidence that increased inflammatory cytokines in the periphery can induce changes in the anterior cingulate cortices linked to negative mood, fatigue, confusion, and reduced connectivity, and the induction of grief is linked both to increasing anterior cingulate cortical activity and increased cytokine production in the periphery. It is interesting in this context that Von Economo neurons and related layer 5 neurons strongly express the receptors for several cytokines, including IL-6 (Tetreault and Allman, unpublished data).

OVERVIEW

Although there is still some debate about the merits of separating schizophrenia from bipolar disorders, the weight of evidence supports the distinction. It is now clear that bipolar disorders are not quite as benign as Kraepelin thought: many patients do not recover completely after an episode of depression or mania. However, it is fair to say that many neuropsychological and electrophysiological anomalies are state dependent. Bipolar disorders can also be distinguished by anomalies in biological rhythms, which do not seem to be affected as much in schizophrenia.

As with schizophrenia, there is overlap between healthy volunteers and bipolar patients in every index of brain structure or function. Although a few genes have emerged, none accounts for a large amount of the variance, and many overlap with schizophrenia. Nevertheless, there are some noteworthy findings that point to a different final common pathway for bipolar disorders. Whereas schizophrenia appears to link to dopamine and glutamate, the links to bipolar disorders are much weaker. Bipolar disorder is much more strongly linked to serotonin and norepinephrine. In fact, there is remarkable consistency across neuropathological studies, where norepinephrine and 5-HT$_{1A}$ receptor abnormalities are reported, to brain imaging studies, where 5-HT$_{1A}$ receptor binding is generally reduced, and genetic studies, where the genes associated with the serotonin transporter and enzymes involved in serotonin and norepinephrine metabolism are associated with the disorder.

One might think at first glance that the brain structures involved in bipolar disorders seem to be the same ones involved in schizophrenia. Certainly there is considerable overlap in structures such as the dorsolateral prefrontal cortex and hippocampus, but there are also some important differences. Whereas schizophrenia is associated with dysfunction in the dorsal anterior cingulate, bipolar disorders are associated with dysfunction in the ventral anterior cingulate and adjacent subgenual prefrontal cortex, evidenced by both gray matter loss and anomalies on functional imaging. Both are part of basal ganglia-thalamocortical neuronal circuits involved in learning new behaviors and integrating affect into behavior. However, as we saw in Chapter 2, the dorsal prefrontal cortex is more likely involved in motivation, error detection, and salience appraisal. It is not surprising, then, that schizophrenia would be associated with amotivation and inappropriate attention to information processing. The ventral anterior cingulate and subgenual prefrontal cortex are more directly linked to sadness and affective processing generally. Consequently, it should be no surprise that these structures would be involved in bipolar disorders.

There are some interesting differences in brain structures connected to the dorsal and ventral anterior cingulate cortices in these conditions. The dorsal anterior cingulate cortex is closely connected with the speech-processing parts of the brain, and both are found to be generally increased in activity during hallucinations. The ventral anterior cingulate and subgenual prefrontal cortex are closely connected to the amygdala. One of the most consistent findings in bipolar disorders is an increase in size and activity of the amygdala. The amygdala, ventral anterior cingulate, and subgenual prefrontal cortex have rich serotonin and norepinephrine innervation. All are connected with the hypothalamus, perhaps explaining vegetative and circadian symptoms. It is interesting that this region may also be particularly vulnerable to inflammation.

Both depressed and schizophrenic subjects are often hyperreactive to stressful situations. The Manaye et al. (2005) study revealed selective neuronal loss in the paraventricular nucleus of the hypothalamus in major depression and bipolar disorder, but not in schizophrenia, which suggests differences in the neural circuitry involved in the stress response between these disorders. The McGowan et al. (2009) study, which showed DNA-methylation changes that reduced the expression of a glucocorticoid receptor resulting in increased stress responses in victims of childhood abuse, also implicates changes in the circuitry of the stress response. Thus, the circuitry regulating the stress response may be part of the final common pathway involved in depression.

What we have so far, then, is an emerging pattern of brain systems. One system, associated with schizophrenia, includes the dorsolateral prefrontal cortex, dorsal anterior cingulate cortex, hippocampus, thalamus, and superior temporal gyrus. Presumably this is a system associated with motivation, cognition, and language processing. Another system, associated with bipolar disorders, includes the dorsolateral prefrontal cortex, ventral anterior cingulate cortex, subgenual prefrontal cortex, hippocampus, and amygdala. Presumably this is a system associated with cognition and affective processing. What about other neuropsychiatric conditions such as autism, which are also associated with affective and language processing abnormalities? The next chapter will address this condition.

6

Autism, ADHD, and Anorexia Nervosa

Autism, attention-deficit/hyperactivity disorder (ADHD), and anorexia nervosa are three conditions that are characterized by serious deficits in social functioning, have a significant degree of comorbidity, and may involve related neural circuits in the prefrontal, cingulate, and insular cortices. There is a strong genetic component to each of these conditions. Each first manifests at a different stage in development: autism in infancy, ADHD in early childhood, and anorexia in adolescence. These conditions may reflect specific developmental defects in recently evolved neural circuitry that supports the capacity to function in complex social environments. Males are far more likely to develop autism and ADHD and females are far more likely to develop anorexia nervosa, which implies an interaction between the sex steroids and the development of these neural circuits.

Autism differs from schizophrenia and bipolar disorders in that symptoms appear before age 3, but many of the impairments have some overlap with these conditions. For example, social interaction is often impaired in children who later develop schizophrenia, although not to the same extent as in autism. Acquisition of language is not usually affected in patients with schizophrenia or bipolar disorder, but both can experience auditory hallucinations; this phenomenon is not characteristic of autism. Repetitive and stereotyped patterns of behavior can be seen in some schizophrenic and bipolar patients who suffer comorbid obsessive-compulsive conditions, but they are not part of the central syndrome. While wide swings of affect, like those seen in bipolar disorders, and flattened affect, like that seen in schizophrenia, are not characteristic of autism, there does seem to be an inability to express emotion in a social context. Thus, autism seems to affect various aspects of social behavior and language common to schizophrenia and bipolar disorder, but in a unique and persistent way.

Since Kanner described autism in 1943, there has been a search for the underlying pathophysiology of the disorder. Up until the past decade or so, the search has not been a fruitful one. However, advances in molecular biology and brain imaging have led to some solid findings that are beginning to shed light on the brain systems involved in this disorder. This chapter will review some of the more relevant findings to our discussion of neuropsychiatric disorders and the nature of the human brain. Indeed, autism afflicts some of the most human functions: language and complex social interactions.

AUTISM

Epidemiology and Natural Course

Incidence and Prevalence

Autism spectrum disorders were once considered to be relatively rare, with an incidence of about 5 per 10,000. One of the most remarkable enigmas related to these disorders has been the dramatic increase (Fig. 6.1) in their reported prevalence over the past 30 years (Newschaffer et al., 2007; Williams et al., 2006b).

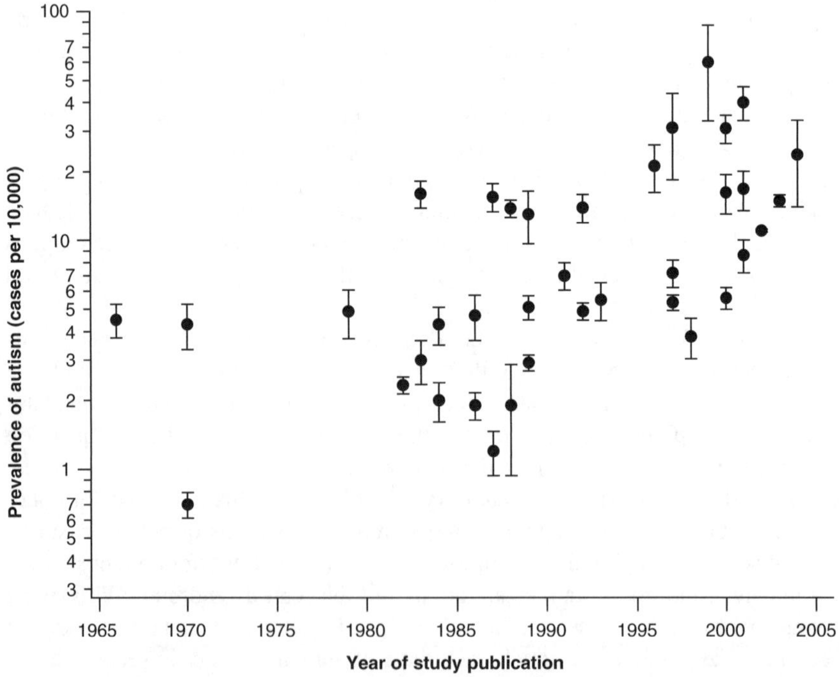

Figure 6.1 Prevalence of autism (cases per 10,000) versus year of study publication. Data from Williams et al. (2006b) log transformed and plotted according to year of publication.

A leading epidemiologist, Dr. Eric Fombonne, has recently observed that this is true for the whole group of pervasive developmental disorders (PPDs), which includes primarily the autism spectrum disorders together with several less common conditions (Fombonne, 2009, p. 597):

> As it stands now, the recent upward trend in estimates of prevalence cannot be directly attributed to an increase in the incidence of the disorder. There is good evidence that changes in diagnostic criteria, diagnostic substitution, changes in the policies for special education, and the increasing availability of services are responsible for the higher prevalence figures. Most of the existing epidemiologic data are inadequate to properly test hypotheses on changes in the incidence of autism in human populations. Accordingly, the possibility that a true increase in the incidence of PDDs has also contributed to the upward trend in prevalence estimates cannot and should not be ruled out based on available data.

Apart from AIDS, obesity, and asthma, there are few other diseases that have dramatically increased in prevalence over the past 30 years; indeed, most diseases have decreased in prevalence. Even cancer, when analyzed by examining rates for successive birth cohorts since 1925, has shown a declining incidence (Kort et al., 2009). Improved diagnostic procedures and increased availability of services apply to virtually all diseases over this period, so we are left with the definite possibility that there has been a real underlying change in incidence that is responsible for at least part of the roughly 20-fold increase in the reported prevalence of autism spectrum disorders. The reason for the increase is not clear, but no doubt better ascertainment and a wider definition of the disorder have contributed to the increased prevalence and variability of findings.

In any case, boys are affected more often than girls by a factor of at least 4 to 1. Between 40% and 55% of autistic patients also suffer from mental retardation. ADHD and mood disorders are frequently associated with autism as well. Although early studies suggested that autism is more frequent in affluent families, more recent studies have not consistently borne this out. All ethnic backgrounds seem to be affected by autism in more or less the same proportion (Newschaffer et al., 2007).

Course of Illness

Despite the fact that autism can now be diagnosed reliably as early as 2 or 3 years of age, there is often a delay of several years between initial symptoms and diagnosis. Early development is normal in many children with autism for about 12 to 18 months. Following a plateau of development, some children regress and actually lose acquired language and social skills. The outcome in children with autism throughout childhood and adulthood varies, particularly with the presence or absence of associated conditions such as mental retardation. The best predictors of functional outcome in autism are age at language acquisition, age at diagnosis, and cognitive status (Newschaffer et al., 2007). Modest degrees of symptom abatement and improvement in skills have been documented in numerous studies of autism patients followed into adulthood. However, most individuals continue to manifest significant symptomatology and dependency, although about 15% have a more favorable outcome in adulthood (Seltzer et al., 2004).

Environmental Factors

Advanced maternal age and paternal age are risk factors for the development of autism. Low birth weight and duration of gestation and intrapartum hypoxia are also associated with an increased risk of autism (Kolevzon et al., 2007). Although there has been much public attention to a possible link between routine childhood vaccinations and autism, the overwhelming majority of studies show no causal association between vaccination and autism (Doja and Roberts, 2006).

Many environmental factors have been implicated in the development of autism. Fetal exposure to teratogens such as valproic acid, thalidomide, and ethanol and pre- and post-natal exposure to heavy metals like mercury and infectious agents have been linked to autism. However, all of these associations are limited by small sample sizes, uncertainties as to exposure timing, dose, and duration, and the time lag between exposure and outcome (Bello, 2007). The causal role in autism of exposure to environmental agents during critical periods in development has not been established but needs to be thoroughly investigated (Landrigan, 2010).

Neuropsychological Findings

A number of social behavioral deficits have been observed in children with autism. Compared to healthy volunteers and mentally retarded children without autism, children with autism are less likely to engage in pretend play, to imitate others, and to follow the gaze and pointing of others. They perform more poorly on tests of facial recognition and emotional recognition from faces and voices (Kasari and Rotheram-Fuller, 2005; Sigman et al., 2006). Not surprisingly, children with autism have difficulty with taking the perspective of others' intentions, knowledge, and beliefs, referred to as the *theory of mind* concept (Baron-Cohen et al., 1985). What these observations suggest is that children with autism have difficulty in conceptualizing social interaction as well as a failure to associate social interactions with reinforcement. It has been suggested that dysfunction of the mirror neuron system could lead to some of the observed deficits in theory of mind and social communication seen in autism (Oberman and Ramachandran, 2007).

Children with autism, like children with ADHD and schizophrenia, have deficits in executive function. However, these deficits tend to be more related to flexibility and planning rather than inhibition (Sigman et al., 2006). Other impairments in skilled motor, complex memory, complex language, and reasoning domains have been reported, while attention, simple memory, simple language, and visual-spatial domains remain intact (Minshew et al., 1997; Williams et al., 2006a). These observations suggest that autism is a disorder of complex information processing with intact or enhanced simple information processing. Thus, autism appears to affect information integration requiring long-distance connections in the brain (Minshew and Williams, 2007).

Psychophysiological Findings

Eye Gaze Abnormalities

Children with autism have impaired gaze monitoring, or looking back and forth from an object to the eyes of another person to determine whether the other person is also looking at the same thing (Baron-Cohen, 1995). When asked to judge averted gaze in whole faces, children with autism fail to show the typical advantage of seeing the whole face, in keeping with facial processing anomalies in these individuals (Wallace et al., 2006). The right superior temporal sulcus plays an important role in gaze processing in healthy individuals. In children with autism, event-related potentials show a failure to selectively activate this region (Senju et al., 2005).

Electrophysiology

Neuropsychological studies have suggested a deficit in tasks that involve long-range connectivity. High-frequency electrophysiological activity in the gamma band is likely necessary for binding information from different regions during these tasks. A preliminary study of gamma activity during an auditory task with magnetoencephalography found that children and adolescents with autism had significantly reduced left hemispheric gamma power compared to controls during the tasks (Wilson et al., 2007). The reduced gamma activity could reflect an underlying connectivity deficit during auditory processing.

Neuroendocrinology

Social withdrawal leads to elevated corticotrophin-releasing hormone levels. Thus, levels tend to be increased in association with depression, as we saw in the previous chapter. Social attachment tends to be correlated with oxytocin levels. It has been suggested that oxytocin may buffer the impact of stress-related events. Lower levels of oxytocin have been found in children with autism. Oxytocin infusions may also improve some behaviors associated with autism, such as repetitive behaviors (Schulkin, 2007).

Neurotransmitter Abnormalities

A number of neurotransmitters have been implicated in the pathophysiology of autism, including serotonin, GABA, and glutamate. These neurotransmitters function not only in signal transduction but also in brain maturation and cortical organization, particularly neuronal migration and positioning. The role of glutamate and GABA is largely supported by pathological, genetic, and brain imaging studies, which are discussed later in this chapter. However, elevated levels of GABA have been reported in autistic patients (Pardo and Eberhart, 2007).

Probably the strongest case for involvement with autism can be made for serotonin. There is interaction between serotonin and brain-derived neurotrophic factor (BDNF), which plays an important role in cortical growth. Interestingly, perinatal stress can lead to long-term alterations in BDNF expression (Pardo and Eberhart, 2007). About 30% of autistic patients have elevated whole blood serotonin levels. Tryptophan, which depletes serotonin, can lead to exacerbation of symptoms in autistic subjects. Conversely, selective serotonin reuptake inhibitors (SSRIs) may improve compulsive and social deficits in autistic patients (Buitelaar and Willemsen-Swinkels, 2000; Scott and Deneris, 2005).

Neuropathological Studies

Autistic patients have a brain growth spurt shortly after birth and then growth slows, so only younger but not older brains are larger in autism than controls (Courchesne et al., 2001; Hazlett et al., 2005; Lainhart, 2006). White matter appears to contribute disproportionately to this volume increase (Herbert, 2005).

Relatively few neuropathological studies have been performed on autistic patients. Early studies found abnormal lamination in the limbic cortex suggestive of migration defects, a reduction in the number of Purkinje cells in the cerebellum, and age-related changes in cell size and the number of neurons in the nucleus of the diagonal band of Broca, the cerebellar nuclei, and the inferior olive (Kemper and Bauman, 1998; Palmen et al., 2004). There is also considerable evidence that signs of neuroinflammation, including microgliosis and astrogliosis, are present in autistic brain tissue from children and adults (Herbert, 2005; Vargas et al., 2005). Tetreault et al (2009) did stereological counts of microglia in fronto-insular cortex in autistic subjects versus controls and found that the autistic brains had significantly more of these cells, thus providing quantitative morphological evidence for inflammation in autism. Inflammatory cytokines, particularly interleukin (IL)-6, are elevated more than 30-fold in the anterior cingulate cortex in autism versus controls (Vargas et al., 2005). IL-6 is also increased in the prefrontal cortex in autism (Li et al., 2009). The nature of the inflammatory process is not known, but several reports have suggested the presence of immunological dysfunction with autism (Ashwood et al., 2006; Pardo and Eberhart, 2007). In a large multicenter study, a family history of autoimmune disease, and especially of thyroid disorders, was significantly related to the risk of regression in functioning of autistic children (Molloy et al., 2006). In a separate study, regression was linked to a family history of autoimmune disease and gastrointestinal symptoms (Valicenti-McDermott et al., 2008). Autistic behaviors in infant monkeys were induced by injecting their mothers during the first trimester of pregnancy with IgG antibodies derived from human mothers who had given birth to autistic children (Martin et al., 2008).

Other studies have focused on minicolumn abnormalities in autism (Casanova et al., 2006). Minicolumns are radially oriented arrays of pyramidal neurons, interneurons, axons, and dendrites that assemble into macrocolumns, where information processing is carried out. Minicolumns have been found to be increased in number and narrower in width, with reduced neuropil and smaller neuronal cell bodies. The anomalies were widespread and possibly related to the increased white matter projections reported in these patients. The reduction of neuropil space was largely related to a deficit in projections from inhibitory interneurons, which could explain why about 30% of autistic patients suffer from seizures (Minshew and Williams, 2007).

Allman et al. (2005) proposed, on the basis of converging lines of evidence, that the Von Economo neurons in the fronto-insular and anterior cingulate cortex are abnormal in autism. An initial stereological study of the numbers of Von Economo neurons in the fronto-insular cortex involving four autistic subjects plus controls did not confirm this conjecture, although one autistic subject had an abnormally high number of Von Economo neurons (Kennedy et al., 2006). However, a second stereological study of Von Economo neurons in the dorsal anterior cingulate cortex involving nine autistic subjects plus controls found that the autistic subjects fell into two groups, one with significantly higher numbers of Von Economo neurons than controls and the other with lower numbers of Von Economo neurons than controls (Simms et al., 2009). In this study the controls occupied a middle zone with respect to Von Economo neuron counts, with practically no overlap with the high or the low group: the autistic subjects either had very large numbers of Von Economo neurons or virtually none. These results suggest that there may be a developmental defect related to Von Economo neuron migration or survival in autism.

Genetic Investigations

The prevalence of autism among siblings of autistic patients ranges from 2% to 6%. Studies of monozygotic twins have found concordance rates of about 60%, greater than those seen in schizophrenia and mood disorders (Andres, 2002; Newschaffer et al., 2007). Linkage studies in autism have identified a number of promising regions of interest (Grice and Buxbaum, 2006; Persico and Bourgeron, 2006; Yang and Gill, 2007). One region that emerges more frequently is the long arm of chromosome 7. This region contains genes linked to language disorders, the serotonin receptor 5-HT2A gene, and the reelin gene, which is involved in neuronal migration. It also contains the MET receptor tyrosine kinase gene that turns on a cell's signaling cascades, leading to increased proliferation, differentiation, and process outgrowth. Anomalies in this gene have been reported in autism; they may be linked to the interneuron and minicolumnar abnormalities found on postmortem examination (Campbell et al., 2006).

As in schizophrenia and mood disorders, there has been increasing sentiment that it is time to give up on a single genetic explanation for autism (Happé et al., 2006). The emerging evidence is that autism can arise from defects in many genes; each of which contributes only a tiny fraction to the total incidence of the disorder. A large number of genes are necessary for normal cell migration, long-distance connectivity, the balance between excitatory and inhibitory neurotransmission, and synaptogenesis. Many of these genes have been implicated in autism spectrum disorders (Geschwind and Levitt, 2007). One gene that may be particularly important in human brain development, the disrupted in schizophrenia gene (DISC1), has recently been associated with autism and Asperger's disorder (Kilpinen et al., 2008). Another commonality with schizophrenia is the striking increase in copy number variations in autism (Bucan et al., 2009;

Marshall et al., 2008; Sebat et al., 2007). Copy number variations occur when there is an increase or a decrease in the number of copies of a particular gene in the DNA. Some of these genes overlap with other disorders. In autism the copy number variations seems to affect neural cell-adhesion molecules, which are important in forming synaptic connections (Glessner et al., 2009; Sebat et al., 2007; Südhof, 2008). One of the most consistently implicated genes in these studies is NRXN1, which we have previously discussed in connection with schizophrenia. NRXN1 makes proteins (the neurexins) that extend from the presynaptic specialization and connect with neuroligins protruding from the postsynaptic membrane to form Velcro-like links at synapses (Südhof, 2008). The RNA for NRXN1 can be spliced to make on the order of a thousand different isoforms that encode different proteins and thus provide great specificity in synaptic connections (Rowen et al., 2002; Ullrich et al., 1995). The neurexins also have a second major function in the Ca^{++}-dependent regulation of synaptic vesicle release of neurotransmitters into the synaptic cleft (Missler et al., 2003). The anomalies in the expression of NRXN1, the neuroligins, and several other genes revealed in these studies could lead to disruption in these neuronal networks, leading to the clinical features of autism.

Brain Imaging Studies

Magnetic Resonance Imaging

An increase in total brain volume has been found in children with autism beginning between 2 and 4 years and persisting until adolescence (Courchesne et al., 2001; Hazlett et al., 2005; Lainhart, 2006). Both white and gray matter differences have been reported. Within the white matter, differences tend to occur in outer zones rather than inner zones, suggesting more short- and medium-range intrahemispheric cortico-cortical connections rather than interhemispheric or cortical-to-subcortical connections (Herbert et al., 2004). In keeping with fewer interhemispheric connections, the corpus callosum has consistently been found to be reduced in size, particularly in the genu and splenium, where fibers from the orbitofrontal cortex cross the brain (Vidal et al., 2006). In contrast to bipolar disorders, there are no consistent structural anomalies in the amygdala in autism (Cody et al., 2002).

Diffusion Tensor Imaging

Several diffusion tensor imaging studies have reported reductions in fractional anisotropy in the corpus callosum. Fractional anisotropy has also been found to be reduced in other white matter regions such as the occipitotemporal and temporoparietal regions, the internal capsule, the cingulum, and the superior temporal gyrus (Alexander et al., 2007; Barnea-Goraly et al., 2004; Ben Bashat et al., 2007; Keller et al., 2007; Lee et al., 2007). Overall, these observations would suggest connectivity anomalies, particularly affecting interhemispheric and long-distance connections.

In Vivo Brain Chemistry

^{1}H Magnetic Resonance Spectroscopy (MRS) There have been relatively few ^{1}H MRS investigations in autism. Although the pattern of abnormalities differs in these studies, widespread reductions in N-acetylaspartate (NAA) are generally reported (Chugani et al., 1999; Friedman et al., 2003; Hashimoto et al., 1997; Hisaoko et al., 2001; Levitt et al., 2003; Otsuka et al., 1999). Widespread reductions in glutamatergic metabolites have been reported in autism as well (DeVito et al., 2007). NAA, a marker of neuronal integrity, has been found to be reduced in a number of neuropsychiatric conditions, including schizophrenia and mood disorders. However, a reduction in NAA and glutamatergic metabolites could be consistent with some of the postmortem findings in autism.

^{31}P MRS Studies A relationship between neuropsychological and language test scores and high-energy phosphates and membrane phospholipids has been reported. As test performance declined in autistic patients, high-energy phosphates and membrane building blocks decreased and membrane breakdown products increased (Minshew et al., 1993). A hypermetabolic state with undersynthesis of neuronal membranes was suggested. While similar membrane differences have been found in schizophrenia, the hypermetabolic state appears to be different in autism.

Functional Brain Imaging Studies

Serotonin In keeping with the serotonin abnormalities reported, a recent single photon computed tomography study has reported a reduction in levels of cortical $5HT_{2A}$ receptor in the total, anterior, and posterior cingulate, bilaterally in the frontal and superior temporal lobes, and in the left parietal lobes in autism spectrum disorders (Murphy et al., 2006). The trajectory of serotonin synthesis has also been found to be abnormal in autistic children on positron emission tomography (PET) (Chugani et al., 1999). Autistic children with left-sided serotonin synthesis deficits generally showed more language impairment (Chandana et al., 2005).

Executive Function and Language Consistent with deficits on complex neuropsychological tasks and long-distance connections, autistic patients showed decreased functional connectivity on functional magnetic resonance imaging (fMRI) between the frontal and parietal areas while performing the Tower of London task. Furthermore, the size of the genu of the corpus callosum was correlated with frontal–parietal connectivity (Just et al., 2007).

Other investigators have found that activity in the prefrontal region was more correlated with the left parietal region in controls, whereas autistic patients had greater correlation with the right parietal region on fMRI (Koshino et al., 2005). During sentence completion tasks, autistic patients showed more activation in Wernicke's area and less activation in Broca's area compared to controls on fMRI (Just et al., 2004). Another fMRI study of sentence comprehension suggested that people with autism are more reliant on visualization to support language comprehension (Kana et al., 2006).

Social Communication Deficits in social communication have been examined by a number of brain imaging studies (Cody et al., 2002; Zilbovicius et al., 2006). While viewing animations that elicited mentalizing, healthy volunteers showed increased activation compared to autistic patients in the mentalizing network: medial prefrontal cortex, superior temporal sulcus at the temporo-parietal junction, and temporal poles (Castelli et al., 2002).

In keeping with the suggestions that the mirror neuron network might be involved in autism, children with autism showed no activity in the inferior frontal gyrus, a mirror neuron region on fMRI, while imitating and observing emotional expressions (Dapretto et al., 2006).

fMRI activation of regions involved in gaze processing, including the superior temporal sulcus region, was not sensitive to intentions conveyed by observed gaze shifts in autistic patients, consistent with gaze anomalies in the disorder (Pelphrey et al., 2005). Autistic patients have been found to have activation deficits on fMRI in facial processing areas when asked to appraise facial expressions, particularly with regard to emotional content (Critchley et al., 2000). In another fMRI study, autistic patients demonstrated a pattern of activity during face discrimination that was consistent with feature-based strategies that were more typical of non-face object perception (Schultz et al., 2000).

ATTENTION-DEFICIT/HYPERACTIVITY DISORDER (ADHD)

ADHD is a common disorder of self-regulation that first appears in childhood but continues into adulthood in 30% to 50% of cases; it is associated with many comorbidities (Brown, 2009). Untreated adults with ADHD often have chaotic lifestyles and may rely on nonprescription drugs and alcohol (Gentile et al., 2006). They commonly have associated psychiatric comorbidities such as autism spectrum, anxiety, antisocial, and bipolar disorders; depression; substance abuse; and learning disabilities (Brown, 2009; Gentile et al., 2006). ADHD appears to be a uniquely human condition and may be, in part, a defect in recently evolved neural capacities for integrating present actions with long-term goals required for the successful participation in culturally mediated social networks. These abilities are crucial for functioning in both school and the workplace. ADHD was first described in a series of three lectures presented in 1902 to the Royal College of Physicians by Sir George Frederick Still, who has been called the father of pediatrics (Barkley, 2006; Farrow, 2006; Still, 2006). In addition to describing the inattentiveness and hyperactivity in these children, Still focused on defects in self-control and volition. He also noted the preponderance of boys, with a ratio of three boys to each girl, which is close to modern observations of ADHD subjects (Barkley, 2006). He also reported that some of the children had aggressive conduct and deficits in their capacity to learn from experience, which are also in accord with modern assessments (Barkley, 2006). ADHD is found throughout the world and typically affects 5% to 10% of children in a population (Faraone et al., 2003). It has an average concordance of 76% in the 20 studies of identical twins done for this disorder and thus is one of the most heritable neuropsychiatric illnesses (Faraone et al., 2005).

ADHD involves far more than simple inattention or fidgeting behavior. Individuals with ADHD are capable of spending many hours focused on playing video games, which are carefully devised to sustain interest by generating continual rounds of excitement. ADHD subjects report that they are able to sustain attention when the task, such as repairing the engine of an automobile, is intensely interesting to them (Brown, 2009). Thus, one aspect of ADHD is a defect in capacity to sustain attention when the prospects of reward are more distant or less motivationally salient, a defect that is characteristic of small children but that in normal development is gradually transcended through learning the connections between current behavior and long-term goals that are socially and culturally mediated. The primary deficit in ADHD might thus be characterized as a *motivation deficit* rather than an attention deficit and may be the consequence of abnormalities in the dopamine reward system discussed below. This defect in the capacity for delayed gratification is linked to a set of executive functions involving prioritizing actions (planning and timing of activities), the adaptive shifting of attention when needed, the exertion of sustained effort, the mounting of adaptive responses to negative feedback, and the management of one's emotions in the face of frustration. Some of these defects in executive functioning are also characteristic of subjects with the behavioral variant of frontotemporal dementia, which has its onset much later in life and involves the anterior cingulate and fronto-insular cortex and the Von Economo neurons located within these areas (Seeley, 2008; Seeley et al., 2006, 2008). Some of these defects in executive functioning can also be seen in the autism spectrum disorders, and there are abnormalities in the anterior cingulate and fronto-insular cortex and in the Von Economo neurons in these conditions as well (Allman et al., 2005; Simms et al., 2009).

A paradox of ADHD is that the most effective drug treatments involve stimulants, typically related to amphetamine. The effectiveness of these stimulants was a serendipitous discovery made by Charles Bradley in 1937 (Bradley, 1937; Brown, 2009). Bradley was seeking a way to treat the severe headaches that followed the passage of air into the space occupied by cerebrospinal fluid to supply a contrast medium in pneumoencephalography in an early brain imaging technique now supplanted by CT and MRI. Bradley reasoned that benzedrine (D- and L-amphetamine) would stimulate the production of cerebrospinal fluid and thus relieve the headaches in children who had undergone this procedure. He did a trial involving 30 children with various neuropsychiatric disorders and found that 14 showed dramatic improvements in their ability to concentrate, their academic performance in school, and their sense of well-being (Bradley, 1937). Their teachers called it the *arithmetic drug* because of the improved performance of some pupils. The stimulants that are effective in treating ADHD all have the property of suppressing the dopamine transporter (DAT), which recycles free dopamine by drawing it back into neurons; this suppression increases the availability of dopamine to act as a reward signal.

Recent work involving the commonly prescribed methylphenidate (Ritalin) in PET experiments in ADHD subjects suggests that this suppressive effect amplifies the stimulus induced by dopamine rather than simply causing a tonic increase in dopamine levels (Volkow et al., 2005). Very recent PET experiments have also shown that both DAT and the dopamine D_2-D_3 receptor are significantly less abundant in the midbrain, hypothalamus, nucleus accumbens, and caudate of subjects with ADHD versus controls, thus strengthening the chain of evidence demonstrating that deficiencies in the dopamine reward signal are part of the causation of ADHD (Volkow et al., 2005). A genetic variant of the D_2 receptor gene known to cause reduced expression of this receptor is linked to difficulties maintaining newly rewarded responses in reversal learning tasks, thus leading to poorer performance in these tasks (Jocham et al., 2009).

The dopamine D_3 receptor is strongly expressed on the Von Economo neurons, and this suggests that they may be involved in ADHD (Allman et al., 2005). The areas that contain Von Economo neurons, the anterior cingulate and fronto-insular cortex, are also linked to ADHD by several lines of evidence. One of the classic probes of executive functioning is the Stroop test, in which subjects are required to ignore highly salient information to arrive at a correct answer. In fMRI experiments, the Stroop and related tests strongly activate the dorsal anterior cingulate cortex in typical subjects, but in ADHD subjects this activation is reduced (Bush, 1999). In a subsequent study it was discovered that the degree of activation of the dorsal anterior cingulate cortex in ADHD subjects was related to the specific polymorphism of the DAT gene they possessed (Brown et al., 2009). The cortex in the dorsal anterior cingulate region is also significantly thinner in ADHD (Makris et al., 2007). In a large-scale meta-analysis of brain areas involved in executive functions in 23 imaging studies done in children and adolescents, the anterior insula, including the fronto-insular cortex, emerged as one of the few brain areas involved in nearly all studies (Houdé et al., 2010). The hemispheric development of the fronto-insular area and surrounding cortex is abnormal in ADHD (Shaw et al., 2009). In a large study involving structural MRIs done in 358 typically developing children and young adults ranging in age from 4 to 20, matched with 218 ADHD subjects, Shaw et al. (2009) found that in the typically developing individuals the cortex involving the fronto-insular area and the nearby anterior insula and posterior orbitofrontal cortex regularly progressed from being about 0.3 mm thicker on the left side at age 4 to being about 0.3 mm thicker on the right side by age 20. By contrast, in the ADHD subjects the fronto-insular area and surrounding cortex was the same thickness at age 4 in both hemispheres, but by age 20 it was about 0.3 mm thicker on the left side (Color Plate 6.1). Thus, the hemispheric specialization for the fronto-insular and adjacent cortex is significantly rightward in typically developing individuals and leftward in ADHD subjects, and the course of postnatal development of these structures differs between ADHD subjects and controls. In normal adult subjects the Von Economo neurons are about 30% more numerous in the right fronto-insular area, which is consistent with the increased thickness of this region in typically developing individuals (Allman et al., 2005, 2010). This rightward enlargement in the fronto-insular and adjacent cortex may be related to the capacity to mount an adaptive response to negative feedback, a subject discussed in more detail in Chapter 10, and a deficiency in this capacity could contribute to the defects in executive functioning characteristic of ADHD.

Although there is considerable evidence linking specific polymorphisms of DAT and the dopamine receptors to ADHD (Sharp et al., 2009), these connections have not been sustained thus far in genome-wide association studies of ADHD, which suggests that many genes contribute small amounts to the disorder (Franke et al., 2009). One interesting suggestion is that ADHD arises from genetic variants associated with cognitive flexibility that favored successful hunting behavior in earlier human populations, where adherence to schedules, long-term goals, and self-control were less important than in complex, densely populated agricultural and industrial societies (Hartmann, 2003).

There are now many long-term follow-up studies of cohorts of children diagnosed with ADHD. There is substantial evidence that a large fraction of them experience significant comorbidities in adulthood, including increased incidences of major psychiatric disorders (especially depression), antisocial disorders, anxiety disorders, and substance abuse (Biederman et al., 2006; see also Brown, 2009 for a book-length compendium of this literature). Figure 6.2 illustrates the first appearances of these disorders as a function of age in a cohort of ADHD subjects compared with a matched cohort of typically developing individuals. The greatly increased incidence in ADHD versus controls suggests that defects in executive functioning predispose these individuals to suffer many other neuropsychiatric disorders as they grow older and face the many challenges of adult responsibilities (Brown, 2009). There is also a significant comorbidity between ADHD and autism spectrum disorders, particularly Asperger's syndrome (Gillberg et al., 2009; Mulligan et al., 2009; Rommelse et al., 2009). One behavior that has been especially studied in adults with ADHD is the operation of motor vehicles, because in this situation defects in focused attention, compliance with social norms, self-control, and the management of frustration can have very severe consequences. There is a large amount of evidence from several studies involving multiple metrics of driving performance that drivers with ADHD present greater hazards than control subjects, but there is also evidence that stimulant therapy reduces these risks (Barkley and Cox, 2007).

In summary, ADHD is a common disorder that arises in childhood but persists into adulthood in many cases. A primary deficit in this disorder seems to be the consequence of the inability to sustain the motivation to achieve longer-term objectives that are essential for living in complex social networks, especially those that require delayed gratification, such as in school and workplace situations. This capacity to participate in complex long-term social networks and their attendant responsibilities is probably recently evolved, and defects in this capacity appear to reduce the threshold for many other neuropsychiatric illnesses, resulting in substantial comorbidities for these individuals. These comorbidities may arise from the severe stress that these individuals suffer as a consequence of their attentional-motivational deficits or possibly from defects in the underlying molecular or neuronal circuitry that exist in common between ADHD and these other disorders.

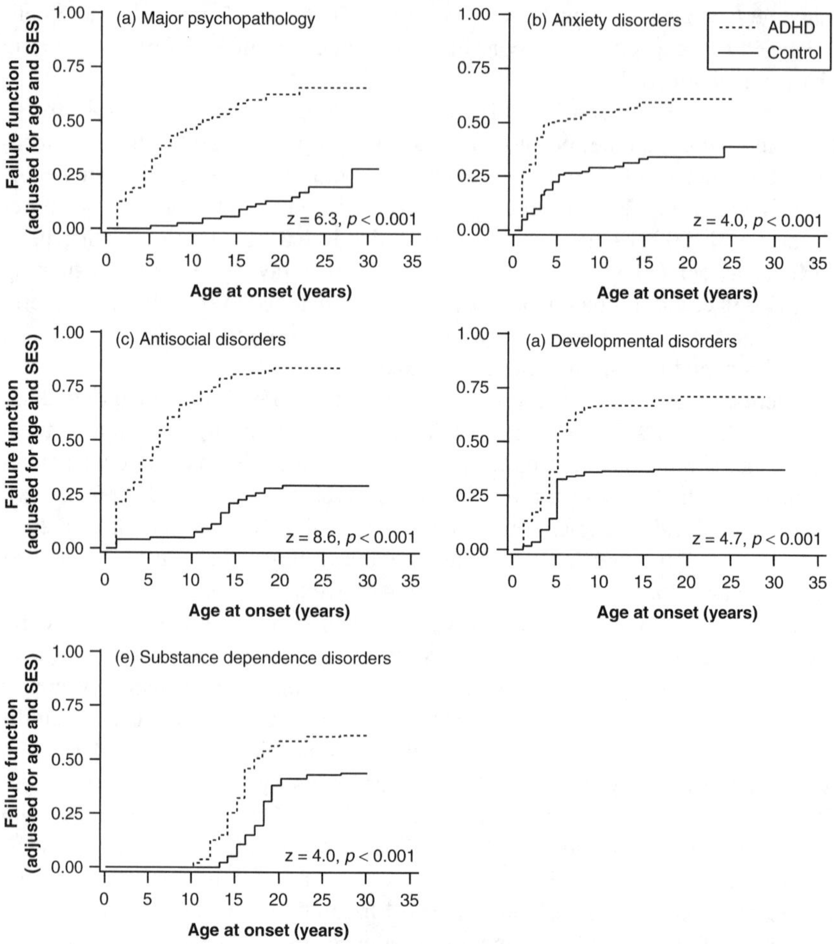

Figure 6.2 Rates of disorders in attention-deficit/hyperactivity disorder (ADHD) subjects (···) compared to controls (-----) for all five composite diagnostic categories: (a) major psychopathology, (b) anxiety disorders, (c) antisocial disorders, (d) developmental disorders, and (e) substance dependence disorders. From Biederman, J., Monuteaux, M.C., Mick, E., Spencer, T., Wilens, T.E., Silva, J.M., Snyder, L.E., and Faraone, S.V. Young adult outcome of attention deficit hyperactivity disorder: a controlled 10-year follow-up study. *Psychological Medicine,* **36**, 167–179, 2006. Copyright Cambridge Journals, published by Cambridge University Press, reproduced with permission.

ANOREXIA NERVOSA, SELF-AWARENESS, AND AUTISM SPECTRUM DISORDERS

Anorexia nervosa involves a profound dysregulation of self-awareness and self-control, with consequent large increases in mortality from suicide, homicide, and respiratory and urogenital disorders documented in carefully controlled epidemiological studies in Sweden and other countries (Papadopoulos et al., 2009).

Patients with anorexia nervosa often have features in common with disorders in the autistic spectrum, such as self-absorption, obsessive behaviors, and diminished empathy (Gillberg, 1992; Wentz et al., 2009; Zucker et al., 2007), and these conditions probably involve disruption of related neural circuitry subserving self-awareness, particularly in the anterior insular cortex (Kaye et al., 2009).

Historical accounts of Saint Margaret of Hungary, who lived in the 13th century, suggest that she had anorexia nervosa (Halmi, 2009), but the earliest clinical description of this disorder was made in 1689 by William Morton (1637–1698), a physician practicing in London. Morton (Pearce, 2004, pp. 191–192) wrote:

> Mr. Duke's daughter, in 1684 and in the eighteenth year of her age, in the month of July fell into a total suppression of her monthly courses from a multitude of cares and passions of her mind...I do not remember that I did ever in all my practice see one that was conversant with the living so much wasted with the greatest degree of consumption (like a skeleton only clad with skin)...A nervous atrophy...wasting of the body without any remarkable fever, cough, or shortness of breath; but it is attended with a want of appetite, and a bad digestion, upon which there follows a languishing weakness of nature, and a falling away of the flesh every day more and more.

The Victorian physician Sir William Gull (1816–1890) observed many such patients and coined the name for the disorder that he described (Pearce, 2006, p. 55) as:

> a particular form of disease...characterized by extreme emaciation....The subjects of the affliction are mostly of the female sex, and chiefly between the ages of 16 and 23. I have occasionally seen it in males of the same age...The patient complained of no pain, but was restless and active. This was in fact a striking expression of the nervous state, for it seemed hardly possible that a body so wasted could undergo the exercise which seemed agreeable. It will be observed that all the conditions in this case were negative, and may be explained by the anorexia which led to starvation, and depression of all the vital functions; viz., amenorrhoea, slow pulse, slow breathing...

Anorexia is sometimes considered a disease that is the consequence of the high social value placed on thinness in young women, but this clearly was not the case in Victorian England and does not explain its occurrence in males. Because it totally suppresses reproduction in women during their period of maximum fecundity and also causes greatly increased mortality, genes related to anorexia must have been strongly selected against in evolution. Nevertheless, studies of identical twins indicate that there is a substantial heritable component in anorexia (Bulik et al., 2007). A polymorphism of the gene BDNF (brain-derived neurotrophic factor, polymorphism RS6265) has been linked to anorexia in eight European populations (Ribasés et al., 2005), which is the most convincing evidence yet for a specific genetic basis for this disorder. In experimental animals, BDNF suppresses appetite and causes body weight reductions (Bulik et al., 2007). The BDNF connection suggests that the genetic basis for anorexia nervosa might have arisen as a mechanism to protect against the effects of starvation, which until recently was commonly experienced in human populations. Perhaps anorexia nervosa results from an inappropriate triggering of this mechanism. The BDNF gene is strongly and preferentially expressed in the anterior insula in mice (Allen Brain Atlas) and is expressed on the Von Economo neurons in humans (Nicole Tetreault and John Allman, unpublished data). We have proposed elsewhere in this volume that the Von Economo neurons are involved in the regulation of appetite because they and related layer 5 neurons in the fronto-insular and anterior cingulate cortex selectively express neuromedin B (NMB) and gastrin-releasing peptide (GRP), which regulate digestive processes and peristalsis in the stomach and intestinal tract and the central mechanisms of appetite regulation in the brain (Allman et al., 2010; Gonzalez et al., 2008). Also discussed elsewhere in this volume is the finding that the number of Von Economo neurons is greatly reduced in frontotemporal dementia and that in a large subset of frontotemporal dementia patients in whom the fronto-insular cortex on the right side is particular affected, the capacity to regulate appetite is severely compromised (Woolley et al., 2007). These patients do not become satiated even after consuming very large amounts of food, and they would thus appear to be the opposite of anorexia nervosa patients. In this context it is interesting that in a long-term study 76% of all patients who were diagnosed with anorexia nervosa as young adults also became bulimic at some stage in their lives (Wentz et al., 2009), pointing again to the severe dysregulation of body image and bodily functions in this disorder. The fact that anorexia nervosa is relatively common (Halmi, 2009; Keski-Rahkohen et al., 2007) suggests how easily the fine-tuned neural circuitry for self-awareness and control can be disrupted, in spite of the fact that such disruptions have disastrous consequences for fitness.

OVERVIEW

Like schizophrenia and bipolar disorders, autism is a complex disorder. Although it shares some features with other conditions such as ADHD, its clinical presentation and course are different. There are no clear causes of autism. Unlike schizophrenia and bipolar disorder, autism has a definite period of onset. By definition, autism onsets prior to the age of 3, when social behavior and language are developing. Thus, more of the neuropsychological, physiological, and brain imaging findings are related to various deficits in brain regions known to mediate social functioning and facial and language processing.

There are a few clues that point to specific anomalies in these brain regions. Minicolumn abnormalities, abnormal brain growth around the time of the onset of symptoms, connectivity abnormalities revealed by diffusion tensor imaging, increased local connections in the frontal cortex, and the reduction in the corpus callosum point to an increase in short- and medium-distance connections and a deficit in long-distance connections in autism. Failure to perform neuropsychological tasks that require these connections and a failure to activate long-distance networks during these tasks provide a very convincing case that this anomaly is fundamental to autism. While connectivity deficits may also underlie schizophrenia and bipolar disorder, they appear to be more regionalized, perhaps owing to the later age of onset.

The central deficits in autism, ADHD, and anorexia nervosa are related to specialized features of human cognition such the capacities for social reciprocity, self-control, and self-awareness. We will next consider another disorder, frontotemporal dementia, which is linked to degeneration of recently evolved circuitry in the brains of apes and humans.

7

Frontotemporal Dementia

Frontotemporal lobar degeneration is associated with many of the same symptoms that are seen in autism, schizophrenia, and bipolar disorder, but it presents much later in life. The most common clinical presentation is a profound alteration in personality and social conduct. Some patients experience emotional blunting and loss of volition, similar to schizophrenia, while others are socially disinhibited and distractible, similar to manic patients. A loss of insight is particularly striking in most cases, and behavior can be stereotyped and perseverative, as in many patients with autism. Occasionally, patients present with psychotic symptoms similar to those seen in schizophrenia.

Behavioral and personality changes are the most common presentation and are generally referred to as frontal-variant, behavior-variant, or just FTD. Other patients present with progressive nonfluent aphasia, in which there are severe problems with word retrieval but preserved word comprehension, or semantic dementia, in which the ability to understand words, faces, objects, and other sensory stimuli is lost. Motor syndromes such as corticobasal degeneration and progressive supranuclear palsy may be associated with frontotemporal lobe degeneration (Boxer and Miller, 2005; Graff-Radford and Woodruff, 2007; Knibb, et al., 2006; Neary et al., 1998, 2005; Roberson, 2006).

EPIDEMIOLOGY AND NATURAL COURSE

Incidence and Prevalence

Frontotemporal lobe degeneration is the second most common diagnosis of dementia in patients under 65 years of age. The prevalence of frontotemporal dementia (FTD) in patients 45 to 64 has been estimated to be 15 per 100,000. One study found that more men are diagnosed with FTD and semantic dementia than progressive nonfluent aphasia, but other studies have found an equal distribution among men and women diagnosed with FTD. Generally socioeconomic features were comparable between the three variants (Boxer and Miller, 2005; Johnson et al., 2005; Neary et al., 2005).

Course of Illness

Patients diagnosed with FTD and semantic dementia had an earlier mean age at onset than patients with progressive nonfluent aphasia. FTD has been diagnosed in persons as young as 21 and as old as 85 (Neary et al., 2005). However, the mean ages for frontotemporal and semantic dementia were 57.5 years and 59.3 years, respectively, in one study, while the age at onset of progressive nonfluent aphasia was 63.0 years (Johnson et al., 2005).

As the disease progresses, symptoms tend to become more widespread. Thus, patients diagnosed with one subtype tend to manifest symptoms overlapping with other syndromes (Roberson, 2006). The median survival for FTD was estimated to be about 6 years, but cases associated with motor neuron disease had a much shorter survival period, in the order of 3 years (Hodges et al., 2003). By comparison, Alzheimer's disease patients survived about 12 years from the onset of symptoms (Roberson et al., 2005).

NEUROPSYCHOLOGICAL FINDINGS

Cognitive Findings

Patients with FTD usually have impaired planning, judgment, problem solving, and organization. Set shifting, concept formation, inhibition of overlearned responses, self-monitoring, and using feedback to guide behavior are particularly affected. In contrast to their poor performance on frontal executive tasks, patients with FTD do well on visuoconstructional tests and memory tests when compared to healthy volunteers and Alzheimer's disease patients (Boxer and Miller, 2005; Harciarek and Jodzio, 2005; Neary et al., 2005; Rahman et al., 1999).

In semantic dementia patients, a somewhat different pattern is seen. The most common presenting problem is a loss of memory for words or a loss of word meaning. Speech is fluent, but there may be frequent paraphasias and an inability to recognize objects. Patients may be aware of their expressive deficits but are often unaware of their comprehension deficits. On formalized testing there is a loss of semantic knowledge. Episodic memory may be relatively preserved, but memory for autobiographical events may be deficient, the reverse of the pattern seen in Alzheimer's disease (Boxer and Miller, 2005; Hodges and Graham, 2001; Perry and Hodges, 2000).

Patients with progressive nonfluent aphasia usually present with deficits in word fluency, pronunciation, or word finding, progressing to agrammatism, phonemic paraphasias, stuttering, apraxia of speech, and agraphia in many cases.

Semantic memory, episodic memory, and visuospatial function and insight can be preserved in the beginning. However, executive function and working memory are often impaired. Depression, social withdrawal, and behavioral abnormalities can also be seen as the illness progresses (Boxer and Miller, 2005).

Emotional Processing and Social Cognition

Patient with FTD have difficulty evaluating both facial and vocal expressions of emotion (Keane et al., 2002; Lavenu et al., 1999; Neary et al., 2005). They also have difficulty inferring what others feel or think in theory of mind tasks, similar to the difficulties seen in autistic patients (Gregory et al., 2002). The brain structures most strongly involved in empathy are the right temporal pole, anterior insula, and anterior cingulate cortex (Rankin et al., 2006).

Nature of Impairment

FTD presents with some findings similar to bipolar disorder. Impulsive behavior, poor judgment, and lack of insight can certainly occur in mania. There are also some similarities to schizophrenia and autism in that patients have difficulty identifying emotions and inferring what others are thinking. In fact, some younger patients with FTD are misdiagnosed with schizophrenia because of apparent loosened associations, amotivation, and disorganization (Velakoulis et al., 2009). Perseveration and executive functioning abnormalities appear to characterize all these conditions to some degree, implicating prefrontal involvement. However, FTD is not usually associated with the obvious mood elevation or racing thoughts seen in mania. Patients with semantic dementia can have language difficulties, but they are clearly different from those seen in schizophrenia. Patients with frontotemporal lobar degeneration rarely hallucinate. Thus, the neuropsychology of frontotemporal lobar degeneration differs in many ways from bipolar disorder, schizophrenia, and autism.

NEUROPATHOLOGICAL STUDIES

Early descriptions of the pathology by Alzheimer included swollen neurons with ubiquitin and/or tau-positive inclusions. The achromatic swollen neurons were later called Pick's cells and the tau-positive inclusions were referred to as Pick's bodies in honor of Arnold Pick. Marked atrophy of both the temporal and frontal lobes was evident on gross examination. On histological examination, widespread gliosis was often found.

Immunohistochemistry

More recent immunohistochemical analysis has revealed four main types of pathological features (Neary et al., 2005): (1) microvacuolation without neuronal inclusions; (2) microvacuolation with ubiquitinated rounded intraneuronal inclusions and dystrophic neuritis within layer 2 of the frontal and temporal cortices and hippocampal dentate gyrus cells; (3) swollen achromatic neurons with Pick bodies; and (4) microvacuolation and tau-positive neurofibrillary tangles or Pick-like bodies in neurons, occasionally associated with tangles in the glial cells of the cerebral cortical white matter. The last two groups are often referred to as tauopathies.

Neurotransmitter Systems

Unlike Alzheimer's disease, there does not seem to be any cholinergic abnormality on postmortem examination. However, serotonin receptors have been reported to be lost from the frontal and temporal cortices in FTD—in contrast to Alzheimer's disease, in which serotonin receptor losses are seen in the temporal and parietal cortices (Proctor et al., 1999). Another postmortem study has found impairment of ascending serotonergic but not adrenergic projections to the forebrain. Serotonergic neurons in the locus ceruleus were preserved (Yang and Schmitt, 2001). Preliminary studies of selective serotonin reuptake inhibitors (SSRIs) have shown promising results for the management of behavioral disturbances in FTD (Graff-Radford and Woodruff, 2007).

Glutamatergic receptors have also been examined. While kainite receptors tend to be unaffected, both alpha-amino-3-hydroxy-5-methyl-4-isoxazole-proprionate (AMDA) and N-methyl-D-aspartate (NMDA) receptors were found to be reduced in the frontal and temporal cortices of patients with Pick's cells and bodies. Patients with FTD without these postmortem findings had only reduced AMPA receptors (Yang and Schmitt, 2001).

Von Economo Neurons

Recent evidence has suggested that FTD specifically targets the Von Economo neurons, which are present in the anterior cingulate and fronto-insular cortex in great apes and humans but not other primates (Allman et al., 2005; Nimchinsky et al., 1999). Seeley et al. (2006) did stereological counts in layer 5 of the anterior cingulate cortex in seven FTD patients, five patients with Alzheimer's disease, and seven age-matched controls (Fig. 7.1, top). FTD was associated with severe and selective losses compared to both the Alzheimer's and the control brains. Relative to control subjects, there was a 74% loss of Von Economo neurons in FTD patients. Surviving Von Economo neurons were often dysmorphic (Fig. 7.1, bottom). Von Economo neuron anomalies were seen across pathological subtypes in frontotemporal lobe dementia patients. The Von Economo neurons are similarly affected in the fronto-insular cortex in FTD brains (Seeley et al., 2007).

GENETIC INVESTIGATIONS

FTD has a strong genetic component. In one study of 42 FTD cases, 19 had at least one other family member with a frontotemporal spectrum disorder. The majority

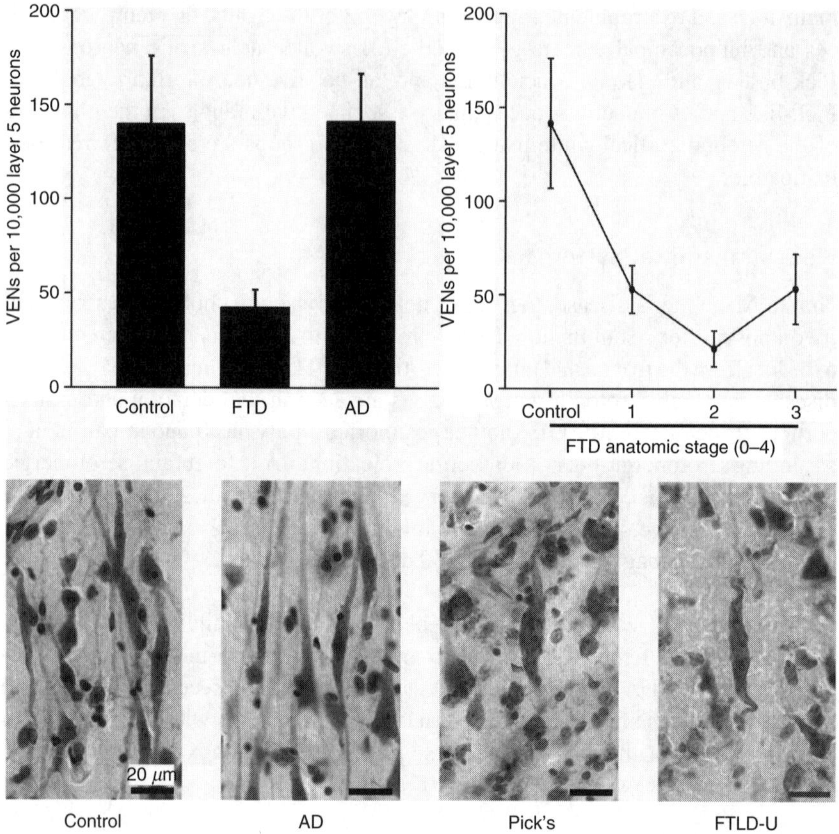

Figure 7.1 *Top*: Severe, selective, disease-specific, and early loss of Von Economo neurons (VENs) in frontotemporal degeneration (FTD). *Left*: Estimates of VEN per 10,000 neighboring neurons indicated selective VEN depletion in FTD compared with non-neurological control subjects and patients with Alzheimer's disease (AD) (**$p < 0.05$, Tukey's tests after F-test for three-group ANOVA). *Right*: Even mild stages of FTD-related atrophy were accompanied by marked VEN dropout. *Bottom*: VEN swelling and dysmorphism in FTD. VENs in normal controls and AD patients showed prominent clustering, smooth contours, and slender, tapering somata. In FTD, VENs were often solitary and swollen (especially in Pick's disease) or showed twisting and kinking of proximal dendrites (both Pick's and FTD with tau-negative and ubiquitin- and TDP-43-positive inclusions due to mutations in progranulin, indicated as FTLD-U). Cresyl violet stain. Scale bars = 20 μm. Photomicrographs are oriented with the pial surface at the top. Reprinted from Seeley, W.W., Carlin, D.A., Allman, J.M., Macedo, M.N., Bush, C., Miller, B.L., and DeArmond, S.J. Early frontotemporal dementia targets neurons unique to apes and humans. *Annals of Neurology*, **60**, 660–667. Copyright 2006, with permission from John Wiley and Sons.

of cases showed a pattern consistent with dominant inheritance (Chow et al., 1999). Mutations in at least four genes are known to cause FTD (Seeley, 2008): (1) MAPT gene, which encodes the tau protein, which stabilizes microtubules and supports axonal transports; (2) PGRN (progranulin), which is a growth factor associated with cell repair; (3) less commonly, VCP (valosin-containing protein), and (4) CHMP2B (charged multivesicular body protein). The tau form of FTD, which corresponds to Pick's disease, is illustrated by the degenerating Von Economo neurons in the bottom of Figure 7.1; the progranulin variant (FTLD-U) is also illustrated by the degenerating Von Economo neurons in this figure. With subtle variations, mutations in each of these diverse genes can all cause the same clinical manifestations, suggesting that their resulting dysfunctions all converge in the same set of molecular and neuronal circuits in the final common pathway that ultimately causes the disease. We think that this principle of diverse genetic defects causing very similar clinical manifestations through the disruption of final common pathways specific to particular disorders may be a key to understanding the mechanisms underlying these disorders. The fact that the different disorders considered in this book have some behavioral features in common suggests that they may also share some parts of these putative final common pathways.

BRAIN IMAGING STUDIES

In keeping with postmortem findings, patients with FTD have structural changes that are clearly visible with most structural brain imaging techniques.

Magnetic Resonance Imaging

MRI studies consistently show frontal and/or temporal atrophy. Volume losses are particularly striking in rostral limbic system regions, including the anterior cingulate and the fronto-insular and orbitofrontal regions (Boccardi et al., 2005). However, a number of other brain structures are involved. Enlargement of the Sylvian fissures and anterior callosal atrophy are often seen. Sometimes hippocampal and entorhinal volume loss can be found in patients with FTD, but the degree of hippocampal loss is much less than in Alzheimer's disease (Harciarek and Jodzio, 2005; Seeley et al., 2007).

Patterns of gray matter loss differ between patients with FTD and semantic dementia. Patients with FTD had atrophy in the right dorsolateral prefrontal cortex and left premotor cortex, whereas patients with semantic dementia did not. Patients with semantic dementia were characterized by tissue loss in the anterior temporal cortex and the amygdala/anterior hippocampal region. Both groups had gray matter loss in the orbital frontal, insular, and anterior cingulate regions (Rosen et al., 2002).

Progression of Volumetric Losses

A number of investigators have examined volumetric correlates of the stage of illness. Early FTD is associated with volume loss in the anterior cingulate cortex, fronto-insular, and orbitofrontal regions. All of these regions are necessary for appropriate, context-sensitive behavior, perhaps explaining why personality changes are often the presenting symptom. As the disease progresses, white matter and posterior gray matter structures interconnected with the earliest sites of injury are affected (Broe et al., 2003; Perry et al., 2006; Seeley et al., 2008).

Clinical Correlations

A number of symptoms of FTD correlate with the degree of volume loss. For example, apathy, disinhibition, eating disorders, and aberrant motor behavior are associated with tissue loss in the ventral portion of the right anterior cingulate cortex and adjacent ventromedial superior frontal gyrus, the right ventromedial prefrontal cortex more posteriorly, the right lateral middle frontal gyrus, the right caudate head, the right orbitofrontal cortex, and the right insula (Rosen et al., 2005). Volume losses on the right side were also found to correlate with performance on a test designed to evaluate empathy. In this study, voxels in the right temporal pole, the right fusiform gyrus, the right caudate, and the right subcallosal gyrus correlated positively with the total empathy score (Rankin et al., 2006).

Functional Brain Imaging Studies

Functional changes on brain imaging may be one of the earliest signs of FTD. In fact, an asymptomatic carrier of a mutation in the tau gene was found to show no abnormalities on computed tomography. The same individual performed normally on cognitive tasks except for letters on the Verbal Fluency Test. However, on brain single photon emission tomography (SPECT), bilateral frontal hypoperfusion was evident (Alberici et al., 2004).

Positron Emission Tomography (PET) and SPECT Studies

There are several imaging studies demonstrating decreased cerebral blood flow and hypometabolism in the ventromedial and inferior frontal cortex and anterior temporal lobes in patients with FTD. Findings are often asymmetrical and lateralized to the left hemisphere. Other regions such as the anterior cingulate, insula, basal ganglia, and thalamus also show decreased cerebral blood flow or hypometabolism in these patients. The metabolic changes are highly correlated with volumetric losses and increase over time (Alexander et al., 1995; Diehl-Schmid et al., 2007; Franceschi et al., 2005; Friedland et al., 1993; Grimmer et al., 2004; Ibach et al., 2004; Ishii et al., 1998; Miller and Gearhart, 1999; Schoeter et al., 2008; Varma et al., 2002; Varrone et al., 2002).

Receptor Binding Studies

The distribution of 5-hydroxytryptamine-2A receptors was examined in 18 patients with FTD. A significant reduction of these receptors was found in the orbitofrontal, frontal medial, and cingulate regions. These findings appear to be consistent with postmortem abnormalities in serotonin and the possible use of SSRIs in these patients (Franceschi et al., 2005).

Clinical Correlations

The relationship between core features of FTD such as apathy and disinhibition and regional metabolic changes has been examined. One study showed that deficits in the overlapping regions of the orbitofrontal cortex correlated with both of these clinical features (Peters et al., 2006). In another study, apathy was associated with a prevalent dorsolateral and frontal medial hypometabolism, whereas disinhibition was associated with hypometabolism in the cingulate cortex, hippocampus/amygdala, and nucleus accumbens perfusion (Franceschi et al., 2005).

Another core feature of FTD is a change in personality associated changes in "self." Miller et al. (2001) reviewed the charts of 72 patients to determine which patients exhibited a dramatic change in their self as defined by changes in political, social, or religious values. In six of the seven patients who were found to have dramatic changes in self, selective dysfunction was found in the nondominant frontal region. Only 1 of the other 65 patients without selective nondominant frontal dysfunction showed a change in self, suggesting that normal nondominant (usually right) frontal function is important for the maintenance of the self.

Specificity

In contrast to functional imaging findings in schizophrenia and bipolar disorder, decreased cerebral blood flow and hypometabolism are found in almost all cases of FTD. Findings even differ from other dementia syndromes such as Alzheimer's disease. Alzheimer's disease is characterized by decreased metabolism in the parietotemporal regions bilaterally, followed by reduction in the frontal regions (Harciarek and Jodzio, 2005). A number of recent investigations have suggested that the differences on PET between Alzheimer's disease and FTD may be useful in the differential diagnosis of these conditions, something that was not possible in other neuropsychiatric disorders (Foster, 2003; Grimmer et al., 2004; Higdon et al., 2004; Jeong et al., 2005).

OVERVIEW

FTD clearly differs from schizophrenia, bipolar disorder, and autism. It typically presents later in life and is associated with variable but more consistent postmortem findings. Neuropsychological findings often overlap with those seen in schizophrenia, bipolar disorder, and autism, but structural and functional deficits in the frontal and temporal regions are much more striking than in any of these conditions.

Despite the obvious differences, FTD affects many of the same brain regions as schizophrenia, bipolar disorders, and autism. Of particular note is the involvement of the medial prefrontal region, which seems to be associated with changes in self-perception and emotional regulation. In fact, patients with FTD demonstrate apathy, as do patients with depression and schizophrenia. They also demonstrate disinhibition, as do patients with mania, but they do not have the same mood cycles, perhaps owing to the more profound structural damage in this condition.

The finding of reduced and dysfunctional Von Economo neurons in patients with FTD is very interesting. These neurons are most abundant in humans. They are found in the anterior cingulate and fronto-insular areas affected in FTD. These same regions appear to mediate social behaviors based on past emotional experience. The following chapters will examine some of the brain networks that support these behaviors. Abnormalities in these different conditions will act as our guide.

8

Self-Monitoring Systems

While there is no doubt that non-human primates have some level of awareness, there is a great deal of debate about whether they have *theory of mind* capabilities. The literature would suggest that the nature of self-monitoring is different somehow in humans. In this chapter, we will examine this capability and its relationship to some of the findings in neuropsychiatric disorders.

We will look at different aspects of self-monitoring, beginning with studies that look at the brain imaging correlates of self-awareness in normal subjects and in patients with neuropsychiatric disorders. Agency and predicted action through corollary discharge systems in normal subjects and in those with neuropsychiatric disorders will then be discussed. Theory of mind and some of the proposed uniquely human capabilities will be examined in neuropsychiatric disorders, and finally we will look at some newly characterized brain networks, such as the default network that may underlie some of these functions.

BRAIN IMAGING STUDIES OF SELF-AWARENESS

Self-Awareness in Normal Subjects

Separating representations of internal states from perceptions of the external world enables behavioral flexibility (Churchland, 2002). In human infants, self-recognition begins at the time when the fibers in the frontal lobe begin to myelinate (Kinney et al., 1988).

Self-Appraisal Studies

There is some evidence to suggest that the right prefrontal cortex is involved in self-representation. When subjects were asked to rate adjectives as to whether they applied to themselves or to others, the right prefrontal cortex activated more with self-ratings (Craik et al., 1999). Activation of the right dorsal medial prefrontal cortex has been associated with self-ratings of traits, regardless of the emotional valence of the trait (Fossati et al., 2003). Similar investigations of self-statements have found activations on both sides in the medial prefrontal cortex, but more often on the right side (Johnson et al., 2002; Kelley et al., 2002). Rating how pictures make you feel leads to both increases and decreases in medial prefrontal activity on both sides of the brain (Gusnard et al., 2001). Thus, self-rating seems to be associated with right-sided activation of many of the same regions of the frontal polar cortex suggested to have undergone specialization in the human brain.

Dorsal and Ventral Anterior Medial Prefrontal Networks

More recent work has suggested that there may be two distinct self-appraisal networks involving the anterior medial (polar) prefrontal cortex. Based on connectivity functional magnetic resonance imaging (MRI) analyses during a self-appraisal decision-making task, both a ventral network and a dorsal network were found. The ventral network consisted of interconnections between the anterior medial prefrontal region and amygdala, insula, and nucleus accumbens. The dorsal network included interconnections between the dorsal medial prefrontal cortex, dorsolateral prefrontal cortex, and bilateral hippocampi (Schmitz and Johnson, 2006). These observations are consistent with the finding that the ventral medial prefrontal cortex interacts with the ventral striatum and amygdala during reward processing (Elliott et al., 2000, 2003; Knutson et al., 2005).

Stuss and Levine (2002) have proposed that the ventral anterior medial prefrontal cortex maintains a mental representation of the self *on-line* in order to guide emotion, reward, and inhibition processing to an appropriate response. The role of the dorsal network may relate to regulatory and inhibitive checks to guide contextually appropriate goal-directed behavior. The connection to the hippocampus may encode personally salient decisions across episodes to maintain a consistent self-schema. Northoff et al. (2006) presented a similar model based on a meta-analysis of studies. However, in this model, a third network, including the posterior cingulate cortex, the retrosplenial cortex, and the medial parietal cortex, was added. This network was seen as a link to past self-referential stimuli.

Other Brain Regions Related to Self-reflection and Self-initiation of Movement

Self-representation is not limited to the medial prefrontal region. Other studies have suggested that self-representation is more widely distributed in the brain. When subjects look at themselves, there is activation throughout the right limbic system (hippocampus, insula, anterior cingulate) and the left prefrontal and superior temporal cortex (Kircher et al., 2000). Other structures are involved as well. When subjects observe a virtual hand that is manipulated to correspond or not correspond to the subject's actual movements, the more the movements were not in the subject's control, the more the right parietal cortex was activated. A reversed pattern of activity was observed in the insula (Farrer et al., 2003).

Self-initiated movement has been associated with cerebellar activation (Blouin et al., 2004). In another study, movement in hypnotized subjects attributed to an external source resulted in higher parietal and cerebellar activation than identical movements correctly attributed to the self. The hypnotic suggestion was proposed to impair the functioning of the cerebellar-parietal network (Blakemore et al., 2003). Thus, the sense of controlling movements or agency appears to be associated with a much wider network of activity, including structures such as the hippocampus, insula, anterior cingulate, parietal, and cerebellar regions.

Abnormalities in Neuropsychiatric Disorders

Schizophrenia

Schizophrenia is associated with a number of internal monitoring deficits. Frith (1987) proposed that hallucinations are associated with an internal self-monitoring deficit that regulates internal speech. Others have suggested that hallucinating patients have a response bias to attribute internal events to an external source (Bentall, 1990). There is some support for internal monitoring anomalies in the brain imaging literature. Hallucinating patients have reduced activation on positron emission tomography (PET) in the left middle temporal gyrus and rostral supplementary areas (both regions involved in monitoring speech) when asked to imagine sentences spoken in another person's voice (McGuire et al., 1995). Schizophrenic patients with active persecutory delusions have shown a marked absence of rostral-ventral anterior cingulate activation, together with increased posterior cingulate activation, during appraisal of neutral and threatening self-referential statements (Blackwood et al., 2004).

The psychological literature provides support for the proposal that schizophrenic patients have a response bias to external attribution of internal events (Brébion et al., 2000; Morrison and Haddock, 1997). However, the psychological literature provides little support for the idea that hallucinators are unable to distinguish inner *imagined* speech from real external speech (Evans et al., 2000). Consequently, the internal self-monitoring deficit associated with schizophrenia may be more related to the *action* of speech than self-representation in a general sense. We will comment more on this below, in the section on corollary discharge systems.

Bipolar Disorder

Patients with bipolar disorder also have disturbances in self-representation, but in a different way than schizophrenic patients. During periods of mania, there is generally an inflated sense of self-importance and even grandiosity. During depression, there is often the opposite: a sense of low self-esteem, sometimes to the point of feeling worthless. This is a very curious phenomenon suggesting that self-monitoring has an affective component that is quite separate from the *action* component seen in schizophrenia. It fits nicely into the recent observations that there are dorsal and ventral self-appraisal networks (Schmitz and Johnson, 2006). If human self-monitoring is organized in this way, it may explain why these patients so often present with disturbed perceptions of themselves.

Autism

Autistic patients have difficulty representing personal and emotional characteristics as well. They perform poorly on tests of facial recognition and emotional recognition from faces and voices (Kasari and Rotheram-Fuller, 2005; Sigman et al., 2006). Autistic patients have been found to have activation deficits on functional MRI (fMRI) when ask to appraise facial expressions, particularly with regard to emotional content (Critchley et al., 2000). Autistic patients seem to use feature-based strategies that are more typical of non-face object perception (Schultz et al., 2000). Thus, these patients have difficulties identifying emotional characteristics in others as well as in themselves. However, this is quite a different disturbance of self-representation, which is more related to theory of mind, which we will discuss below.

Frontotemporal Dementia

Patients with frontotemporal dementia have also have difficulty evaluating both facial and vocal expressions of emotion, which seem to go beyond their difficulties with set shifting, concept formation, and inhibition of overlearned responses (Keane et al., 2002; Lavenu et al., 1999; Neary et al., 2005). A core feature of frontotemporal dementia is a change in personality often associated with changes in self. As we saw in Chapter 7, patients who exhibited a dramatic change in their self, as defined by changes in political, social, or religious values, were found to have selective dysfunction in the nondominant frontal region (Miller et al., 2001). The involvement of this region in these patients is consistent with the suggestion that the right prefrontal region is associated with representations of self.

Neuropsychiatric disorders are associated with disorders of self-representation. However, the most intriguing aspect of these anomalies is that they are subtly different in each disorder. In mood disorder, affective representations predominate. In autism, there is predominantly a deficit in representation of the characteristics of others. In frontotemporal dementia, we see self-attribution errors and deficits in the representations of the characteristics of others. Finally, in schizophrenia, we see a deficit in agency. We will look at the concept of action and agency more closely in the next section.

COROLLARY DISCHARGE SYSTEMS

Corollary discharge systems are integrative mechanisms that prepare for the consequences of self-initiated action, allowing the distinction to be made between

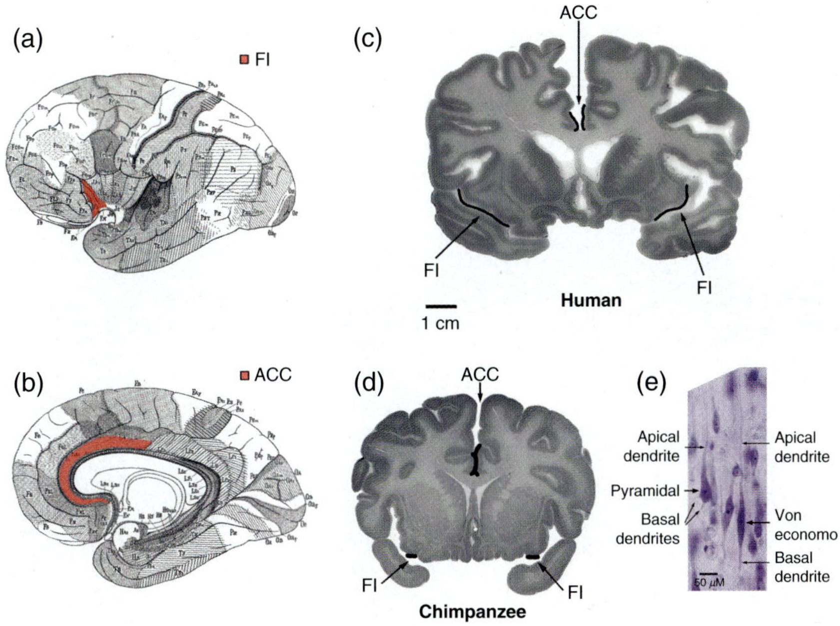

Color Plate 3.1 Regions of the brain containing Von Economo neurons. (a) A lateral view of the brain, with fronto-insular cortex (FI) shown in red. (b) A medial view of the brain, with anterior cingulate cortex (ACC) shown in red. (c) FI and the spindle-cell–containing region of ACC indicated on coronal sections through a human brain (50-year-old woman) and (d) a common chimpanzee brain (sections shown with the right hemisphere of the brain on the right of the figure). Note that FI is much larger in the human than in the chimpanzee. (e) A Von Economo neuron and a pyramidal neuron in layer 5 of FI. Both types of neuron have a single apical dendrite, but note that the Von Economo neuron also has only a single basal dendrite, in contrast to the pyramidal neuron's multiple basal dendrites. Photomicrograph by the authors of a section from the 50-year-old human brain shown in part (c). Reprinted from Allman, J.M., Watson, K.K., Tetreault, N.A., and Hakeem, A.Y. Intuition and autism: A possible role for Von Economo neurons. *Trends in Cognitive Sciences*, **9**, 367–373, Copyright 2005, with permission from Elsevier.

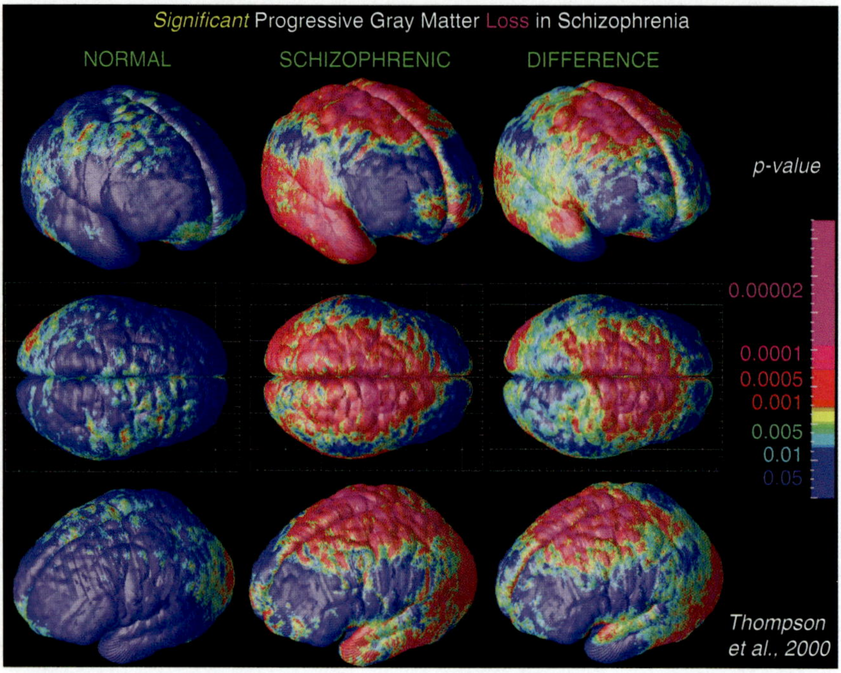

Color Plate 4.1 Significance of dynamic gray matter loss in normal adolescents and in schizophrenia. Highly significant progressive loss occurs in schizophrenia in parietal, motor, supplementary motor, and superior frontal cortices. Broad regions of temporal cortex, including the superior temporal gyrus, experience severe gray matter attrition. By comparing the average rates of loss in disease (middle column) with the loss pattern in normal adolescents (first column), the normal variability in these changes can also be taken into account, and the significance of disease-specific change can be established (last column). Reprinted from Thompson, P.M., Vidal, C., Giedd, J.N., Gochman, P., Blumenthal, J., Nicolson, R., Toga, A.W., and Rapaport, J.L. Mapping adolescent brain change reveals dynamic wave of accelerated gray matter loss in very early-onset schizophrenia. *Proceedings of the National Academy of Sciences of the USA*, **98**, 11650–11655. Copyright 2001, with permission from the National Academy of Sciences, U.S.A.

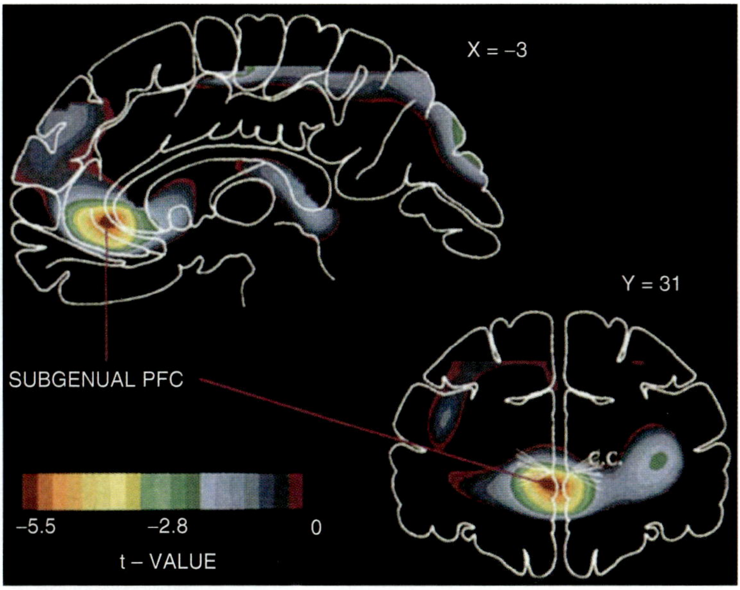

Color Plate 5.1 Coronal ($y = 31$ mm) and sagittal ($x = -3$ mm) sections showing negative voxel t values where metabolism is decreased in depressed patients relative to controls. This image, generated post hoc to provide optimal localization of the subgenual prefrontal cortex (PFC) abnormality, compares all unmedicated depressed patients scanned with bipolar and unipolar depressed patients with controls. The spatial resolution of positron emission tomography precludes clear laterality distinctions. Anterior, or left, is to the left. Reprinted from Drevets, W.C., Price, J.L., Simpson, J.R., Todd, R.D., Reich, T., Vannier, M., and Raichle, M.E. Subgenual prefrontal abnormalities in mood disorders. *Nature*, **386**, 824–827, Copyright 1997, with permission from Nature Publishing Group.

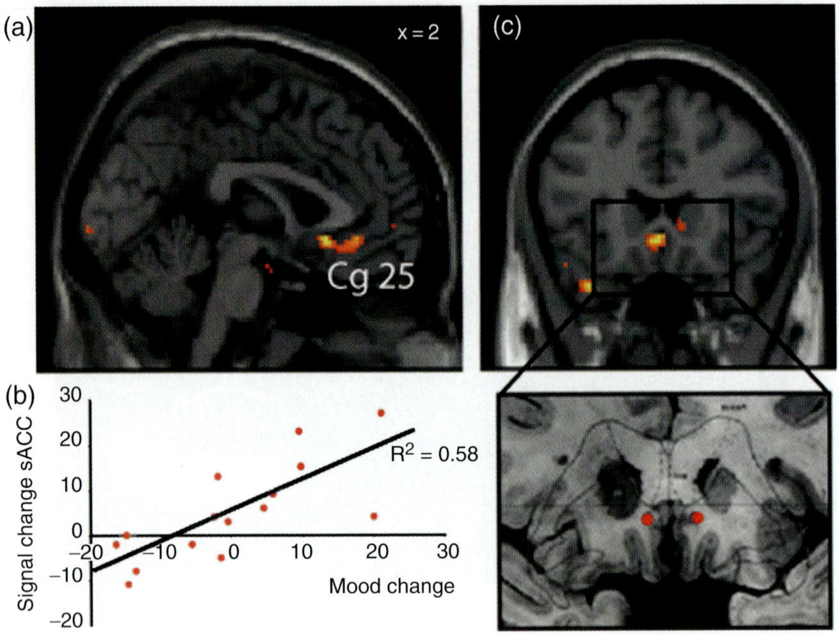

Color Plate 5.2 Subgenual cingulate (subgenual anterior cingulate cortex [sACC], Cg25) activity predicts inflammation-associated total mood change. (a) Region of subgenual cingulate (Cg25) that shows the strongest prediction of inflammation-associated deterioration in total mood. (b) Correlation of activity in an 8-mm-diameter region of interest centered on the peak subgenual cingulate voxel (ordinate) with inflammation-associated total mood change (abscissa). (c) Area of placement of deep brain stimulation electrodes for the treatment of primary depression showing relative position with respect to activation shown in (a). Reprinted from Harrison, N.A., Brydon, L., Walker, C., Gray, M., Steptoe, A., and Critchley, H.D. Inflammation causes mood changes through alterations in subgenual cingulate activity and mesolimbic connectivity. *Biological Psychiatry*, **66**, 407–414, Copyright 2009, with permission from Elsevier.

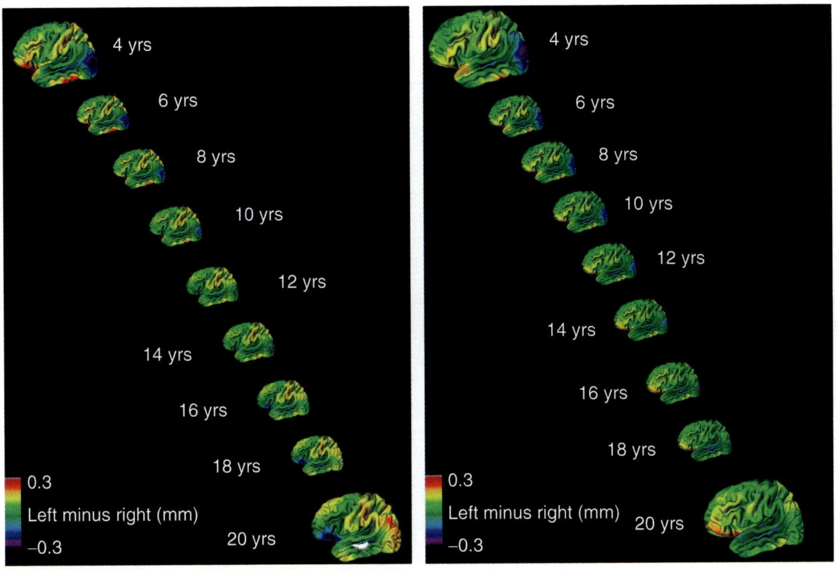

Color Plate 6.1 *Left*: Differences between left and right cortical thickness at each age. Red and yellow areas indicate a thicker left cortex, blue and purple areas a thicker right cortex. Note the changing asymmetries in the right orbitofrontal and inferior frontal regions and in the left posterior temporo-occipital cortex. *Right*: Differences between left and right cortical thickness at each age for the right-handed attention-deficit/hyperactivity disorder cohort. Red and yellow areas indicate a thicker left cortex, blue and purple areas a thicker right cortex. From *Archives of General Psychiatry*, **66**, 888–896. Copyright 2009, American Medical Association. All rights reserved.

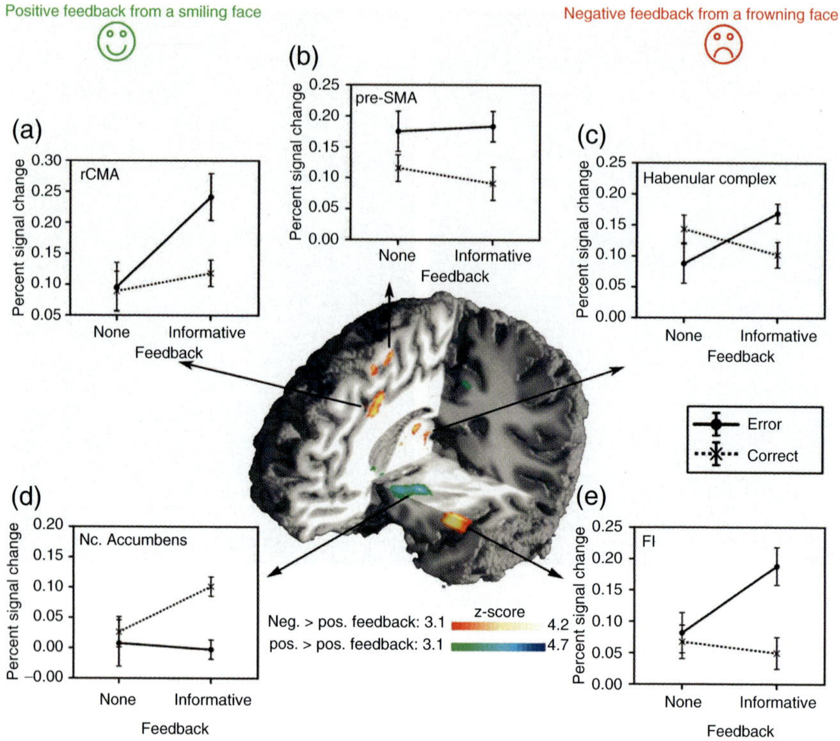

Color Plate 10.1 Brain activation associated with smiling and frowning faces presented during a complex task. The central picture shows the *z*-map resulting from contrasting negative and positive informative feedback. Signal change of the hemodynamic response is shown for correct and error trials with and without informative feedback at the motor component of the anterior cingulate cortex (rCMA) (a), presupplementary motor area (pre-SMA) (b), habenular complex (c), ventral striatum (nucleus accumbens) (d), and left fronto-insular cortex (FI) (e), modified from Ullsperger, M., and von Cramon, D.Y. Error monitoring using external feedback: Specific roles of the habenular complex, the reward system, and the cingulate motor area revealed by functional magnetic resonance imaging. *Journal of Neuroscience,* **23**, 4308–4314. Copyright 2003, with permission from Society for Neuroscience.

self-produced and externally produced events. Most of these systems have been studied in motor responses, but it is likely that there are comparable analogues in cognitive systems (Graybiel, 1997). It has been suggested that a disruption in these *cognitive pattern generators* could explain hallucinations and delusions in schizophrenia (Feinberg and Guazzelli, 1999).

Feinberg and Guazelli (1999) provided some interesting evidence of the existence of these cognitive pattern generators from Penfield's neurosurgical studies. When Penfield stimulated the temporal lobes of patients, the patients experienced past memories but indicated that they thought that the surgeon caused them to have the thought. Clearly their ability to distinguish internally from externally produced experiences was intact. Graybiel (1997) suggested that the basal ganglia and their loop circuits with the prefrontal cortex and thalamus are essential for the retention and expression of cognitive pattern generators in the motor systems of thought. Schizophrenic patients may lack the circuitry to make the distinction (Frith, 1995; Frith et al., 2000).

In the case of delusion of control, there may be a disconnection between the regions initiating actions in the prefrontal cortex and parietal regions involved in predicting the sensory consequences of action. Movement is perceived as being produced by someone else in the absence of its predicted path. There is some evidence in support of this in imaging studies where the observation of movement is experimentally distorted. When subjects do not feel in control, the inferior parietal cortex is activated (i.e., the image of their self-initiated movement has been distorted). Schizophrenic subjects do not show parietal activation, suggesting that there could be a disconnection between parietal and prefrontal regions (Farrer et al., 2004).

Studies using distorted feedback about movements have further illustrated monitoring difficulties in schizophrenic patients. When schizophrenic patients performed simple wrist and finger movements while watching an image of either their own hand or an alien hand executing the same or different movements, they were more impaired on discriminating their own hand from the alien one. They also tended to misattribute the alien hand to themselves (Daprati et al., 1997). Patients who felt delusionally influenced by others or an outside force were particularly impaired on this task (Franck et al., 2001). This could suggest that in schizophrenia, the problem is not so much monitoring internal events but a problem with the *who* system (Georgieff and Jeannerod, 1998), which involves the structures activated during self-representation and self-initiated tasks. A similar failure of self-monitoring of subvocal speech has been suggested, but we will discuss these issues further in Chapters 9 and 11 (Frith and Dolan, 1996).

These studies raise the question of whether self-processing has a unique substrate in the brain. Recent reviews (Gillihan and Farah, 2005; Legrand and Ruby, 2009) suggest that the sense of agency related to physical movements may have a specific neural localization. However, other aspects of self-processing, such as trait appraisal, autobiographical memory, and the awareness of first-person perspective, do not seem to be related to a unitary system, despite the individual's experience of a unified self. How do humans appraise others?

THEORY OF MIND

The term *theory of mind* was coined by Premack and Woodruff (1978). It arises from the observation that emotions, desires, plans, and beliefs are not directly observable; in this sense they are a *theory*. In humans, at least, these mental states are representations about internal states and the internal states and intentions of others. This capacity is sometimes referred to as *mentalizing*. The ability to explain and predict the behavior of ourselves and others by attributing mental states through this capacity allows us to consider the consequences of various action alternatives before acting. Many have suggested that the emergence of this capacity was the origin of cultural cognition (Tomasello et al., 2005).

More recently, it has been suggested that theory of mind is just one form of self-projection ability. When we think about the future (prospection), remember the past, or conceive the viewpoint of others (theory of mind), we are using the same core brain network. All of these processes involve the use of past experience to imagine perspectives and events beyond those associated with the immediate environment. All these forms of self-projection seem to emerge at about the age of 4 years (Buckner and Carroll, 2007).

It has been proposed that humans go through three stages of representational development. In infants, primary representations faithfully model reality. By the second year, representations can model hypothetical situations that do not necessarily correspond to reality. An example of this stage of representational development would be a child using a stick as a gun. By about the age of 4, representations of representational relations emerge. At this stage, the child becomes aware of the intentions of others and is able to detect deception, the acid test of theory of mind (Perner, 1991).

Do Animals Have Theory of Mind?

Darwin (1886) suggested in *Descent of Man* that there was no fundamental difference in the psychological abilities between humans and other species. This idea has had considerable support over the years with observations about the social behavior of many animals, particularly primates. Chimpanzees can even recognize themselves in the mirror (Gallup, 1970). It was assumed that if other species exhibited similar behaviors to humans, they must have similar psychological processes. For example, if a chimpanzee looks at what his trainer is looking at, does this suggest the chimpanzee thinks that the trainer is looking at something important, so maybe he should look too? In a carefully constructed series of experiments Povinelli et al. (2000) showed that this is likely not the case; in fact, they concluded that chimpanzees do not harbor representations of mental states in general, not just in this particular situation.

Not all investigators have agreed that primates do not harbor representations of mental states. While there is agreement that there is no convincing evidence of deception in other species, a strong case has been made for the presence of secondary representations. A chimpanzee has been observed to act as if she were pulling a toy on a string and would use appropriate movements when the pretend string apparently became stuck on a real object. Another chimpanzee traveling with his pregnant mother picked up a log and carried it for hours, treating it like a baby (Suddendorf and Whiten, 2001).

Thus, there is good reason to believe that some primates are capable of secondary representation equivalent to 2-year-old humans. Chimpanzees understand to some degree the goals, knowledge, and intentions of others. However, there is no convincing evidence that they understand false beliefs (Call and Tomasello, 2008). Consequently, chimpanzees have some but not all qualities of theory of mind seen in humans. It is likely that humans alone have the ability to reminisce about the past and imagine the future (Suddendorf and Busby, 2003).

What Brain Regions Are Associated with Theory of Mind?

Most commentators have suggested that theory of mind is a cognitive specialization related to an evolutionary change in the medial prefrontal cortex (Amodio and Frith, 2006; Povinelli and Preuss, 1995). Brain imaging studies have shown that other regions are likely involved. Three regions are consistently activated during theory of mind tasks: the anterior paracingulate cortex, the superior temporal sulci, and the temporal poles bilaterally (Gallagher and Frith, 2003). It is of note that these are regions that have undergone some specializations in the human brain.

It is interesting that these areas tend to be activated during other forms of self-projection, such as prospection and remembering past autobiographical events. As we have discussed previously, midline frontal regions are also activated during self-referential tasks. Consequently, there appears to be a core network that supports remembering, prospection, theory of mind, and tasks that require complex problem solving and imagination (Buckner and Carroll, 2007).

Abnormalities in Neuropsychiatric Disorders

There is no doubt that schizophrenic and bipolar patients have difficulties with theory of mind tasks (Bora et al., 2005, 2009; Brüne, 2005; Lahera et al., 2008; Olley et al., 2005; Sprong et al., 2007). In some cases, performance on theory of mind tasks correlates with gray matter loss in patients with schizophrenia in regions associated with theory of mind, such as the right temporal pole (Herold et al., 2009). However, it is difficult to separate theory of mind deficits from generalized cognitive deficits. Deficits in patients with autism and frontotemporal dementia are often more striking. These deficits are particularly striking in autistic patients (Baron-Cohen et al., 1985). These patients also have impairment on complex tasks, which may involve self-projection brain regions (Minshew et al., 1997; Williams et al., 2006a). Brain imaging during theory of mind tasks has also revealed deficits in brain activation in autistic patients in the medial prefrontal, superior temporal, and temporal pole regions (Castelli et al., 2002).

Patients with frontotemporal dementia also have impairment on complex tasks that involve self-monitoring and concept (Boxer and Miller, 2005; Harciarek and Jodzio, 2005; Neary et al., 2005; Rahman et al., 1999). They have difficulty evaluating both facial and vocal expressions of emotion (Keane et al., 2002; Lavenu et al., 1999; Neary et al., 2005). On theory of mind tasks, they have similar difficulties to those seen in autistic patients (Gregory et al., 2002). Both patients with frontotemporal dementia and semantic dementia have impaired cognitive empathy, while only patients with semantic dementia have deficits in the emotional components of empathy (Rankin et al., 2005). On structural brain imaging, loss of volume in the right temporal pole was found to correlate with ratings of empathy in these patients (Rankin et al., 2006). Patients with frontotemporal dementia have a striking reduction in the number of Von Economo neurons as well, as the disease progresses.

Thus, there is now mounting evidence that both autism and frontotemporal dementia are associated with deficits in theory of mind. Furthermore, the anomalies in brain structure and function in these patients overlap to some degree with brain regions known to be associated with this capacity in normal subjects.

DEFAULT NETWORK

It has been pointed out that many of the same regions associated with prospection, remembering the past, and theory of mind overlap with the *default network* (Buckner et al., 2008). The default network refers to brain regions that are active at rest. The network was originally referred to as the default mode network, but we will use the simpler label. The network includes the posterior cingulate and retrosplenial cortices, the lateral parietal cortices, the ventral and dorsal medial prefrontal cortices, and the parahippocampal gyri. These regions were suggested to be associated with internally generated *stimulus-independent* thought as well as self- and salience-monitoring. The default network is deactivated during attention-demanding tasks. During performance of these tasks, *task-related network* is activated in the dorsolateral prefrontal cortices, frontal eye fields, inferior parietal lobules, middle temporal region, and insula. Thus, it has been suggested that activities in these two functional networks are negatively correlated or *anticorrelated* (Fox et al., 2005; Fox and Raichle, 2007; Gusnard et al., 2001; Raichle and Snyder, 2007).

The default network has been defined by functional connectivity analysis on conventional resting MRI (Greicius et al., 2003) and spontaneous low-frequency fluctuations of the blood oxygen level-dependent (BOLD) signal over time (Fox et al., 2005; Fransson, 2005). The latter are thought to reflect neural synchrony of gamma activity, possibly related to consciousness. The default network has been demonstrated by a number of independent investigators using different techniques. Considering these different approaches, it is remarkable that resting state is so consistently associated with the medial prefrontal, posterior cingulate, and temporal lobe structures. However, some investigations have found that the network extends to other structures, such as the thalamus, inferior frontal cortices, and angular and parahippocampal gyrus on the left side (Fox et al., 2005; Fransson, 2005; Greicius et al., 2003). Others suggest that there are a number of different intrinsic networks that can be distinguished from the default network (De Luca et al., 2006; Seeley et al., 2007, 2009).

What controls the switch from the default network to the task-activated network is not known. Some have speculated about thalamus involvement in the switch, but more recent work has shown that the right fronto-insular and anterior cingulate cortices seem to control the switch from the default network to the task-activated network (Sridharan et al., 2008). This is particularly interesting because both of these regions are rich in Von Economo neurons (Sridharan et al., 2008; Williamson, 2007).

There has been some controversy about the concept of a "resting" network (Morcom and Fletcher, 2007). However, there is some evidence that mind-wandering is associated with activity in the default network (Mason et al., 2007). Lesion studies also seem to be consistent with the concept. Patients with damage to the medial prefrontal cortex and anterior cingulate sometimes describe the feeling of an "empty mind" and suggest that they have "nothing to say" (Damasio and Van Hoesen, 1983). As discussed above, the medial prefrontal cortex and posterior cingulate cortex on one or both sides are often activated with self-representational tasks. However, it is also likely that other brain structures, such as the insula, right parietal cortex, and cerebellar parietal network, are important in self-representation. Some of these structures are more closely related to the task-related network.

Fransson (2005) suggested that the medial prefrontal cortices, posterior cingulate cortices, angular gyrus, and temporal lobe structures sustain a memory-retrieval system for autobiographical events (Maddock et al., 1999; Maguire and Mummery, 1999). Retrieval of autobiographical events seems to be consistent with a role for these structures in stimulus-independent thought. It is also consistent with Raichle and Gusnard's (2005) proposal that the default mode may be essential for manipulation of past events in order to consider a course of action. However, stimulus-independent thought might be expected to be associated with language processing. The medial prefrontal cortex and cingulate cortices have not typically been associated with language, but the anterior cingulate is closely connected with speech areas and may regulate their activity during silence (Barbas et al., 1999, Hunter et al., 2006). Consequently, there is reason to believe that this network is involved with stimulus-independent thought with other associated networks.

The default network can be seen in light sleep and anesthesia, but in deeper states of sleep there is an altered correlation between regions. In particular, correlations between the posterior regions and the anterior cingulate and medial prefrontal regions seem to be much less prominent in deep sleep. Some have interpreted this to suggest that the default network may play a role in the sustenance of conscious awareness (Horovitz et al., 2009).

Development of Resting State Networks

There is now some evidence to suggest that the default network undergoes considerable revision during postnatal development. The infant brain has been shown to have five unique resting state networks. These networks included all the same regions involved in the adult default network, but there was a striking difference: the anterior network involving the medial prefrontal cortex was not associated with activity in the posterior cingulate and precuneus regions, suggesting that these connections develop over time (Fransson et al., 2007).

By age 2 years, healthy children show clear connections between the principal regions of the default network (Gao et al., 2009). However, there appears to be considerable revision of these connections to adulthood. A study of 7- to 9-year-old children, adolescents, and adults showed clear differences with brain maturation. Children had less connectivity of the ventral medial prefrontal cortex than adults. Over time, increasing long-range and posterior connections were apparent (Fair et al., 2007, 2008). These findings are particularly relevant to the development of self-monitoring systems, which depend on the medial prefrontal cortex.

The Default Network in Other Species

An interesting question to ask would be whether species that do not have theory of mind have a default network. If they do, it would be difficult to conclude that this network is associated with these functions. We now have some data in rats, monkeys, and chimpanzees.

There is reason to believe that resting-state spontaneous low-frequency fluctuations of the BOLD signal are conserved across species. Long-range correlations of these low-frequency fluctuations have been demonstrated across somatosensory and visual regions in rats in the absence of external stimuli (Pawela et al., 2008). Low-frequency fluctuations of the BOLD signal have been observed in the visual cortex in monkeys during various behavioral states (Leopold et al., 2003). However, it is difficult to evaluate differences from human studies without information about frontal regions.

A recent study used PET to examine resting-state networks in chimpanzees and humans (Rilling et al., 2007). Both humans and chimpanzees showed high levels of activity in most anterior and posterior default regions. However, chimpanzees differed from humans by showing higher levels of activity in the ventromedial prefrontal cortex and lower levels of activity in left-sided cortical regions involved in conceptual processing and language in humans.

Abnormalities in Neuropsychiatric Disorders

Resting-state abnormalities have now been described in a number of neuropsychiatric conditions (Williamson, 2007). In a study of connectivity across the default network in chronic schizophrenic patients, generally decreased connectivity was found, particularly in the insula, temporal lobe, corpus striatum, and prefrontal regions (Liang et al., 2006). Another group (Garrity et al., 2007) found significant spatial differences between schizophrenic patients and controls in the frontal, anterior cingulate, and parahippocampal regions, all regions associated with the default network. Using methodology based on Fransson (2005), marked deficits in connectivity were found in a number of default regions, including the posterior cingulate, medial prefrontal, and cerebellar regions (Bluhm et al., 2007). Other investigators have found decreased connectivity with the prefrontal cortex and hippocampus in schizophrenic subjects during the resting state (Zhou et al., 2007, 2008).

Bluhm et al. (2007) found a positive symptom-dependent correlation between the posterior cingulate and the auditory cortex. This suggests that hallucinations may be associated with activity in the auditory cortex and posterior cingulate. Without activity in the anterior cingulate and prefrontal regions, this may lead to the perception that the hallucination is not internally produced. This is consistent with other studies of the time course of hallucinations showing that hallucinations are preceded by both middle temporal activity and deactivation of the anterior cingulate (Hoffman et al., 2008). More recent investigations have suggested that increased deactivation in specific regions of the default network, including the medial prefrontal cortex and precuneus, is associated with positive symptoms, while reduced deactivation of the anterior cingulate is associated with reduced attentional control (Broyd et al., 2009). Thus, there is considerable evidence of anomalies in multiple regions of the default network in schizophrenia, although patterns vary according to the methodologies employed.

Anomalies in the default network have also been found in other neuropsychiatric conditions. Autistic patients failed to deactivate the medial prefrontal, rostral anterior cingulate, posterior cingulate, and precuneus cortices during cognitive tasks (Kennedy et al., 2006). Another investigation of neurotypical adults found a relationship between autistic traits and the pregenual anterior cingulate cortex-insula social network in the resting state (Di Martino et al., 2009). Chronic depressed patients, with and without psychosis, demonstrated significantly greater resting-state subgenual cingulate and thalamic functional connectivity with the default network (Greicius et al., 2007). Alzheimer's patients showed decreased resting-state activity in the posterior cingulate and hippocampus, suggesting abnormal connectivity between these structures (Greicius et al., 2004). More recently, Seeley et al. (2009) have shown that different neurogenerative disorders, including frontotemporal dementia, cause circumscribed atrophy in regions associated with several intrinsic connectivity networks.

Thus, anomalies in the default network are not specific to schizophrenia, but there are some differences between disorders. In mood disorders, we see abnormal connections between the default network and the subgenual prefrontal cortex. The subgenual prefrontal cortex is implicated in mood disorders in many brain imaging studies. Similarly, the default network with the hippocampus is affected in Alzheimer's disease, which is also associated with structural deficits in this region. What these differences may suggest is that there are several subsystems in the default network.

OVERVIEW

There are many aspects to self-monitoring: self-appraisal, agency, autobiographical memories, prospection, and theory of mind. Many of these capacities overlap with the default network. In fact, a recent quantitative meta-analysis of neuroimaging studies found a common neural basis of autobiographical memory, prospection, theory of mind, and the default network (Spreng et al., 2009). There is some evidence that most of these capacities are uniquely human. If they are uniquely human, then it is difficult to see how the default network could underlie these capacities, as there seems to be at least a modified form of this network in chimpanzees. Do neuropsychiatric disorders help us understand this problem?

Amodio and Frith (2006) have suggested that there are three divisions to the medial prefrontal cortex: the dorsal division monitors action, a middle or rostral division is related to social cognitive processes, and an orbital division is related to reward and punishment. It is likely that all of these regions are involved in unique self-monitoring subsystems. Neuropsychiatric disorders may point to the nature of these subsystems. For example, schizophrenia may be related to a dorsal subsystem that controls action and agency. Bipolar disorder may be related to an orbital subsystem that relates to mood. Both autism and frontotemporal dementia may be related to failures of the rostral subsystem at different stages of life. However, before we try to put these things together, there is another human capability that we need to account for: language. The next chapter will look at the human brain structures that might be involved in this ability.

9

Language Systems

An obvious difference between human and non-human primates is the capacity for language. This chapter will look at what is associated with this capacity in the human brain from several perspectives. We will look at the nature of language and whether there is a universal language structure. What we know about the brain regions involved in language processing will also be discussed. Whether primates have some language capabilities will also be examined.

Anomalies in brain asymmetry have been suggested to underlie some neuropsychiatric disorders. This possibility will be critically examined, particularly with reference to schizophrenia. Other anomalies in speech perception in autism and frontotemporal dementia have been described. How do these disorders help us understand language systems in the brain? This and other questions related to language will be discussed in this chapter.

THE NATURE OF LANGUAGE

What happens when an individual speaks to another individual? The speaker not only utters sounds but also follows the rules of sentence structure (syntax). The listener interprets these sounds to extract meaning (semantics) at not only a content level but also an emotional level. Language is a representational process that requires theory of mind—that is, the listener has to appreciate that there is another person who has an idea or feeling that is being communicated to the listener (Wise, 2003).

Is Language an Instinct?

Interestingly, speech can be filtered into as little as three broad-frequency bands and still be intelligible, although some subtle information such as the age, sex, and identity of the speaker is lost (Shannon et al., 1995). How does this happen? Some theorists such as Pinker (1995) suggest that language is a "human instinct." In other words, there are modular processing units in the human brain that lead to the capacity for language. Other theorists argue that there are innately specified attentional biases and linguistic predispositions. However, the innate predisposition does not fully explain language. To understand how linguistic representations become flexible and manipulable, several levels of *representational redescription* are required, and this goes far beyond the basic use of symbols of which some higher primates are capable. Indeed, the use of language itself in different cultural contexts may shape our cognitive biases (Haun et al., 2006).

Language Regions in the Human Brain

What do we know about the brain regions involved in language in the human brain? Between the cochlea and the auditory cortex, there is some early processing of auditory signals in the cochlear nucleus, the superior olivary complex, the inferior colliculus, and the medial geniculate body of the thalamus (Patterson and Johnsrude, 2008). The auditory cortex is much more complicated than Wernicke's area; in fact, it extends down the whole length of the superior temporal gyrus (Pandya, 1995). There are two main streams of processing that arise from the auditory core. An anterior (ventral) stream projects to the ventrolateral and dorsolateral frontal cortex, suggesting a role in processing meaning. A posterior (dorsal) stream involves the parietal cortex and the ventrolateral and dorsolateral prefrontal cortex. The posterior stream is thought to process articular-gestational representations of speech acts. Like vision, speech is likely processed as both a sound and as an action (Scott and Johnsrude, 2003). Connections between Broca's area and the superior temporal region are particularly prominent in adult humans compared to children and non-human primates (Friederici, 2009).

Brain Asymmetry

Asymmetry can be seen in the human brain at both a macroscopic and a cytoarchitectural level in the human brain. In Chapter 3, we noted a longer left sylvian fissure and a larger left planum temporale. The auditory cortex has also been found to have bigger pyramidal cells, thicker myelinated fibers, and wider cortical columns (Dehaene et al., 2006). Some might argue that these findings are associated with an innate capacity for speech, but this is far from clear. Others point out that many of the changes could be effect rather than cause. During fetal development there is a longer left sylvian fissure and a larger left planum temporale, but in the first year of life there is no left–right difference in cerebral blood flow. There is also considerable plasticity in the immature brain. Damage to the dominant hemisphere in childhood leads the nondominant hemisphere to take over language with almost no ill effects (Dehaene et al., 2006).

The genetic basis of brain asymmetry is not known, but it has been suggested that a translocation occurred from the ancestral X chromosome to the Y chromosome, resulting in duplication of the *Protocadherin 11X* gene such that it is represented on the X and Y chromosomes in man. This translocation has been dated to 6 million years ago, about the same time as the chimpanzee–hominid bifurcation. This translocation has been proposed to account for the development of cerebral asymmetry and language in humans (Williams et al., 2006c).

Language Networks

Language involves complex networks of brain activity linking the frontal, temporal, and parietal regions. It has been pointed out that no one region holds the key to a specific language function: there has to be a time-dependent connectivity between several regions. Syntactic processing requires an intact network of left hemisphere regions, including the left inferior frontal cortex (including Broca's area) and regions of the posterior temporal and parietal cortex. Semantic processing engages a more anterior region of the left medial temporal and superior temporal gyri and the left inferior frontal cortex (Tyler and Marslen-Wilson, 2008). The right hemisphere is also involved in language to some degree. Patients with left hemisphere damage can process simple words but are not capable of fluent speech (Tyler and Marslen-Wilson, 2008).

DO PRIMATES HAVE LANGUAGE?

Monkeys, chinchillas, and birds can be trained to perceive speech syllables categorically like humans, but they are unable to generalize these behaviors to other contexts (Dehaene-Lambertz et al., 2006). Even attempts to teach speech to chimpanzees have failed.

Teaching Chimpanzees Language

Some fascinating early work in this area was done by Savage-Rumbaugh (1986). After several failed attempts at teaching chimpanzees speech, a visual symbol approach was taken by developing a graphic symbol keyboard. Reared in a primate research center, chimpanzees named Sherman, Austin, Nim, and Kanzi were eventually able to use graphic symbols on a keyboard to communicate such things as what food they wanted on an outdoor cookout. Kanzi was also able to indicate which person was to be the agent and which was to be the recipient by a pointing gesture after touching graphic symbols such as "Sue [Dr. Savage-Rumbaugh] bite person [the person to which Kanzi pointed]" (Savage-Rumbaugh, 1986). By 46 months, Kanzi was able to produce about 800 unique non-imitated combinations of these symbols.

While the chimpanzee studies showed that it was possible for non-human primates to map concepts to arbitrary symbols one to one with extensive training, some have argued that this is not language (Karmiloff-Smith, 1992). The symbols are not signs within a structured system. Even a long list of lexical items is not naming and not even close to the linguistic competence of a 2- or 3-year-old child. Chimpanzees are not capable of representational redescription. Children have (Karmiloff-Smith, 1992) "explicit representations which allow them to reflect on component parts of words and to progressively build linguistic theories." So what makes the human brain unique in this regard?

Evolutionary Basis of Language

It was suggested that one of the unique features of humans is a descended larynx, but we now know that several other mammalian species have a descended larynx (Hauser et al., 2002). Others have suggested that imitation might be the key, but mammals such as dolphins and birds such as parrots have remarkable imitative capacities. Surprisingly, monkeys do not imitate, and chimpanzees are only slightly better, despite the presence of mirror neurons (Hauser et al., 2002). This may be because monkeys lack a direct connection between the primary motor cortex and the nucleus ambiguus, the site of laryngeal motor neurons (Jurgens, 1995).

Where the capacity to recombine meaningful units into an unlimited number of larger structures with unique meaning came from is not known. From an evolutionary perspective such unique abilities are usually adaptations of structures used for something else. One of the possible precursors for recursive abilities is the brain structures used by many species for navigation, but this hypothesis has not yet been fully tested (Hauser et al., 2002). Others have proposed that speech arises from the neural substrate that controls complex orofacial movements in Broca's area in non-human primates (Lieberman, 1985; Petrides et al., 2005). This substrate may involve a closer connection between the superior temporal region and the inferoparietal region and/or the development of direct connections between the precursor of Wernicke's region and areas 44, 45, and 46 (Aboitiz and García, 1997).

Is Long-term Auditory Processing Unique to Humans?

The observation that non-human primates can use visual but not auditory symbols to communicate may be related to the ability of humans to hold auditory information on-line in order to rehearse a possible response (Aboitiz and García, 1997; Wise, 2003). In fact, a recent study (Fritz et al., 2005) has demonstrated that monkeys do not seem to have the capacity to place auditory stimuli into long-term storage. In contrast, monkeys appear to be able to utilize long-term visual information, perhaps explaining how they can manipulate visual symbols (Colombo and Graziano, 1994; Wright, 1998). In this study, monkeys were trained on a task designed to evaluate auditory recognition memory. After surgery to remove the rostral superior temporal gyrus or the medial temporal lobe, performance was impaired on the memory task. Both these brain structures are associated with short-term working memory. After surgery to remove the rhinal cortex, a brain structure associated with long-term memory, performance was unaffected, suggesting that they relied only on short-term memory to do the task. Similar findings have been reported in dogs (Kowalska et al., 2001). The authors proposed that language is unique to humans not only because brain structures are related to speech but also because it requires long-term auditory memory.

IMAGING LANGUAGE

Brain imaging studies have questioned the classical view that language is processed by a single neural system involving the inferior frontal cortex (mostly Broca's area), the posterior temporal cortex (mostly Wernicke's area), and the white matter tract that connects them (arcuate fasciculus). While these regions are still considered to be important in translating sound to meaning, it is clear that there are multiple parallel processing streams extending outward from the auditory cortex in both posterior and anterior directions. There is also an increasing recognition that language is processed in both hemispheres, although some aspects of language processing show clear asymmetries (Patterson and Johnsrude, 2008; Scott and Johnsrude, 2003; Scott and Wise, 2004; Tyler and Marslen-Wilson, 2008; Wise, 2003).

Dorsal and Ventral Language Streams

The classical view of language processing focuses only on a dorsal stream between Wernicke's area and Broca's area. It is now evident that there is also a ventral stream that extends from the posterior temporoparietal region to the superior and middle temporal cortex and the anterior temporal and orbitofrontal regions via the inferior longitudinal fasciculus and uncinate fasciculus. Essentially, the ventral stream is an auditory "what" system (Hickok and Poeppel, 2004). Curiously, the macaque lacks the middle temporal gyrus, which is a prominent part of this stream (Tyler and Marslen-Wilson, 2008). Diffusion tensor imaging studies in humans have revealed considerable asymmetries in some of these white matter tracts. For example, white matter composition appears to be increased in the left arcuate fasciculus and inferior longitudinal fasciculus (Büchel et al., 2004). Other investigators have suggested that the arcuate fasciculus is found in both hemispheres but the ventral stream is seen only in the left hemisphere (Parker et al., 2005).

Functional Imaging Studies

Speech is associated with a complex pattern of activations. The motor act of articulation is associated with bilateral cerebellar activation. Left-lateralized regions adjacent to the Sylvian sulcus are also activated by both propositional (responding to a question) and non-propositional speech (counting or reciting overlearned nursery rhymes). Propositional speech is also associated with activation in the left posterior inferior parietal, anterolateral and medial temporal, and medial prefrontal regions. Thus, the process of communicating involves many regions beyond

Wernicke's and Broca's areas (Blank et al., 2002). Not surprisingly, some of these regions are involved in theory of mind and the default network.

Functional imaging studies have generally shown bilateral activation of speech-processing regions in the temporal lobes (Scott and Wise, 2004; Zatorre and Gandour, 2008). It has been proposed on the basis of functional imaging studies that there are three subsystems for the processing of inflectional morphology, sentence-level syntactical analysis, and sentence-level semantic interpretation that involve both sides of the brain (Tyler and Marslen-Wilson, 2008).

On the basis of functional connectivity analysis, the key network supporting regular inflectional morphology includes the left inferior frontal region, the anterior cingulate cortex, and the left middle temporal gyrus. The network supporting syntactical processing includes the left inferior frontal region and the posterior temporal and parietal regions. The syntactical network overlaps with areas involved in semantic processing, which includes the bilateral anterior middle and superior temporal gyrus (Hickok and Poeppel, 2007; Tyler and Marslen-Wilson, 2008). These studies suggest that no one region is associated with language capacity; rather, the capacity for language depends on the co-activation of several overlapping regions within the inferior frontal, temporal, and parietal regions on both sides of the brain.

LANGUAGE ANOMALIES IN NEUROPSYCHIATRIC DISORDERS

Language is affected in some way in almost all neuropsychiatric disorders. Language is least affected in bipolar disorder, but even in this disorder there are subtle impairments. Depressed patients' thoughts are often slowed; in rare cases, they can be almost mute. The reverse characterizes manic patients, where speech is often pressured, with some patients demonstrating a *flight of ideas*. However, speech itself is usually normal. This not the case in frontotemporal dementia associated with temporal lobe involvement. As we saw in Chapter 7, semantic dementia patients commonly present with a loss of memory for words or a loss of word meaning. These patients have fluent speech, but there may be frequent paraphasias. Often they are aware of their expressive deficits but are unaware of their comprehension deficits. Dysfunction of the anterior temporal lobes appears to mediate semantic representational difficulties in these patients. In fact, temporary semantic difficulties can be induced in normal subjects with repetitive transcranial magnetic stimulation over the anterior temporal lobe (Pobric et al., 2007). Patients with progressive nonfluent aphasia usually present with deficits in word fluency or pronunciation progressing to agrammatism, stuttering, and apraxia of speech. Considering the structural changes found in the temporal lobes of these patients, none of these symptoms are surprising.

Autism is associated with more striking language deficits; in fact, one of the key criteria for the diagnosis is a qualitative impairment in communication. There may a delay in or a total lack of the development of spoken language. In individuals with adequate speech, there is often a marked impairment in the ability to initiate or sustain a conversation with others. Patients can show stereotyped or repetitive use of language or idiosyncratic language.

Schizophrenia is also associated with language abnormalities, but they are of a different type. In schizophrenia, there can be a disorder of the flow of thought: one idea does not follow from the previous one, and in some patients this can reach the point of *word salad*. Another feature of schizophrenia is auditory hallucinations. One of the most characteristic symptoms is hearing a voice commenting on one's actions. The voice is not under the patient's control and is usually perceived as coming from someone else, although patients can also hear their own thoughts aloud such that someone standing next to them could also hear them.

Auditory hallucinations are usually associated with activity throughout the limbic system and the auditory cortex (see Chapter 4). Frontal activity does not usually seem to be associated with hallucinations. Many have suggested that auditory hallucinations are just the patient's thoughts that have failed to be labeled as such. As we saw in the previous chapter, schizophrenic patients who experience auditory hallucinations have increased correlations of low-frequency oscillations between the posterior cingulate and temporal regions associated with language (Bluhm et al., 2007). These same patients have a deficit in correlations between the posterior cingulate and medial prefrontal regions associated with the default network. If the anterior cingulate and medial prefrontal regions participate in labeling a thought as being internally generated, it is possible that parts of the language network have become disconnected in schizophrenia, resulting in thoughts or voices that are not perceived as being internally generated.

Another recent brain imaging study has found that aberrant patterns of hemodynamic coherence in the temporal lobe can differentiate schizophrenic patients from controls with a 97% level of accuracy at the initial assessment (Calhoun et al., 2004). The fact that language seems to be so central to schizophrenia has led some to suggest that anomalies in the development of language and brain asymmetry must underlie this disorder. We will consider this possibility in more detail.

Schizophrenia as a Failure of Hemispheric Dominance for Language

Recent interest in asymmetry in schizophrenia began with Flor-Henry's (1969) observation that schizophrenia-like psychosis is more common in temporal lobe epilepsy when there is a left-sided focus. Later, Gruzelier (1984) proposed the hemispheric imbalance model. In this model, symptoms reflecting relatively transient excitation were associated with the right hemisphere dysfunction, whereas symptoms reflecting more persistent withdrawal were associated with underactivity of the left hemisphere. Some support for the model was found in a number of postmortem, skin conductance, evoked potential, and electroencephalographic investigations in schizophrenic patients (Gruzelier and Flor-Henry, 1979). While neuropsychological investigations have found bilateral hemispheric impairment, deficits were more prominent on tests sensitive to left temporal and parietal function (Abrams and Taylor, 1979). Subsequent CT studies found that ventricular enlargement was greater on the left than the right side. In some cases, even a reversal of asymmetry was evident (Nasrallah, 1986).

Crow (1990a, 1990b, 1995, 1997a, 1997b, 1998) developed the idea further. He argued that there is genetic diversity in the evolution of the uniquely human characteristic of language that has developed as a result of progressive hemispheric specialization. Because schizophrenic patients often show lesser structural and functional asymmetries, symptoms may reflect a failure of hemispheric dominance for language. His position was that hemispheric specialization allowed acoustically coded information to be retained for a few seconds in the dominant hemisphere so that a visuospatial sketch pad could be activated in the nondominant hemisphere to determine the direction of thought. If callosal connections were impaired between the hemispheres, the result would be a disrupted train of thought and a breakdown in the distinction of *you* and *I*. The most likely location for the cerebral dominance gene (and schizophrenia gene) was suggested to be the pseudoautosomal region of the sex chromosomes.

Crow was not the first to go down this path. Jaynes (1977) argued that at one time humans were not truly conscious. The brains of early humans were essentially split in two. The executive part in the nondominant hemisphere was called "god" and the other part in the dominant hemisphere was "man," which followed god. Sometime around 1200 b.c. the nondominant hemisphere came to be inhibited by the dominant hemisphere, leading to true consciousness. Schizophrenia was attributed to a throwback to the *bicameral mind*, in which the voice of the nondominant hemisphere would be experienced as god. Another suggestion was offered by Nasrallah (1985), who argued that split-brain patients who had commissurotomies to treat their epilepsy actually have two distinct and separate selves. With defective interhemispheric integration, the right hemisphere could become an alien intruder, leading to thought insertion and delusions of passivity. Interestingly, there is a report of a paranoid patient who went into complete remission following callosotomy.

A recent postmortem study has reported that pyramidal cells in area 9 of the dorsolateral prefrontal cortex are denser on the left than on the right in normal subjects. This pattern is reversed in schizophrenic patients. Asymmetries of cell size and shape seem to be lost in schizophrenic patients (Cullen et al., 2006). Structural brain imaging studies have also provided some evidence for impaired hemispheric specialization and/or interhemispheric communication in schizophrenia. A meta-analysis of 28 studies confirmed the presence of reduced callosal area in schizophrenia (Arnoane et al., 2008). Crow (1990b) cited seven computed tomography (CT) and magnetic resonance imaging (MRI) studies where there was significant diagnosis by hemisphere interaction in temporal regions. Subsequent MRI studies have found some support for reduced or reversed cerebral asymmetries (Bilder et al., 1999; Bullmore et al., 1995; DeLisi et al., 1997; Sharma et al., 1999). However, there is considerable evidence against the lateralization hypothesis. The strongest contrary evidence comes from the National Institute of Mental Health (NIMH) MRI study of discordant twin pairs, which found bilateral changes in lateral ventricular and hippocampal volumes (Suddath et al., 1990). Detailed postmortem and brain imaging studies of the planum temporale have failed to find convincing evidence of reduced or reversed asymmetry (Shapleske et al., 1999). An MRI investigation of cerebral asymmetry in familial and non-familial schizophrenic patients and their unaffected relatives has failed to replicate earlier findings as well (Chapple et al., 2004).

The results of functional imaging studies have been somewhat stronger but still mixed. Gur et al. (1994) found impaired lateralization during verbal tasks sensitive to left hemisphere function and facial memory tasks sensitive to right hemisphere function. There is evidence of a lack of left–right asymmetry of dopamine transporter in the striatum in schizophrenic patients (Hsiao et al., 2003; Laasko et al., 2000). However, investigations of verbal fluency have found both lateralization anomalies (Artiges et al., 2000; Lewis et al., 1992) and normal lateralization during verbal tasks (Dye et al., 1999; Spence et al., 2000). A decrease in cerebral blood flow on fMRI on the left side along with an increase on the right was reported in schizophrenic patients listening to speech (Woodruff et al., 1997). Another fMRI study of discordant monozygotic twins has found decreased language lateralization for both affected and unaffected twins. Anomalies in both affected and unaffected twins might be expected if a gene predisposing to schizophrenia is related to the development of language lateralization (Sommer et al., 2004).

Thus, there is some support for anomalies of language lateralization and/or impaired interhemispheric transfer in schizophrenia, but the evidence is not conclusive. Thus far, no gene in the pseudoautosomal or other region has emerged that might link schizophrenia to a failure to develop cerebral dominance for language. There is also the problem that schizophrenic patients usually develop language capabilities in a normal way before the onset of the illness; if there is a defect in asymmetry, one might expect some difficulties. A more plausible hypothesis is that disturbed lateralization is present in some patients as a manifestation of an early neurodevelopmental insult of various etiologies that disturbs the normal process of hemispheric specialization, among other effects (Bullmore et al., 1997).

LANGUAGE CANNOT BE CONSIDERED IN ISOLATION

Songbirds have complex auditory and vocal processing, but it is not combined with the same complexity of meaning. What seems to be different in humans is that this action system became teamed up with other parts of the brain such as the medial prefrontal cortex and parietal cortex to produce language as we know it. It is interesting that the structure of language bears some resemblance to theory of mind. In language there is a subject, a verb, and an object. In theory of mind there is me, you, and the relationship between us. Curious, isn't it? Perhaps the same adaptation of the human brain led to both capacities. In this regard it is interesting that propositional speech activates not just classical language areas but also areas involved in the default network and theory of mind.

The key difference between monkeys and humans seems to be that humans have access to long-term auditory processing. This is not easy to explain. However, if humans have a unique adaption of the prefrontal cortex that supports theory of mind and language that involves the medial prefrontal cortex, then this may provide a clue. The medial prefrontal cortex is part of a network that supports autobiographic memories. The network includes the medial temporal, temporoparietal, dorsolateral prefrontal, and retrosplenial regions. This type of extended network could support long-term auditory processing. It might also explain why patients with frontotemporal dementia and autism have both language and social deficits. Schizophrenia could also be related to this network, but in a fundamentally different way. In schizophrenia, not just affect and language are affected but also agency, suggesting that a particular subsystem of this network is affected. Before we speculate further on this, let's look at ideas about the so-called *social brain* and how the brain processes emotion.

10

Affective Processing and the Social Brain

The focus of this chapter is to look at the nature of affective processing in humans. Not much is known about what is unique to human emotional processing. However, we will look at the neural pathways associated with emotions in both animals and humans. It seems likely that humans experience many of the same emotions as animals, but there are notable differences. There are also differences in the way that emotions are represented in the human brain that differ from animals.

Emotions play an important role in social behaviors. In recent years, there has been increasing interest in the concept of a *social brain*, which brings together many aspects of emotional processing and communication. We will examine some of the brain regions involved in the social brain from a neuroanatomical and evolutionary perspective. Our thesis is that the adaptations that led to the social brain in humans may also have made it vulnerable to some of the neuropsychiatric disorders we have been discussing.

EMOTIONAL PROCESSING IN ANIMALS

Much of what we know about emotional processing in animals (and humans) comes from work on fear. LeDoux (1996) highlighted two pathways involved in a fear response (Fig. 10.1). The direct pathway is through the thalamus to the amygdala. Because the cortex is not involved, there is only a crude representation of the stimulus. However, the direct pathway is quick, so action can be taken to avoid danger before the stimulus is fully appraised. The indirect pathway allows

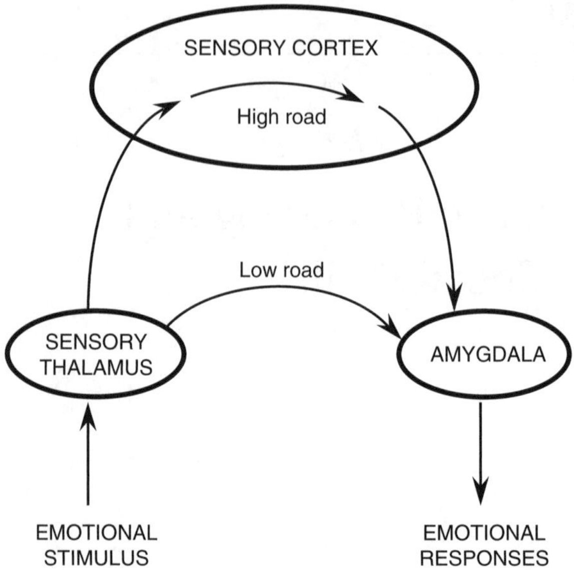

Figure 10.1 The low and the high roads to the amygdala. Information about external stimuli reaches the amygdala by direct pathways from the thalamus (the low road) as well as by pathways from the thalamus to the cortex to the amygdala. The direct thalamo-amygdala path is a shorter and thus a faster transmission route than the pathway from the thalamus through the cortex to the amygdala. However, because the direct pathway bypasses the cortex, it is unable to benefit from cortical processing. As a result, it can provide the amygdala with only a crude representation of the stimulus. It is thus a "quick and dirty" processing pathway. The direct pathway allows us to begin to respond to potentially dangerous stimuli before we fully know what the stimulus is. This can be very useful in dangerous situations. However, its utility requires that the cortical pathway be able to override the direct pathway. It is possible that the direct pathway is responsible for the control of emotional responses that we don't understand. This may occur in all of us some of the time but may be a predominant mode of functioning in individuals with certain emotional disorders. Reprinted from LeDoux, J. *The Emotional Brain: The Mysterious Underpinnings of Emotional Life*. New York, 1996, with permission from Simon and Schuster Paperbacks.

for full appraisal from cortical centers. Many anxiety disorders that occur in humans can be seen in lower animals. One of the reasons that this may happen is that the direct pathway may be primarily involved.

It is now fairly widely accepted that there are innate emotions in both the animal world and in humans. Based on facial expressions, Ekman (1984) distinguished six primary emotions: surprise, happiness, anger, fear, disgust, and sadness. Plutchik (1980) suggested that emotions were like colors and could be placed on a wheel. Primary emotions like joy and fear could be mixed to make guilt based on cognitive operations. Basic emotions can be seen in lower animals, but pride, shame, and gratitude might be uniquely human (Smith and Lazarus, 1990). It is not surprising that emotions unique to humans are associated with higher cortical processing regions. For example, fearful faces evoke amygdala activation, but faces showing disgust evoke activity in the anterior insula and the caudate-putamen

(Phillips et al., 1998). Guilt was associated with activity in the bilateral anterior temporal poles, anterior cingulate, and left anterior insular cortex/inferior frontal region (Shin et al., 2000). Emotions that are internally generated also seem to be associated with insular activity (Reiman et al., 1997).

NEUROBIOLOGY OF EMOTIONS IN HUMANS

The early theories proposed by Cannon and James saw emotion as the perception of a bodily response in a particular context: for example, fear is your heart pounding as you face an impending threat. Later theorists suggested that the emotional response is preceded by an appraisal process, which may be conscious or unconscious (Lazarus, 1991). More contemporary investigators have suggested that there are distinct processes related to the regulation of the affective state and emotional behavior (Lane and Nadel, 2000; LeDoux 1996; Phillips et al., 2003a).

Animal studies have highlighted the role of the amygdala in the initial emotional response to a stimulus. However, the anterior insula may also be involved. The anterior insula is connected with the amygdala, hypothalamus, periaqueductal gray matter, and ventromedial cortex. All of these structures form a network that appraises threatening stimuli and initiates an autonomic response (Augustine, 1996; Davis and Whalen, 2001; Ongur and Price, 2000).

Functional neuroimaging studies in human subjects have largely confirmed the importance of the amygdala in the modulation of vigilance to emotionally salient information. Generally, amygdala activation is associated with negative emotional states, whereas positive emotional states may be associated with both activation and deactivation. The insula appears to be associated with delay fear conditioning and anticipation of aversive events, suggesting a role in the representation of aversive stimuli (Phillips et al., 2003a).

The amygdala and insula have also been implicated in the production of an affective state and emotional behavior. Amygdala lesions in both monkeys and humans lead to decreased autonomic responses and impaired fear conditioning in anxiety-provoking situations. Lesions to the insula in rats lead to reduced fear reactivity to contextual stimuli (Phillips et al., 2003a). The ventral anterior cingulate and orbital and ventromedial prefrontal cortex may also play a role in the production of emotional responses. These regions are closely connected with the amygdala and anterior insula. Blood flow is usually increased in the subgenual anterior cingulate during induction of a sad mood (Mayberg et al., 1999). Lesions of the ventral anterior cingulate impair autonomic responses in fearful situations and lead to reduced aggression and emotional blunting in both humans and animals (Bush et al., 2000; Devinsky et al., 1995; Paus, 2001). Orbitofrontal lesions in monkeys lead to impaired ability to break a learned association between a stimulus and a reward. The orbital cortex inhibits sympathetic autonomic behaviors elicited by amygdala stimulation (Phillips et al., 2003a).

Other brain regions have been implicated in reward processing. The ventral striatum seems to be critical in the perception of reward. Dopamine may also play a role (see Chapter 2). In fact, a positive correlation has been found between the euphoric response to dextroamphetamine and the magnitude of dopamine release in the ventral striatal region in a positron emission tomography study of healthy subjects (Drevets et al., 2001).

Regulation of emotional behavior is likely associated with the medial prefrontal cortex. Two compartments within the medial prefrontal cortex seem to have distinct roles. The ventrolateral compartment is capable of responding to unconscious stimuli via direct and indirect connections with the hypothalamus, amygdala, thalamus, ventral striatum, and brainstem nuclei. The mediodorsal compartment, derived from the hippocampus, has been implicated in the inhibition of the stress response. It has been suggested that there is a reciprocal relationship between the ventral network, including the medial prefrontal cortex and subgenual anterior cingulate, and the dorsal network, including the dorsal anterior cingulate and dorsolateral prefrontal cortex (Mayberg et al., 1999; Phillips et al., 2003a).

THE SOCIAL BRAIN

The concept of the social brain was proposed by Brothers (1990). In her review, it was argued that social knowledge is operationally distinct from other knowledge. Drawing from psychoanalytical thinking, Brothers observed that infants perceive the world in the crude representations of pleasure and displeasure. However, human infants are particularly focused on facial expressions and can imitate facial gestures at 36 hours of age. Later, social smiling develops even in blind infants. Clearly, there seems to be an innate disposition on the part of human infants to establish and maintain rapport, and gradually the child develops representations of this dyadic relationship with the caregiver. After piecing together information largely from lesion and brain stimulation studies in humans, it was proposed that there are specific brain regions associated with this process: the orbitofrontal cortex, temporal cortex, and amygdala, all regions associated with emotional processing.

The social brain proved to be a very useful concept, pulling together ideas from many different disciplines. The concept has been thoughtfully reviewed in two recent papers, and we will summarize the contents of those reviews (Adolphs, 2003; Frith, 2007). Brothers' suggestions for the regions involved in the social brain have held up well, but there have been some new developments. The first of these is the concept of mirror neurons, which we have referred to in previous chapters. Looking back on Brothers' original paper, her comments on imitation seem to anticipate these neurons, which have since been found to be throughout the brain and involved in emotional as well as motor functions (Gallese, 2007; Rizzolatti and Craighero, 2004). Another development is that the adjacent regions of the anterior cingulate cortex have been added to the list of social brain regions (Amodio and Frith, 2006).

Frith (2007) argued that the function of the social brain is to enable predictions during social interactions. Without such predictions, complex social interactions would not be sustainable. However, he goes a step further and suggests that *theory of mind* is the "most important attribute" of the social brain. Without this capacity, it would not be possible to make predictions on the basis of mental states. What are the roles of each brain region in this predictive process? Frith (2007) suggests that the amygdala is part of a system that learns to associate value with stimuli. Thus, the amygdala is involved with prejudice and conditioning (i.e., Is this face trustworthy?). The temporal poles provide more information of trustworthiness based on life experience or scripts (Damasio et al., 2004; Funnell, 2001). Further support of this role has been reported by Zahn et al. (2007). The posterior superior temporal sulcus/temporoparietal junction predicts movement trajectories and perspective taking. Perspective taking is important in social cognition because it allows one to imagine one's body in another position in space.

The role of the medial prefrontal cortex is a bit more complex. A number of investigations have reported an association between mentalizing activity and medial prefrontal activity (Gregory et al., 2002; Mitchell et al., 2005a; Rowe et al., 2001; Stuss et al., 2001). However, it has recently been shown that a patient who had a lesion in the medial prefrontal cortex could do theory of mind tasks (Bird et al., 2004), so it is likely that other regions are involved in mentalizing as well. There may also be some specialization within these regions—for example, attending to one's own emotions and the mental states of others tended to be associated with medial activations (Gilbert et al., 2006). Other roles attributed to the medial prefrontal cortex include the ability to store individual dispositions and attitudes with regard to self and others.

Although emotional information is represented on both sides of the brain, it has been suggested that the right brain plays a particularly important role in processing social emotions. Schore (2003) has proposed that emotional regulation is related to mother–child interactions early in life in which internal, possibly medial prefrontal, representations lead to control of fear responses in the child. In this way the parasympathetic nervous system is enhanced while the sympathetic nervous system involved in "fight-or-flight" responses is suppressed. There is certainly some evidence that there are lateralized aspects to emotional response, but as we saw in Chapter 8, self-representation is bilateral, so it is difficult to see how emotional self-representation could be right-sided.

It is likely that the social brain is not limited to primates. Whales, carnivores, and at least some insectivores have been suggested to show some aspects of a social brain (Dunbar and Shultz, 2007). Nevertheless, there is convincing evidence that the frontal polar cortex (area 10) has undergone considerable enlargement and specialization during hominid evolution (Semendeferi et al., 2001). How evolutionary changes translate into the functional social brain is not known. Some have suggested that the capacity for social cognition has arisen from the mirror neuron system (Gallese, 2007), but some shortcomings of this approach have been pointed out (Frith, 2007; Mitchell et al., 2005b). While the mirror system is well suited to monitoring continually changing states of emotions and intentions of others, it does not represent the stable attitudes and predilections of others that are essential for social interactions.

SELF-AWARENESS, EMPATHY, AND INTUITION

While the social brain is not limited to primates, the circuits for self-awareness are to a large extent specific to primates, and particularly human specializations arise from separate classes of neurons located in lamina I of the spinal cord. According to Craig (2003, p. 305):

> Ascending lamina I activity is integrated mainly in several brainstem sites in non-primates, but in primates there is a direct thalamocortical homeostatic afferent pathway to the dorsal posterior insular cortex. There, a discrete field provides a topographic, modality-selective representation of all interoceptive afferent activity from lamina I (i.e., sympathetic afferent input) and from the solitary nucleus (i.e. parasympathetic afferent input). This pathway is just visible in monkeys but in humans it is greatly enlarged, and microstimulation, lesion and functional-imaging studies provide convergent evidence confirming its role in pain, temperature, itch, muscle sensation, sensual touch, hunger, thirst, cardiorespiratory activity. In humans, this interoceptive cortical image engenders discriminative sensations, and it is re-represented in the middle insula and then in the right (non-dominant) anterior insula. This seems to provide a meta-representation of the state of the body material self as a feeling (sentient) entity—that is, emotional awareness.

A branch of this ascending pathway proceeds via the median dorsal nucleus of the thalamus to the anterior cingulate cortex (Fig. 10.2). The Von Economo neurons, discussed in detail elsewhere in this volume, are located in layer 5 of the anterior cingulate cortex and in the fronto-insular cortex, which is a portion of the anterior insula. The Von Economo neurons transmit the processed information from the highest levels in these pathways and like other components of this system have undergone expansion in the brains of humans.

The activity of both the fronto-insular cortex and the anterior cingulate cortex increases with the uncertainty of the decision (Critchley et al., 2001), and the activity of the fronto-insular cortex is very selectively activated when the subject receives a risk prediction error signal when learning the outcome of a wager in a gambling task (Preuschoff et al., 2008). Damage to the insular cortex in patients causes deficits in their capacity to learn from such risk prediction errors in gambling tasks, resulting in poor decision making (Clark et al., 2008). Note that these studies are not explicitly social, and it is likely that this circuitry probably evolved with respect to the interaction of the individual with his or her total environment, both social and non-social. The close association of these circuits with the basic mechanisms for physiological homeostasis (hunger and thirst) suggests that they evolved to support adaptive decision making during foraging for food. However, these circuits were also very well suited for navigating the social world, since decision making in a social context typically involves incomplete knowledge, risk, and uncertainty. Thus, the social brain circuitry is derived from this more basic circuitry, which is engaged when coping with an uncertain world.

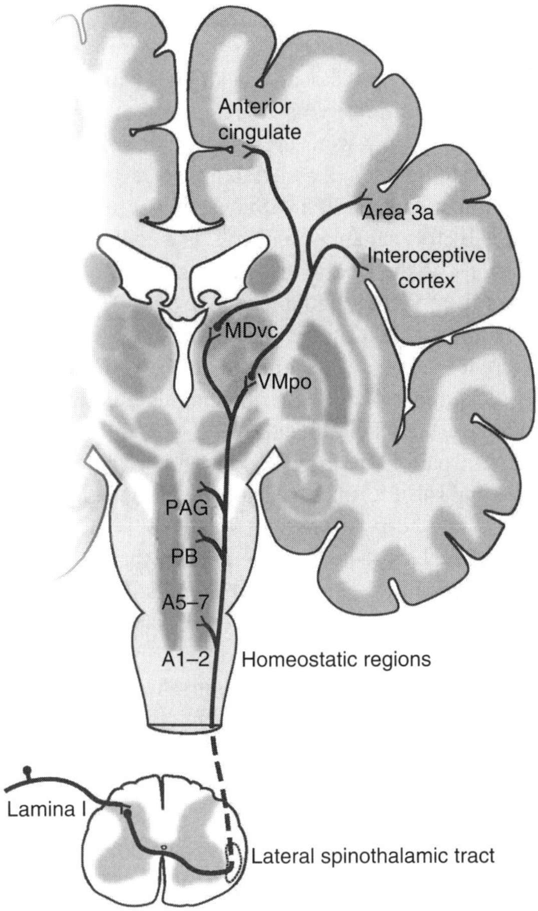

Figure 10.2 Summary of the projections of the lamina I system in primates. Modality-specific lamina I neurons project first to autonomic sites in the spinal cord (not shown) and to homeostatic sites in the brainstem, (including the noradrenergic cell groups A1-A2 and A5-A7, the parabrachial nucleus (PB), and the periaqueductal gray (PAG). In primates, lamina I neurons also project by way of the crossed lateral spinothalamic tract to two sites in the thalamus: the posterior part of the ventral medial nucleus (VMpo) and the ventral caudal part of the medial dorsal nucleus (MDvc). The VMpo provides a high-resolution, modality-specific sensory representation of the physiological condition of the body in interoceptive cortex at the dorsal margin of the insula, and it sends a corollary projection to area 3a in the sensorimotor cortex. The MDvc integrates lamina I input with brainstem homeostatic activity (from PB and PAG) and produces behavioral drive in limbic motor cortex (anterior cingulate). These generate the feeling and the motivation, respectively, that constitute the homeostatic emotion of pain. Reprinted from Craig, A.D. A new view of pain as a homeostatic emotion. *Trends in Neurosciences,* **26**, 303–307. Copyright 2003, with permission from Elsevier.

One striking feature of the fronto-insular and anterior cingulate cortices is the capacity of these structures to respond to social error signals. For example, Ullsperger and Von Cramon (2003) scanned subjects while they performed a complex task in which they received feedback in the form of smiling or frowning faces (Color Plate 10.1). When they were presented with a smiling face, the nucleus accumbens was activated, which is associated with reward. When they were presented with a frowning face, area FI and the habenular nuclei in the posterior thalamus were activated by this negative feedback. The lateral habenula projects to the dopaminergic neurons of the midbrain and its activation suppresses the reward circuitry that arises from them (Bianco and Wilson, 2008; Christoff et al., 1986; Matsumoto and Hikosaka, 2007); this habenular circuit appears to be dysfunctional in schizophrenic patients (Shepard et al., 2006). Frowning faces also activated the motor component of the anterior cingulate cortex, where it probably suppresses ongoing movement commands.

The observation of pain in others is a powerful signal of error in one's social network. When normal subjects observe another person being injured in a particular part of their body, they respond with a reduction in the motor evoked potentials in the muscles vicariously affected by the pain in their own bodies, which has been called the *embodiment of empathy* (Minio-Paluello et al., 2009). Singer et al. (2004a) investigated the neural correlates of empathy in couples where the female partner was scanned while she observed her male partner receiving a mild injury. This elicited strong activation of the anterior insula, including the fronto-insular cortex, and the anterior cingulate cortex. The magnitude of these responses in the different subjects in this experiment was well correlated with individual differences in empathy as a trait in these subjects as measured by two different tests, the Empathy Concern Scale and the Balanced Emotional Empathy Scale (Singer et al., 2004a). These results support the hypothesis that the fronto-insular cortex and the anterior cingulate cortex register social error and that this function is an extension of the mechanism for homeostatic regulation of one's own body to that of others. There is also compelling evidence that these structures are also activated during experience of many other types of social error, including deception, embarrassment, guilt, and resentment (Berthoz, 2002; Sanfey et al., 2003; Shin et al., 2000; Spence, 2001). These mechanisms for the recognition and processing of social error are a prerequisite for social reciprocity in generating context-appropriate responses to the behavior of social partners. They are notably deficient in the autism spectrum disorders and many other neuropsychiatric disorders.

While these processes are often conscious, they can proceed covertly without the subject's direct awareness. For example, when subjects gaze into the eyes of others, if the size of the pupils of the eyes of the observed subject change in a way that is discordant with the changes in pupil size in the subject, both the fronto-insular and the anterior cingulate cortices are activated (Harrison et al., 2009). This discordance in pupil size change is reflective of differences in autonomic arousal and emotional experience between the observed individual and the subject, which is a covert signal that there is a discordance in their feelings about the social transaction that they are conducting, another type of social error signal.

Yet another powerful social error signal, which is definitely conscious and may be uniquely human, is humor. Watson et al. (2007) scanned subjects while they rated 100 cartoons for how funny they felt they were (Fig. 10.3). In both the fronto-insular and the anterior cingulate cortices, activity increased as a function of how funny the subjects judged the cartoons to be. Humor is a powerful way of updating information about social interactions, to reinforce learning between social partners, and to allow future social interactions to proceed more smoothly. The experience of humor and laughter relaxes the body, create positive feelings, and relieves social tension. The lack of socially shared humor is a deficit in autism spectrum disorder and many other neuropsychiatric disorders.

Many of the processes just described operate through the cognitive mechanism commonly known as intuition. We define intuition as a form of cognition in which many variables are rapidly evaluated in parallel and compressed into a single dimension. This compression facilitates fast decision making. Typically we are not aware of the logical steps or assumptions underlying this process, although intuition is based on experience-dependent probabilistic models. Instead, we

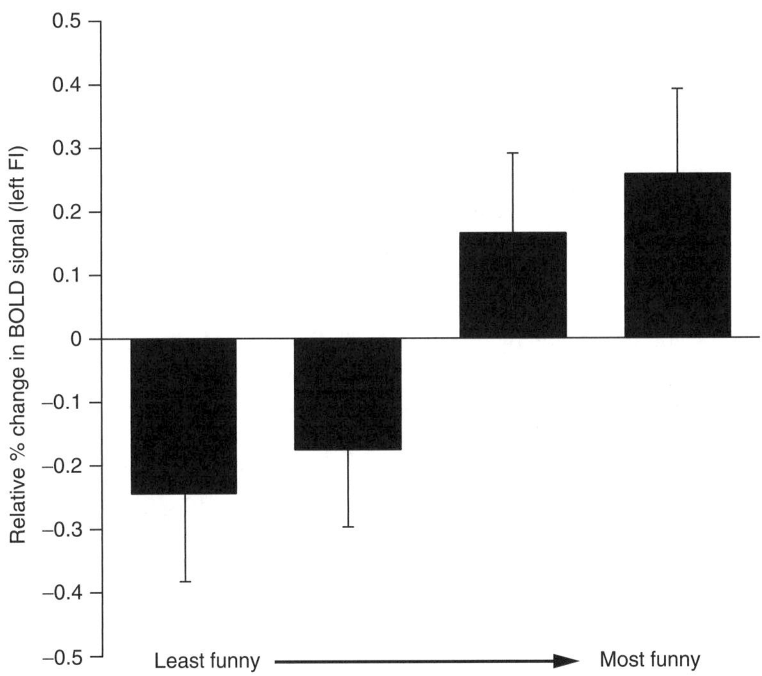

Figure 10.3 Area FI responds to the degree of perceived humor in cartoons. Relative % change in the brain oxygen level-dependent (BOLD) signal in left fronto-insula across all subjects versus subjective rating of funniness. Error bars represent standard error of the mean. Reprinted from Watson, K.K., Matthew, B.J., and Allman, J.A. Brain activation during sight gags and language-dependent humor. *Cerebral Cortex,* **17,** 314–324. Copyright 2007, with permission from Oxford University Press.

experience the intuitive process as visceral sensations ("gut feelings"). Intuition operates largely in the social domain but can also be applied to purely physical situations. Intuition is plastic; it is not instinct, although instinctive feelings may contribute to it. Emotional value judgments contribute to both intuition and deliberation. Intuition involves the rapid comparison of a current transaction with previously experienced similar events and a visceral assessment of the probability of a favorable or unfavorable outcome for the current transaction. By contrast, deliberation is much slower and involves serial processes of inductive and/or deductive reasoning. Many lines of evidence suggest that the fronto-insular and the anterior cingulate cortices and the specialized Von Economo neurons are involved in the neural mechanisms of intuition (Allman et al., 2005). Intuition is crucial for timely and effective social decision making and is deficient in autism spectrum disorders and other neuropsychiatric disorders.

EATING TOGETHER AND THE COMPLEX SOCIAL EMOTIONS

Like sharing humorous experiences, eating together is an important way that we establish and strengthen social bonds, which derives from the functions of the fronto-insular and anterior cingulate cortices. The regulation of food intake is expressed in the primordial opposed emotions of *lust*, arising from the consumption of the nutritious and appetizing, and *disgust*, which induces the spitting out or vomiting of the toxic (Woodward and Allman, 2007). Disgust means literally *bad taste*, and facial expressions of disgust powerfully activate the fronto-insular and the adjacent anterior insular cortices (Mataix-Cols et al., 2008; Phillips et al., 1997), demonstrating the social component to this insular processing. Remarkably, Jabbi et al. (2008) found that the same lateral part of area FI in the right hemisphere was activated by disgusting tastes, by observing someone else's facial expressions of disgust and by imaginating disgust. Thus, these structures register both the disgust we feel when something distasteful is ingested *and* our social partner's experience of disgust. Our partner's expression of disgust can arise from a social experience as well as a gustatory one. Our language is full of food-based metaphors that we use to describe social interactions. The neural substrate for lust–disgust served as the evolutionary template for the circuitry for the complex social emotions that tend to occur in polar opposites, such as love–hate, gratitude–resentment, self-confidence–embarrassment, trust–distrust, empathy–contempt, approval–disdain, pride–humiliation, truthfulness–deception, and atonement–guilt (Woodward and Allman, 2007). The first of each of these pairs generally favors the formation of social bonds and the second tends to disrupt bonds. They thus range from the poles of prosocial to antisocial. Many of these complex social emotions are known to activate the fronto-insular and anterior cingulate cortices. The social emotions for which this has been demonstrated thus far include lust (Karama et al., 2002), love (Bartels and Zeki, 2004), resentment (Sanfey et al., 2003), embarrassment (Berthoz et al., 2002), trust (Singer et al., 2004b), empathy (Singer et al., 2004a), deception (Spence et al., 2001), and guilt

PROSOCIAL		ANTISOCIAL
Lust	⟷	***Disgust***
Love	⟷	***Hate***
Gratitude	⟷	***Resentment***
Self-confidence	⟷	***Embarrassment***
Trust	⟷	Distrust
Empathy	⟷	Contempt
Approval	⟷	Disdain
Pride	⟷	Humiliation
Truthfulness	⟷	***Deception***
Atonement	⟷	***Guilt***

Emotions in bold italics typeface activate anterior insular cortex

Figure 10.4 Prosocial and antisocial emotions based on Woodward and Allman, 2007. Italicized emotions activate the anterior insular cortex.

(Shin et al., 2000), and it is likely that the others will be found to activate fronto-insular and anterior cingulate cortices as well (Fig. 10.4).

There is a tendency for the prosocial emotions, such as love and trust, to be linked to the activation of the fronto-insula and the adjacent parts of the anterior insula in the left hemisphere, while the antisocial emotions, such as disgust, arise more from activation of these structures in the right hemisphere (Craig, 2009; Mataix-Cols et al., 2008). This lateralization may arise from a skewing toward the right hemisphere of the circuitry for mounting active responses and associated sympathetic autonomic arousal, and a skewing toward the left hemisphere for calming responses associated with parasympathetic quietude (Craig, 2005; Rogers and Andrew, 2002). The capacity to differentiate among the complex social emotions is likely to be the product of relatively recent evolution, though arguably they do occur in animals. This capacity to differentiate and to introspect upon these complex emotions is an essential component of healthy psychological functioning, which breaks down in many neuropsychiatric disorders.

IMPLICATIONS FOR NEUROPSYCHIATRIC DISORDERS

Almost all neuropsychiatric disorders are associated with some anomalies in affective processing and social functioning, but the nature of these anomalies is quite different in each condition. We will first consider autism and frontotemporal dementia, both of which are clearly associated with social deficits. We will then look at schizophrenia and bipolar disorders with regard to both affective processing and social functioning.

Autism

Brothers (1990) singled out autism as the best example of a selective absence of social cognition. As we saw in Chapter 6, the literature largely supports this observation. Patients with autism do not tend to pretend play or imitate (Kasari and Rotheram-Fuller, 2005). They also perform very poorly on theory of mind tasks (Baron-Cohen, 1985). In fact, in most cases, they prefer their own company to playing with other children.

The imaging literature implicates social brain regions in autism. While short connections are preserved, long connections, including those between regions associated with the social brain, are deficient (Herbert et al., 2004). During mentalizing tasks, autistic patients also show impaired activation in brain regions associated with the social brain, such as the medial prefrontal cortex and temporal poles (Castelli et al., 2002).

Some have suggested that many of these deficits could be explained by anomalies in the mirror neuron system (Oberman and Ramachandran, 2007). This idea has some appeal because the mirror neuron system does participate in imitative behavior. However, the idea that autism is primarily related to a mirror neuron deficit has been challenged (Southgate and Hamilton, 2008). The mirror neuron system is involved in matching the actions of self and others. The case for abnormalities in this process is weak in autism. It is also likely that the imitation abnormalities in autism extend beyond the mirror neuron system. Lack of attention to social or communicative cues associated with brain regions beyond the mirror system could lead to a failure to imitate. Many of these brain regions are associated with the social brain.

Thus, Brothers' (1990) observation that autism is associated with a deficit in the social brain has received considerable support from the psychological and brain imaging literature, providing both support for the concept of a social brain and insight into which brain regions might be involved. However, autism is not the only disorder associated with social behavioral abnormalities: at the other end of the lifespan is frontotemporal dementia.

Frontotemporal Dementia

Like autistic patients, patients with frontotemporal dementia have difficulty evaluating both facial and vocal expressions of emotion (Keane et al., 2002; Lavenu et al., 1999; Neary et al., 2005). They also have difficulty inferring what others think or feel, and they perform poorly on theory of mind tasks (Gregory et al., 2002). Frontotemporal and semantic dementia patients have gray matter loss in the orbital frontal, insular, and anterior cingulate regions, all regions associated with the social brain (Rosen et al., 2002). Apathy, lack of empathy, and disinhibition are associated with social brain regions such as the medial prefrontal cortex, orbitofrontal cortex, insular cortex, temporal poles, and anterior cingulate cortex (Rankin et al., 2006;

Rosen et al., 2005). Several imaging studies demonstrating decreased cerebral blood flow and hypometabolism in the medial prefrontal and anterior temporal lobes in patients with frontotemporal dementia were discussed in Chapter 7. These metabolic changes are highly correlated with volumetric losses and increase over time (Alexander et al., 1995; Diehl-Schmid et al., 2007; Franceschi et al., 2005; Friedland et al., 1993; Grimmer et al., 2004; Ibach et al., 2004; Ishii et al., 1998; Miller and Gearhart, 1999; Schroeter et al., 2008; Varma et al., 2002; Varrone et al., 2002).

It might not be surprising that two different conditions occurring at opposite ends of the lifespan affect social functioning if they both affect similar brain regions. Although there are some notable differences between these conditions. there are also some similarities. Among the differences are the occurrence of progressive nonfluent aphasia and semantic dementia in some patients with frontotemporal dementia. While semantic deficits and nonfluent aphasia are not typical features of autism, language is usually delayed. This suggests a close relationship between brain structures mediating language and those mediating social behaviors more generally.

Schizophrenia

Brothers (1990) pointed out that the paranoid psychoses involve a distortion of other people's intentions and motivations. As the evaluation of other people's intentions is key to the understanding of the social brain, it was suggested that these disorders might also be related to the social brain. Whether this is the case or not, there is no doubt that social functioning is impaired in schizophrenia; in fact, it is one of the requirements for the *Diagnostic and Statistical Manual of Mental Disorders, Fourth Edition, Text Revision* (DSM-IV-TR) diagnosis of the disorder.

There are now many studies showing that schizophrenic patients have deficits in social cognition and facial processing not unlike those seen in other conditions, such as autism and frontotemporal dementia (Brüne, 2003; Brunet-Gouet and Decety, 2006; Phillips et al., 2003b; Russell and Sharma, 2003). The impairments are on a number of social cognition tests, not just the theory of mind tasks (Bertrand et al., 2007). They do not seem to be related to intelligence levels but may be state dependent to some degree (Bertrand et al., 2007; Brunet-Gouet and Decety, 2006). It is also possible that social cognition may be affected by dopamine levels, especially during mentalizing (Brunet-Gouet and Decety, 2006).

It has been proposed that schizophrenia arises as a consequence of social brain evolution (Burns, 2004, 2006). Burns (2004) argued that paleoanthropological and comparative primate research suggest that hominids evolved complex frontotemporal and frontoparietal connectivity for social cognition and the intellectual demands of living in a group. The ontogenetic mechanism of the schizotypal spectrum was suggested to be a sequential "hypermorphosis" that preceded the migration of *Homo sapiens* out of Africa. The phenotype carried certain advantages such as creativity but was not necessarily adaptive in reproductive terms. Because the disorder shared a common genetic basis with the evolving circuitry of the social brain, it persisted.

Burn's (2004, 2006) argument is appealing in some ways. Schizophrenia is a human disorder, and one would expect some connection with unique human characteristics. However, we have little understanding of the genetic basis of schizophrenia, let alone the social brain. Information is beginning to emerge, but slowly (see Chapter 11). Another problem is that anomalies in social cognition can be found in several disorders, not just schizophrenia. In fact, a better case can be made for social brain abnormalities in autism and frontotemporal dementia than schizophrenia. A further problem is that the postmortem, brain imaging, and neuropsychological deficits found in schizophrenia are widespread (see Chapter 4). Some social brain regions do show abnormalities in schizophrenia, but the anomalies are more striking in other regions. Consequently, it is difficult to see how the social brain is the focus of what makes the human brain vulnerable to schizophrenia.

Bipolar Disorders

A recent meta-analysis of 330 emotion induction and cognitive task imaging studies in normal subjects showed a segregated involvement of the prefrontal cortex in these tasks (Steele and Lawrie, 2004). Emotion induction resulted in inferior medial activation, whereas cognitive tasks were associated with dorsolateral activation. These results are consistent with the suggested role of the orbitofrontal cortex in decoding and representing primary reinforcers and in controlling and correcting reward-related and punishment-related behaviors (Rolls, 2000). Nevertheless, the question arises as to whether there are separate regions in the orbital and medial prefrontal cortex associated with rewarding versus punishing stimuli. Initial work had suggested that the medial prefrontal cortex was more activated after rewarding feedback and the lateral prefrontal cortex was more activated by punishment (Gottfried et al., 2002; O'Doherty et al., 2001; Small et al., 2001). However, not all studies have found this pattern (Elliott et al., 2003; O'Doherty et al., 2003). Other brain regions seem to be important in signaling reward contingencies, in particular the caudolateral orbitofrontal cortex and the insula. The ventral striatum, anterior cingulate, and amygdala are also involved in responding to rewarding versus punishing feedback (Budhani et al., 2007; O'Doherty et al., 2003).

As we saw in Chapter 5, major depressive and bipolar disorders are associated with dysfunction in the orbital and medial prefrontal cortex (Drevets, 2007; Phillips et al., 2003b). The posterior lateral and medial orbitofrontal cortex is associated with gray matter volumetric reductions, histopathological abnormalities, and activation anomalies during the presentation of emotional stimuli and in reward paradigms. Depression severity is inversely correlated with physiological activity in parts of the posterior lateral and medial prefrontal cortex. In contrast, activity in the anteromedial orbitofrontal cortex situated in the ventromedial polar cortex is increased in depression. Effective antidepressant treatment is associated with a reduction of activity in this region (Drevets, 2007).

Drugs used to treat mood and anxiety disorders alter the function of serotonin, norepinephrine, and dopamine. The serotonin pathway arises from the raphe nuclei in the brainstem and targets the thalamus and basal ganglia. Another serotonergic pathway projects to the amygdala, hippocampus, and hypothalamus and eventually winds around the corpus callosum to target much of the cortex. The noradrenergic pathways arise in the locus ceruleus and lateral brainstem tegmentum to target many of the same structures. The dopamine pathway projects from the ventral tegmentum in the brainstem to the nucleus accumbens in the ventral striatum. Thus, serotonin, noradrenergic, and dopaminergic pathways are well placed to modulate mood-processing regions; dopamine may mediate reward signals that are represented and regulated by these brain regions (Drevets, 2007; Mega et al., 1997; Phillips et al., 2003b).

Drevets (2007) proposed that some regions in the orbitofrontal cortex appear to inhibit or modulate emotional expression while others appear to facilitate emotional expression. Major depressive disorder results from dysfunction within a network including the orbitofrontal cortex, medial prefrontal cortex, amygdala, structures in the temporal lobe, striatum, thalamus, and brainstem. It is very interesting that the anterior medial prefrontal cortex is involved in mood disorders. This region is very close to regions associated with the social brain. What this suggests is that the social brain may be regulated by orbital frontal and subgenual prefrontal regions.

NEUROPSYCHIATRIC DISORDERS AND GENETIC IMPRINTING

Crespi and Badcock (2008) have proposed a novel approach to understanding neuropsychiatric disorders: they argue that autism involves a pattern of constrained overgrowth, whereas schizophrenia involves undergrowth during development of the social brain. As a result, social cognition is underdeveloped in autism spectrum conditions and hyperdeveloped in psychotic spectrum conditions. The reason for these neurodevelopmental abnormalities is proposed to be due to genomic imprinting—that is, in psychosis there is a bias toward increased relative effects from imprinted genes with maternal expression that engender a pattern of undergrowth. An increased bias toward paternally expressed genes is seen in autism spectrum disorders, leading to overgrowth.

Essentially what Crespi and Badcock (2008) are suggesting is that psychosis and autism are diametrical disorders of the social brain. There are some problems with this idea. First, it is now well accepted that there is an excess of short connections and a deficiency of long connections in autism (see Chapter 6), so the idea of overgrowth is misleading. Similarly, the suggestion that the social brain is hyperdeveloped in schizophrenia is not supported in the literature. These patients show widespread social cognition deficits (see above). Finally, there is really no evidence that genes associated with imprinting are more affected in schizophrenia than genes not associated with schizophrenia. However, other genes may be more closely connected to both the social brain and neuropsychiatric disorders. We will look at these more closely in the next chapter.

OVERVIEW

Affective processing is not something that is limited to humans: it is very clear that animals have very similar emotions to humans, with the possible exceptions of shame and guilt. We know a lot about the pathways involved in processing affect in both humans and non-humans. The emotional response derives largely from the amygdala and the fronto-insular cortex, particularly with complex emotions such as shame and guilt. The medial and orbital prefrontal cortex and subgenual prefrontal cortex participate in emotional response and regulation. It might be expected that these same regions would be part of the social brain, which regulates behavior. The social brain also includes parietal and temporal regions that allow emotions to be mapped in space and time from a personal perspective.

All neuropsychiatric disorders are associated with dysfunction of social brain regions. Deficits in social cognition are most striking in autism and frontotemporal dementia but are also present in schizophrenia. Mood disorders do not seem to be associated with the same degree of impairment of social cognition. However, social functioning can be severely affected in these disorders. Depressed patients often withdraw from social interactions and lose all sense of enjoyment. The opposite is often associated with manic states. Bipolar patients do have difficulty performing theory of mind tasks and often have a deficit in emotional regulation, which impairs social interactions. Thus, each neuropsychiatric disorder seems to be associated with different aspects of emotional representation and control. In the next chapter, we will discuss some of the neuronal systems that might underlie these disorders.

11

Why Do We Have These Disorders?

Many investigators have noticed that the same regions are activated no matter what the task. Variously referred to as the *central circuit of the mind*, *cognitive control network*, and *global workspace*, this network of brain regions includes the dorsal anterior cingulate, dorsolateral prefrontal, and anterior insular cortices (Anderson et al., 2008; Cole and Schneider, 2007; Dehaene et al., 1998; Dosenbach, et al., 2006; Duncan and Owen, 2000). This is not to say that there are not specific networks for specific tasks. There clearly are differences in brain activation patterns in different tasks (Cabeza and Nyberg, 2000). However, the human brain seems to approach a task in the same way.

We have reviewed many of the functions at which the human brain excels: theory of mind, language, and social cognition. There is a certain similarity between these different functions as well. Theory of mind is just that, a theory of mind. It is a representational model of you and me that allows predictions across time. Language is really quite similar: subject, verb, and object, a way of representing two things and the relationship between them. Even the social brain is a way of representing emotional information between two or more people. As Karmiloff-Smith (1992) points out, the human brain is capable of representational redescription. So how does the human brain do this?

The prefrontal cortex, which is activated during most tasks, has to have a central role. There are several approaches to understanding prefrontal cortex function, which have been carefully reviewed elsewhere (Wood and Grafman, 2003). We will not discuss these in detail but will look at some aspects of the prefrontal cortex and the human brain that might be pertinent to our discussion of what makes the human brain vulnerable to neuropsychiatric conditions. Non-human primates have a frontal cortex and can do delayed response tasks. Yet non-human primates do not have language or theory of mind, at least at the same level as humans. Our suggestion is that the reason for this is that the prefrontal cortex has developed networks adapted for these unique functions. Let us look at some possible configurations of these networks.

REPRESENTATION IN THE HUMAN BRAIN

The human brain is all about representation, or more specifically representational redescription. "Representational redescription" strikes us as an awkward term, so we will refer to the representational brain. As Karmiloff-Smith (1992) pointed out, chimpanzees are not capable of representational redescription (see Chapter 9). We are unable to accomplish representational redescription at birth; it develops throughout childhood. As we saw in Chapter 8, 2-year-olds can model hypothetical situations that do not necessarily correspond to reality; for example, a stick can represent a gun. By age 4, representations of representational relations emerge, and with that the awareness of the intentions of others (Perner, 1991). It is these tertiary representations that characterize the human brain. In a sense, theory of mind, language, and social cognition are all related to this capacity. Let us look at how this capacity is expressed.

Perceiving action and planning action activate the same brain regions (Prinz, 1997). To plan an action, we usually call upon representations of past actions, which correspond to some of the regions that are common to most cognitive tasks—that is, the dorsolateral prefrontal, dorsal anterior cingulate, and medial prefrontal cortices. If it is a new task, the dorsal anterior cingulate cortex is activated. However, as it becomes learned, activation in this structure is replaced by activation in the anterior insula (Raichle et al., 1994). As we saw in Chapter 2, learning new behaviors is associated with changes in basal ganglia-thalamocortical neuronal circuits that connect the prefrontal cortex with subcortical structures controlling movement. The dorsal anterior cingulate cortex directs attention to the regions involved in the task and monitors for possible errors, which is particularly important when learning a new task.

The big question is how the activity in the five main basal ganglia-thalamocortical neuron networks is coordinated. You will recall that there are two *cognitive* circuits originating from the dorsolateral prefrontal and lateral orbitofrontal cortices, a *limbic* circuit originating in the anterior cingulate and medial prefrontal cortices, and two motor circuits, one for eye movements and one for other motor responses. Consciousness is unitary and widely distributed across the cortex, so how do we learn to combine the cognitive, perceptual, and emotional aspects of experience into a representation of self and others? As we saw in Chapter 3, some have argued that *binding* likely occurs at the subcortical level, perhaps through changes in the reticular activating nucleus of the thalamus. We would agree that integration has to occur at this level, but it does not explain human consciousness. Human consciousness is associated with the capacity for time travel and tertiary representations. This must depend on brain structures that have undergone evolutionary changes.

Several brain regions are associated with mental time travel. The dorsolateral prefrontal cortex seems to play a central role in holding information over time, but other regions are also involved. When one recalls a past event, a large bilateral network is activated, including the temporal lobes, temporo-parieto-occipital junction, dorsal prefrontal cortex, medial prefrontal cortex, and retrosplenial cortex (Steinvorth et al., 2006). Construction and elaboration of future events is associated with activation of the right frontopolar and left ventrolateral prefrontal cortices (Addis et al., 2007). Interestingly, the anterior prefrontal cortex is specifically activated by internally generated information (Christoff et al., 2003). Thus, the frontal pole (area 10) is increasingly seen as a possible substrate for tertiary, self-generated representations (Burgess et al., 2007; Ramnani and Owen, 2004). This would certainly fit with the observation that the brain tends to mature posterior to anterior. As the prefrontal cortex matures, progressively higher orders of control are achieved (Badre, 2008). We have already noted in Chapter 3 that the medial prefrontal cortex has undergone substantial adaptation in the human brain. However, the temporal pole has undergone adaptations in the human brain and is also associated with social cognition, as we saw in Chapter 10.

Another feature of the human brain is a large number of Von Economo neurons, which are distributed in both the dorsal and ventral aspects of the anterior cingulate and fronto-insular cortices. Von Economo neurons may play a role in bridging these regions by virtue of their structure: they have very little dendritic branching and are designed for fast signal integration, important characteristics if distant parts of the brain are to be synchronized. Synchronization is critical to conscious appreciation of stimuli. Memory is only facilitated by the hippocampus; it is not stored there. Perception and recollection are associated with coordinated activity across the cortex, which is independent of hippocampal activity: we can be conscious and recall events even if we do not have a hippocampus. Von Economo neurons may have other functions as well.

Allman et al. (2001, 2005) speculated that Von Economo neurons may be an evolutionary interface between emotion and cognition. Because they are capable of fast signaling, they could be involved in fast intuitive judgments of complex situations. Thus, outputs from the anterior cingulate and fronto-insular cortex are relayed to parts of the frontal and temporal cortex associated with theory of mind and social cognition. The Von Economo neurons are present in species that demonstrate advanced social behaviors. However, humans have much larger numbers of these neurons.

SCHIZOPHRENIA

Specific functional systems are affected in schizophrenia: systems that initiate action to seek reward and those that initiate speech seem to be most affected. Patients are often flat and unmotivated, suggesting a deficit in the system that initiates action. There are other symptoms associated with deficits in the initiation of action and speech. As Kraepelin so astutely observed, many patients feel that their thoughts are not their own and are being influenced by outside forces.

One of the common symptoms Kraepelin observed was hearing one's thoughts aloud such that others could hear them, or hearing a voice that no one else can hear. Often the voice was carrying on a running conversation with the patient. Patients tend to show some consistency in their symptoms. For example, it is usually the same voice or voices that emerge with each relapse. In some patients the voices are male, while in others they are female; sometimes they are someone from the patient's past. One of us (P.W.) treated a very unfortunate man who constantly heard *Mr. Panocus* talking to him from a certain place in the wall of his rented room. *Mr. Panocus* would at times just comment on what he was doing—making tea, reading, or whatever. At other times he would ridicule him and scold him for past misdeeds. This went on for years despite treatment with antidopaminergic drugs. Fortunately, other patients respond better to these medications.

Where would we look for a system that is associated with initiating new actions or behaviors and initiating internal speech? The most likely candidate is the anterior cingulate cortex. The anterior cingulate is associated with learning new behaviors. Patients who have damaged this region are flat and unmotivated and describe a feeing of nothing being on their mind (Damasio et al., 1983). We know that this region is closely connected with speech areas and may regulate the activity of speech areas during silence (Barbas et al., 1999; Hunter et al., 2006; Yukie and Shibata, 2009). We also know that the anterior cingulate cortex is closely connected with the medial prefrontal cortex and dorsolateral cortex. Decreased glutamatergic input from the anterior cingulate to the dorsolateral prefrontal cortex could lead to reduced dopaminergic activity in the prefrontal cortex and increased dopaminergic activity in the striatum via projections between the brainstem and the dorsolateral prefrontal cortex (Lewis and Gonzales-Burgos, 2006). Propositional speech is associated with activation in the medial prefrontal region as well as the left posterior inferior parietal, anterolateral, and medial temporal prefrontal regions (Blank et al., 2002). The anterior cingulate cortex is further connected to the hippocampus. Deficits in anterior cingulate glutamatergic inputs to the hippocampus could further compromise dopaminergic regulation in basal ganglia-thalamocortical neuronal circuits (O'Donnell and Grace, 1998).

The anterior cingulate cortex is divided into a dorsal cognitive division and an affective ventral division (Devinsky et al., 1995). It is difficult to evaluate structural and functional imaging studies, as most were done in chronic patients. Findings such as decreased gray matter and increased ventricular volumes seen in chronic patients are not as prominent in first-episode patients (DeLisi, 2008). However, cortical thickness in the anterior cingulate may predict onset of psychosis in high-risk individuals (Wood, et al., 2008). Loss of both dorsal and ventral anterior cingulate volume has also been reported in a large group of first-episode patients. In contrast, first-episode patients with mostly bipolar disorder had only decreased ventral anterior cingulate volumes (Koo et al., 2008). Increased glutamatergic activity in first-episode patients has been reported in the dorsal anterior cingulate cortex, followed by decreased glutamergic activity (Théberge et al., 2002, 2003). Increased glutamatergic metabolites have been found in closely connected structures such as the thalamus in first-episode patients as well. Curiously, decreased glutamatergic metabolites correlated highly with gray matter loss in temporal speech-processing areas (Théberge et al., 2007). Decreased anterior cingulate and medial prefrontal activity has also been reported in the default network in schizophrenic patients (Bluhm et al., 2007). Thus, there is considerable support for the involvement of the anterior cingulate and medial prefrontal cortices early in schizophrenia.

If one accepts that the dorsal anterior cingulate, dorsolateral prefrontal, and medial prefrontal cortices are part of a network associated with control of directed effort, then dysfunction of this network in schizophrenia might be expected to be associated with volitional deficits, thought disorder, thought insertion, and delusions of passivity. Because these regions (particularly the dorsal anterior cingulate) are closely connected with speech areas, dysfunction in the initiation and control of speech might also be expected, as propositional speech is associated with medial prefrontal activity. In some ways, Hughlings Jackson's ideas about levels of control may come into play in that speech areas are released. Dysfunction of the anterior cingulate cortex could lead to either excitatory or plastic changes in the auditory cortex, allowing it to essentially go off-line. When this happens, speech is no longer perceived as being internally produced and is experienced as auditory hallucinations. It is not difficult to imagine how the loss of control over thoughts could be elaborated into paranoid or grandiose delusions in an effort to make sense of them. Only humans would be vulnerable to this disorder, as only humans have developed complex brain structures to support language and social representation.

BIPOLAR DISORDER

Bipolar disorders present with a different constellation of symptoms, suggesting a different pathophysiology. The difference in this disorder is in the regulation of emotional response: there is enhanced response with agitation and mania and diminished response in depression. Although psychotic symptoms can occur in both states, they are not typical of the condition; in fact, delusions of passivity, thought disorder, and commenting voices are very uncommon in these disorders. There does not seem to be a problem with agency in this disorder. As we saw in Chapter 5, cognitive and executive deficits do occur, but they tend to be more prominent during acute episodes, suggesting that dorsolateral prefrontal dysfunction may be common to both schizophrenia and bipolar disorders. Bipolar patients do have difficulty with theory of mind tasks, but it is difficult to dissociate this deficit from a generalized cognitive deficit. There is not much work on social cognition in bipolar disorders, but clinical experience would suggest that this aspect is much less affected than in other neuropsychiatric conditions.

Where would we look for a system involved in emotional regulation? As we saw in Chapter 10, there is such a system in the human brain: it includes the ventral anterior cingulate cortex, the orbitofrontal cortex, medial prefrontal cortex, and amygdala. Major depressive and bipolar disorders are clearly associated with anomalies throughout this network. As we discussed in Chapters 5 and 10, the posterior lateral and medial orbitofrontal cortex is associated with histopathological abnormalities, gray matter volume reductions, and activation anomalies during the presentation of emotional stimuli and in reward paradigms (Drevets, 2007; Phillips et al., 2003b). Depression severity is inversely correlated with physiological activity in parts of the posterior lateral and medial prefrontal cortex. In contrast, activity in the anteromedial orbitofrontal cortex situated in the ventromedial polar cortex is increased in depression. Effective antidepressant treatment is associated with a reduction of activity in this region (Drevets, 2007).

Drevets (2007) suggested that some regions in the orbitofrontal cortex appear to inhibit or modulate emotional expression while others appear to facilitate emotional expression. It is interesting that there is a difference in activity between anterior and posterior regions in the ventral prefrontal cortex. This suggests that the orbitofrontal cortex may be the ventral input to the representational brain. This makes sense because emotion is critical for social relationships; however, it may also make it vulnerable. In depression, for example, enhanced inhibition from anteromedial structures may lead to changes in the emotional response system mediated by the amygdala. In mania, the reverse situation may occur. The fact that ventromedial polar cortex activity predicts response to medication suggests that this may be the case. These patients are not just experiencing a grief/loss reaction like that seen in less evolved species; they are experiencing a more human experience characterized in many cases by human emotions such as guilt and remorse. We have previously commented on the association of these emotions with the anterior insula, which is part of the extended emotional processing network in humans, in Chapter 10.

If the extended emotional processing network in the prefrontal cortex fails to inhibit the amygdala, one would expect symptoms such as those seen in mania. One would also expect some changes in the structural and functional features of the amygdala. As we saw in Chapter 5, this seems to be the case. The amygdala is one of the few structures found to be increased in size in some patients with bipolar disorders. Thus, the extra layer of control associated with the representational brain once again leads to vulnerabilities. Complex emotional relationships can be coded, but when this system breaks down for any number of reasons, emotional control is lost.

AUTISM

In contrast to schizophrenia, autism is not often associated with disorders of the initiation of action. Patients are not really flat or uninterested; on the contrary, they can become enormously preoccupied by objects. Language is affected to varying degrees, but autistic patients do not often suffer from hallucinations. Like patients with schizophrenia and bipolar disorder, they show deficits in social cognition and theory of mind. In contrast to patients with bipolar disorder, however, autistic patients do not usually have difficulty with regulating emotion, at least in the sense of suffering periods of depression or mania. The deficit in autism is primarily a social deficit: these individuals are not usually very interested in developing social relationships and have difficulty conceptualizing their emotions and the emotions of others.

Where would we look for a system in the brain that is associated with representing relationships and emotion? The medial prefrontal cortex and polar frontal cortex (area 10) have to be involved in some way. However, the evidence for the direct involvement of these regions is limited. Deficits in the mentalizing network have been reported in autistic patients. Areas showing deficits included the medial prefrontal and temporal pole regions (Castelli et al., 2002). However, postmortem and structural imaging studies have shown more widespread anomalies. Minicolumns, which are essential for higher cortical processing and long-distance cortico-cortical connections, were found to be abnormal in autistic patients (Casanova et al., 2006; Herbert et al., 2004). The nature of these anomalies suggests a structural abnormality in regions associated with mentalizing rather than an abnormality in the control of these regions. This disorder assaults the very core of the representational brain. However, it is interesting that not all representations are affected. Language is largely intact in some patients, suggesting that language skills are dependent on other brain regions.

FRONTOTEMPORAL DEMENTIA

The symptoms of frontotemporal dementia overlap to some degree with autism. Both patients have deficits in theory of mind and social cognition. They do not usually have delusions of passivity, thought disorder, or hallucinations. However, they can have disorders of emotional regulation, like bipolar disorder patients. Some patients are found to be apathetic, while others have impulse control problems. Many patients also have abnormalities with language. It is not a problem of identifying the source of a thought or internal voice as in schizophrenia; rather, it is a problem with either producing speech or understanding speech. This unusual collection of symptoms becomes even more interesting when it occurs later in life in people who did not previously show anomalies in social functioning or language.

Where would we look for a part of the brain associated with social cognition, emotional regulation, and language processing? Like autism, the medial prefrontal and polar frontal cortex would likely be involved, but the addition of difficulties with emotional regulation and language production and understanding would implicate other brain regions. As we saw in Chapter 7, the imaging literature appears to bear this out. Volume losses are particularly striking in the anterior cingulate, fronto-insular, and orbitofrontal regions (Boccardi et al., 2005). Patients with semantic dementia demonstrated tissue loss in the anterior temporal cortex and the amygdala/anterior hippocampal region (Rosen et al., 2002). Apathy and disinhibition were associated with tissue loss in the ventral portion of the right anterior cingulate cortex and adjacent ventromedial superior frontal gyrus, the right ventromedial prefrontal cortex more posteriorly, the right lateral middle frontal gyrus, the right caudate head, the right orbitofrontal cortex, and the right insula (Rosen et al., 2005). Several functional imaging studies demonstrated decreased cerebral blood flow and hypometabolism in the ventromedial and inferior frontal cortex and anterior temporal lobes, which are highly correlated with volumetric changes in patients with frontotemporal dementia (Alexander et al., 1995; Diehl-Schmid et al., 2007; Franceschi et al., 2005; Friedland et al., 1993; Grimmer et al., 2004; Ibach et al., 2004; Ishii et al., 1998; Miller and Gearhart, 1999; Schroeter et al., 2008; Varma et al., 2002; Varrone et al., 2002).

If any disorder might shed light on the human brain, one would think that it might be frontotemporal dementia. So, what is causing these profound changes in a previously normal brain? The best answer so far appears to be Von Economo neurons. Seeley et al. (2006) found a 74% loss of Von Economo neurons in frontotemporal dementia patients across pathological subtypes. Surviving Von Economo neurons were often dysmorphic. The reduction in the number of Von Economo neurons is evident even in the early stages of the disease, when the first defects in social functioning, such as the loss of empathy, emerge (Seeley et al., 2006; see also Fig. 7.1). The fact that a loss of these neurons could so severely affect social cognition, emotional regulation, and language processing suggests that they must play a role in the representational brain. Do these disorders tell us anything else about the representational brain?

NEUROPSYCHIATRIC DISORDERS AND THE REPRESENTATIONAL BRAIN

Neuropsychiatric disorders tell us something about how the normal human brain is constructed. In psychiatry, as in neurology, the brain breaks down in discrete ways, often along functional lines. Conditions like schizophrenia tell us about the systems that control directed effort and initiate action and speech. It is likely that the key regions are the anterior cingulate, particularly the dorsal aspect, speech areas (Wernicke's and Broca's), hippocampus, and dorsolateral prefrontal cortex in schizophrenia. This dorsal control system is mirrored by a ventral control system for encoding emotion in a social context, which is involved in bipolar disorders. This system includes the ventral anterior cingulate, subgenual prefrontal cortex, the orbital prefrontal cortex, amygdala, and dorsolateral prefrontal cortex. Both of these control systems interact with a representational system that particularly developed in humans. This system includes the frontal pole, anterior insula, and temporal pole. The representational system is particularly affected in autism and frontotemporal dementia. A simplified diagram showing these structures is shown in Figure 11.1.

Several authors have previously commented on some aspects of this model. Frith (1992) was one of the first to suggest that schizophrenia was a disorder of meta-representation (or what others have referred to as representational redescription). Meta-representation was associated with some of the above regions, including the dorsolateral prefrontal cortex and anterior cingulate. Some similarities to meta-representational anomalies in autism were also noted. Amodio and Frith (2006) have commented on the dorsal and ventral divisions of the anterior cingulate, the connection with the medial prefrontal cortex, and its role in mentalizing. den Ouden et al. (2005) have demonstrated that the medial prefrontal cortex, superior temporal region, and temporal poles participate in intentional tasks. Abraham et al. (2008)

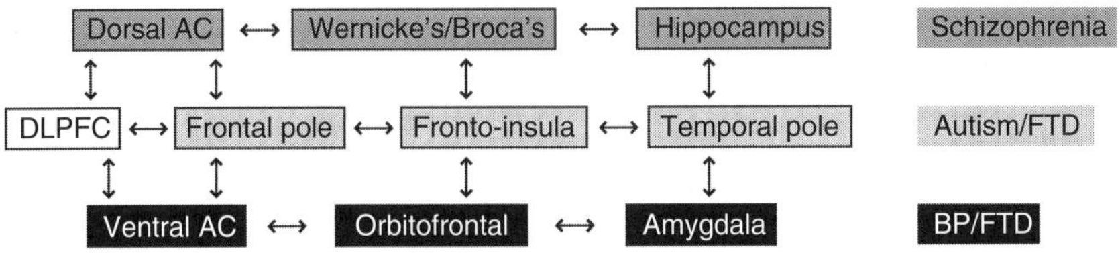

Figure 11.1 The representational brain and neuropsychiatric disorders. The dorsal-directed effort control system implicated in schizophrenia is shown in dark gray. The ventral emotional encoding system implicated in frontotemporal dementia (FTD) and bipolar disorder (BP) is shown in black. Both interact with the representational social cognition system (shown in light gray), which has been associated with autism and FTD. The dorsolateral prefrontal cortex (DLPFC) interacts with all three systems and is shown in white. Interactions between these regions likely involve many more than those indicated by the arrows. AC = Anterior cingulate.

have suggested that the medial prefrontal cortex, temporal poles, and precuneus are involved in intentional tasks. These findings suggest an overlap between the networks associated with theory of mind, intentional action, and the default network.

Ochsner (2008) has highlighted the role of the dorsal and lateral prefrontal cortex and the dorsal medial prefrontal cortex in *description-based* regulation. *Outcome-based regulation* was seen as depending more on the ventral and medial prefrontal cortex. These functional systems were seen as cutting across diagnostic boundaries. This view differs from our approach in that neuropsychiatric disorders are seen as overlapping to some extent. However, we believe, as Kraepelin did, that they can be separated functionally and anatomically.

Phillips et al. (2003b) suggested that there is a ventral system for emotional processing that includes the amygdala, insula, ventral striatum, ventral anterior cingulate, and prefrontal cortex. This system identifies emotional significance and is involved in the production of affective states and autonomic regulation of emotional responses. A dorsal system including the hippocampus, dorsal anterior cingulate gyrus, and prefrontal cortex is for effortful regulation of affective states and subsequent behavior. Psychotic symptoms are largely attributed to faulty emotional appraisal systems. Bipolar disorders are attributed to an oversensitive but dysfunctional neural system for the identification of emotional significance, production of affective states, and regulation of emotional behavior. In our view, this model fails to appreciate the role of brain structures associated with tertiary representations of language and emotional relationships.

Buckner et al. (2008) have proposed two brain systems. The first is the default network, discussed in Chapter 8, for internally focused tasks, autobiographical memory, envisioning the future, and conceiving the perspectives of others. The second is the medial temporal lobe system for information about prior experiences, which is used for mental simulations in the medial regions. Both converge on the posterior cingulate cortex. They attribute autism to anomalies in the development of the default network and provide some evidence of disordered default network functioning in autism to support their suggestion. While the default network overlaps some parts of the medial prefrontal cortex, it is difficult to see how this is specific to autism. In fact, the same network can be seen in monkeys, which do not have theory of mind capabilities. Schizophrenia was attributed to overactivity of the default network. This area of investigation is new, but we have not found support for this contention. If anything, there is less connectivity between the posterior node and the anterior node, which is associated with the medial prefrontal cortex and mentalizing (Bluhm et al., 2007). Although we would agree that the default mode network is related in some way to the representational brain, we do not believe that they are the same thing. We believe that a more useful way to construct mentalizing is to consider the frontal and temporal poles as part of the same system controlled by converging input from a dorsal and ventral prefrontal system.

Our approach does not exclude the possibility of interactions between the dorsal and ventral control systems. Mayberg et al. (1999) suggested that the dorsal attentional–cognitive networks are in balance with a ventral vegetative–autonomic network. An imbalance between these networks is associated with depression. This is quite consistent with findings in this disorder and is consistent with our approach. An updated version of this model (Holtzheimer and Mayberg, 2009) suggests that the anterior cingulate may be central to many neuropsychiatric disorders. However, our model differs in that we view neuropsychiatric disorders as arising from primary lesions to the representational brain or the networks that control it (i.e., the dorsal-directed effort or ventral, emotional encoding networks).

Another aspect that should be acknowledged is that there are lateralized differences in these structures. Schore (2003) has pointed out the importance of the right medial prefrontal cortex in the development of emotional regulation and mentalizing. There are also lateralized aspects of language processing, which we have discussed in Chapter 9. Consequently, it is quite possible that emotional encoding may be partially lateralized to the right while directed effort and language are partially lateralized to the left. However, it is clear that both emotional encoding and language are not completely lateralized.

One thing that this model might help with is the puzzle of how only humans are capable of long-term auditory memory processing, which we commented on in Chapter 9. The reason may be related to the nature of this network. As we saw in Chapter 9, language processing involves regions beyond Wernicke's and Broca's areas, including regions associated with long-term memory processing. Only humans are capable of tertiary representations, and these representations are by nature rooted in the past as well as the present and future.

GENETIC CORRELATES

The search for the genes that led to *Homo sapiens* has been a frustrating one. As we noted in Chapter 3, about 10% of genes differ in their expression between humans and chimpanzees in at least one region of the brain (Khaitovich et al., 2004). Do studies of unique human capabilities and their disorders help to narrow the search? There are some genes that may be more likely than others to be associated with the representational brain and possibly some neuropsychiatric disorders. Unfortunately, there has been very little work on the overlap between human genes and the genes associated with neuropsychiatric disorders.

It is interesting that both chimpanzees and humans showed particular differences from gorillas in the gene expression related to aerobic energy metabolism in the anterior cingulate region, a region associated with the default network and the representational brain (Uddin et al., 2004). There are promising correlations between the genes associated with neurodevelopment and neurotransmitter systems. Genes involved in glutamatergic signal transduction are linked to schizophrenia, and genes involved in serotonergic signal transduction are linked to bipolar disorders (Harrison and Weinberger, 2005; Lasky-Su et al., 2005; Rapoport et al., 2005). Both neurotransmitter systems play an important role in the development and regulation of the dorsal and ventral prefrontal systems discussed above. Genes affecting the cell's signaling cascades are associated with increased proliferation, differentiation, and process outgrowth. Anomalies in one of these genes have been reported in autism and may be linked to interneuron and minicolumnar abnormalities found on postmortem examination (Campbell et al., 2006).

One of the most interesting genes (see Chapter 4) that may be associated with neuropsychiatric disorders, brain development, and human adaptations is the disrupted in schizophrenia gene (DISC1). DISC1 is involved with neuronal migration, neurite outgrowth, and neuronal maturation as well as synaptic transmission and plasticity in adults (Ross et al., 2006). Very promising linkages between anomalies in this gene and both schizophrenia and autism have been reported by several groups (Harrison and Owen, 2003; Harrison and Weinberger, 2005; Kilpinen et al., 2008; Perlman et al., 2004). DISC1 is also expressed in Von Economo neurons. It has been suggested that this gene is associated with the control of dendritic branching, perhaps explaining the reduction of dendritic branching in these cells. As Von Economo neurons seem to be present in key locations throughout the representational brain, this could be an important clue to both the development of the human brain and some neuropsychiatric conditions. In the case of frontotemporal dementia, at least, Von Economo neurons play a central role in the pathophysiology.

OVERVIEW

The human brain is more than the social brain. The human brain is a representational brain capable of representing and communicating through language the views and feelings of others. It is also capable of reflecting on past events and anticipating future events. It is likely that many of these functions overlap in the human brain. The representational brain is not the midline structures alone, although midline structures code unique time-dependent information that is essential for representational redescription. We propose that the control of the representational brain is accomplished by a dorsal action-oriented system and a ventral emotion-oriented system. It is the elaboration of these connections that gives the human brain its unique capabilities.

We further propose that it is the unique configuration of the representational brain that makes the human brain vulnerable to neuropsychiatric disorders. While lower species may share many of these brain structures, they do not have the next level of complexity introduced by tertiary representations in the frontal and temporal poles. The evolutional changes that led to the adaptations in these brain regions are far from clear, but we suggest that the proliferation of Von Economo neurons and genes associated with this cell type might play a central role by linking medial prefrontal regions with affective and speech areas in a unique way early in brain development.

The way these networks break down determines the nature of the neuropsychiatric disorder. We have argued that it makes sense to think of schizophrenia as being associated with a dysfunctional dorsal-directed effort/language control system consisting of the anterior cingulate, hippocampus, and language areas. Bipolar disorders (and perhaps frontotemporal dementia) are associated with a dysfunctional ventral emotional encoding system consisting of the ventral anterior cingulate, amygdala, and orbitofrontal cortex. Both interact with the representational brain, including the frontal and temporal polar cortices and insula. Dysfunction of these brain regions is associated with autism and frontotemporal dementia. We will look of some of the implications of this approach in the next chapter.

12

Implications

Have we really made any progress since the remarkable observations of Jackson, Kraepelin, Kanner, and Pick? The clinical entities that they described have stood up well. We still argue about the cases that have features of more than one disorder, but for the most part, the concepts are still intact. In fact, most find the original descriptions of these disorders easily recognizable in the patients of today: they have the same constellation of symptoms and clinical course. Since the original descriptions, we have come to know that they also have some differences in pathology, differences on brain imaging, and differences in treatment response.

Unfortunately, the misplaced hope that each neuropsychiatric disorder might have a specific cause has met with disappointment. An enormous amount of money has been spent on looking for the smoking-gun gene for these disorders. A miracle is always possible, but we are not likely to understand the extremely complex interactions among the hundreds of genes and environmental events that underlie these disorders in our lifetime. We argue that the challenge of our time is to figure out the final common pathways of these disorders.

THE SEARCH FOR FINAL COMMON PATHWAYS

Psychiatry is at the that stage medicine was about 400 years ago before William Harvey came along. His description of the circulatory system allowed us to understand the symptoms of heart failure such as edema, liver enlargement, and shortness of breath. When the pump breaks down, fluid backs up. One could think of the brain in a similar way: it is simply a machine to integrate affect, cognition, and perception. When it breaks down, you do not see edema, but you do see things like hallucinations, delusions, and problems with affective regulation. If we can figure out the systems that integrate affect, cognition, and perception, we might be able to move our interventions from the level of bloodletting to digitalis.

William Harvey had an important clue to the nature of the circulatory system. While he was studying with Fabricius in Italy, he became aware of venous valves. These valves allowed blood to flow in only one direction, back to the heart. Once he understood these, he realized that the teaching of the time was wrong: blood did not flow away from the liver; rather, it flowed to the liver and the heart, where it was pumped full of nutrients, to the lungs, where it acquired oxygen, and then was pumped back to the tissues. It was a simple idea but a powerful one. Do we have any comparable clues in our search for the brain systems that integrate affect, cognition, and perception? We argue that we do. These are human disorders, so the nature of the human brain is our best clue.

We are not the first to point this out. Tim Crow and many others have argued passionately that the asymmetry of the human brain, which allows language, leaves the human vulnerable to schizophrenia. As we discussed in Chapter 9, there is some support for this suggestion. However, we believe that it is only part of the story. The human brain is not just about language: it is about representation, or, as Karmiloff-Smith (1992) argues, representational redescription. Theory of mind, time travel, and complex emotional relationships are as much a part of being human as language.

SHOULD WE GIVE UP ON GENETIC STUDIES?

We argue that we should give up looking for the gene that explains schizophrenia or any other psychiatric disorder. However, this does not mean that we should give up on genetic studies. On the contrary: a better understanding of the final common pathway of these disorders might inform the search for candidate genes. Since so many genes have been linked to these disorders, finding the ones that are linked to the final common pathway is a large step forward, even if individually they do not contribute a lot to the variance overall. Already there are suggestions that intrinsic networks have some genetic associations (Glahn et al., 2010; Seeley et al., 2009).

One gene that shows particular promise is DISC1, which has been linked to schizophrenia, mood disorders, and autism (Hennah et al., 2009). DISC1 plays many roles in brain development, which may lead to anomalies in the representational brain. Curiously, it is expressed in Von Economo neurons. As we have discussed in Chapters 4 through 7, a number of other genes, particularly the neurexins and neuroligins, that are involved in brain development have been linked to these neuropsychiatric disorders. Copy number variations are also clearly abnormal in many neuropsychiatric conditions. It is interesting that many of the genes involved in the duplications or deletions are related to the formation of synapses and the formation of neuronal networks. Consequently, anomalies in duplication of genes may be another pathway to dysfunctional neuronal networks.

As it became increasingly clear that molecular genetic studies were not going to come up with simple answers to neuropsychiatric and other disorders, molecular geneticists started to argue that understanding how a gene works may help identify new treatment approaches even if that gene is associated with a particular disorder. This may be a reasonable approach to many medical conditions like atherosclerotic heart disease, but some caution is required when applying the argument to brain disorders. The brain develops through a cascade of epigenetic steps, each dependent on the other. Any genetic anomaly, and there has to be a substantial number in any neuropsychiatric condition, could have the same overall effect on a functional network. Thus, correcting the effect of that gene would be possible only during brain development, not once the individual reaches maturity. The fact that many carry the genes associated with these conditions and do not develop the condition raises an ethical and practical dilemma as to whether intervention would be feasible.

WHAT DO NEUROPSYCHIATRIC DISORDERS TELL US ABOUT THE HUMAN BRAIN?

Neuropsychiatric disorders can tell us a number of other things about the human brain. We propose that there are three unique networks: (1) one related to representation, including the medial prefrontal cortex and fronto-insula and temporal poles; (2) one related to control of directed effort and language, including the dorsal anterior cingulate, auditory processing regions, and hippocampus; and (3) one related to emotional encoding, including the orbitofrontal cortex, subgenual anterior cingulate, and amygdala in the human brain. All three networks interact and also interact with the dorsolateral prefrontal cortex (Fig. 12.1). What do neuropsychiatric disorders tell us about these networks?

Schizophrenia may tell us that initiation of action and language are linked. This may not come as a surprise: we already know that other perceptual systems such as vision are organized into an action and identification system, and there is no reason to think about the representational system as being anything more than a *sense* designed to evaluate and respond to the outside world. The medial prefrontal cortex (see Chapter 9) is activated during speech, suggesting that this part of the representational brain is involved in language as well. In fact, the anterior default network, which includes much of the medial prefrontal cortex in humans, is associated with internal speech and stimulus-independent thought. It is quite possible that the posterior cingulate is also involved in the control of directed effort and language. We noted in Chapter 9 that non-human primates seem to process short-term representations of auditory information but do not seem to be capable of long-term auditory storage. One of the unique substrates for long-term auditory processing in humans may be through the posterior cingulate cortex, and there is some evidence of impaired connections between the anterior and posterior cingulate cortices in schizophrenia (Williamson, 2007).

One might ask why patients who have had a stroke or tumor affecting the medial prefrontal cortex do not develop hallucinations or delusions of passivity.

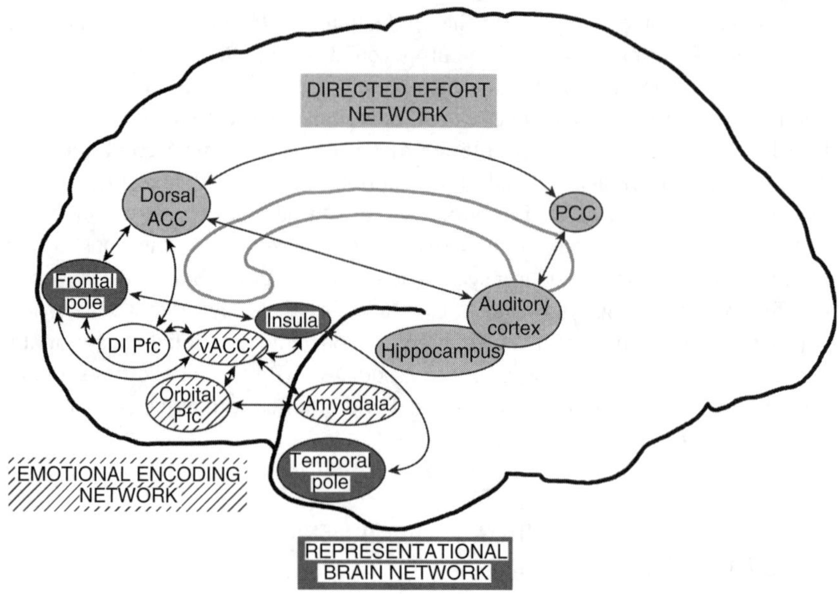

Figure 12.1 The representational brain. The representational brain network (dark gray) includes the frontal pole, insula, and temporal pole. The directed effort network (light gray) includes the dorsal anterior cingulate cortex (ACC), posterior cingulate cortex (PCC), auditory cortex, and hippocampus. The emotional encoding network (lined) includes the orbital prefrontal cortex (Pfc), ventral anterior ACC (vACC), and amygdala. The networks interact and also interact with the dorsolateral prefrontal cortex (Dl Pfc, not shaded).

They are certainly flat and almost mute, like many schizophrenic patients, but they do not have hallucinations (Damasio and Van Hoesen, 1983). One of the reasons may be the time of the lesion. The evidence is overwhelming that schizophrenic patients have had an early neurodevelopmental lesion. This lesion probably affects the development of the directed effort network and is uncovered with the cortical pruning that occurs around adolescence. An early insult to this network affects not only regions associated with the network but other regions involved in representation. Patients who experience a stroke or tumor later in life do not have this vulnerability and therefore may not be prone to its effects, which in this case may be the development of hallucinations and/or delusions of passivity.

Autism and frontotemporal dementia illustrate that there are parts of the brain devoted to processing social information and emotions. The findings in these disorders point to some of the regions that might be involved in these functions. In the case of frontotemporal dementia, the role of Von Economo neurons in these behaviors is highlighted by the striking loss of these neurons in this condition.

Bipolar disorders illustrate that dysfunction of certain regions of the medial and orbital prefrontal cortex and amygdala lead to profound changes in mood regulation, experienced as clinical depression and mania. Although some patients do experience hallucinations, most do not, suggesting that these networks are separate from those involved in schizophrenia.

The brain breaks down in discrete ways. That these disorders exist at all tells us that there are discrete functional systems: one related to self-monitoring and initiation of action and language, one for the representation of social information, and one for the regulation of affect. It is easy to see how the first two functions would be important to living in large groups. However, the regulation and representation of affect are also important: without representation of affect within a specific context, it would not be possible to interpret social cues.

WHAT ABOUT OTHER NEUROPSYCHIATRIC DISORDERS?

We chose to focus on a few neuropsychiatric disorders, but there may well be implications for several other disorders. While posttraumatic disorders have been described in elephants (Bradshaw et al., 2005), there may be some unique features in humans. In fact, an emerging brain imaging literature has implicated many of the regions involved in representation as well as emotional processing (Lanius et al., 2001). Lanius et al. (2004) showed that patients who had been exposed to trauma but did not develop a posttraumatic stress disorder were able to activate their prefrontal cortex during a script recreating their trauma. This would be expected, as the prefrontal cortex is associated with recall of episodic memories. However, patients with posttraumatic stress disorder did not activate the prefrontal cortex; instead, they activated posterior brain regions associated with implicit memory during a script recreating their trauma. Implicit memories tend to be visual and locked out of time, much like the flashbacks that these patients experience. Thus, posttraumatic stress disorders may represent a temporary failure to activate the representational brain caused by overwhelming fear.

Another disorder that may be relevant is psychopathy. Many patients with this disorder are highly attuned to another's thoughts and feelings; in fact, they are able to exploit this ability. However, they also demonstrate emotional hyporesponsiveness (Blair and Mitchell, 2009), suggesting that unlike patients with autism they are able to represent the emotions of others, but their own emotions to any particular situation may be deficient, suggesting a disorder of emotional responsiveness in these patients. One might also think about a number of anxiety syndromes, but it is likely that higher-level processing plays a less significant role in these disorders, as many can be found naturally in the animal kingdom.

THE DEFAULT NETWORK AND THE REPRESENTATIONAL BRAIN

The default network shares many features with the representational brain, but they are not the same thing. It is clear that certain aspects of the default network can be seen in primates not capable of representational redescription, albeit in qualitatively and quantitatively different configurations from humans in frontal and language regions (Rilling et al., 2007). In humans, we see evidence of an anterior and posterior default system in neonates, but they are not connected (Fransson et al., 2007). In children, we see a progressively increasing connection between the anterior and posterior default regions, particularly involving social brain regions (Fair et al., 2008). Thus, experience seems to play a large role in the development of these brain regions. Something has to synchronize these brain regions. The Von Economo neurons, which are found in these regions and are abundant in the human brain, may be involved. By linking brain regions such as the medial prefrontal cortex with attentional, affective, and speech areas, Von Economo neurons may have enabled the default network to evolve into its present form in humans.

Anomalies in the default network in neuropsychiatric disorders may shed some light on unique connections in the human brain. Although most disorders have been associated with anomalies, the most striking feature is that each disorder is associated with aberrant connections between the default network and parts of the brain that might be expected to be involved in these disorders. For example, the medial prefrontal and anterior cingulate regions often show disordered connections in schizophrenia. In mood disorders we often see abnormal connections between the default network and the subgenual prefrontal cortex, while connections between the default network and the hippocampus can be found in Alzheimer's disease. Each may reflect a unique adaption of the default network in the human brain that has become dysfunctional.

THE REPRESENTATIONAL BRAIN, ATTENTIONAL NETWORKS, AND HUMAN AWARENESS

As we discussed in Chapter 11, many have noticed the regional similarities between different cognitive functions unique to humans. The default network overlaps with regions associated with theory of mind, the social brain, and prospection. These regions are deactivated when attention-demanding tasks are required. What we do not know much about is how these networks relate to attentional and task-related networks. Theory of mind and the social brain may be based in midline structures, but it is likely that this information is dependent on input from task-activated regions, particularly the prefrontal cortex. It is likely that it is the synchronous activity of both the default network and the task-activated networks that makes representational redescription possible.

The regions involved in attention-demanding tasks are not unique to humans but clearly have a dorsal and ventral organization. The dorsal attentional system includes the intraparietal cortex and superior frontal cortex on both sides of the brain, while the ventral attentional system includes the temporoparietal cortex and inferior frontal cortex mostly on the right side (Corbetta and Shulman, 2002; Fox et al., 2006; Seeley et al., 2007). The dorsal attentional system applies goal-directed, top-down control that can be overridden by the ventral attentional system, which attends to salient events.

What we do not know is how the medial prefrontal and temporal pole regions, which seem to be particularly well developed in humans, interact with cortical regions associated with language and attention-demanding tasks. There has to be some mechanism that allows the medial prefrontal cortex to be deactivated yet connected enough to store information during attention-demanding tasks.

Perhaps the prefrontal region suppresses the default network (Greicius et al., 2003; Knight et al., 1999); perhaps it is another brain region such as the thalamus (Greicius et al., 2003; Sherman, 2001). More recent work has suggested the right fronto-insular and anterior cingulate cortices are responsible for the switch (Sridharan et al., 2008). The exact mechanism of the switch is not known, but the mechanism may have something to do with neuropsychiatric disorders.

Craig (2009) has suggested that the fronto-insula is central to human awareness, possibly as a result of connections between the fronto-insula and anterior cingulate by Von Economo neurons. We do not know exactly where Von Economo neurons project, but the idea that the fronto-insula acts to coordinate activity across the cortex leading to conscious awareness is an appealing one. In fact, it is reminiscent of the suggestion by Crick and Koch (2005) that the claustrum acts in a similar way. As indicated in Chapter 2, the claustrum, which surrounds and projects to the fronto-insula, is exquisitely topographically organized and in an ideal position to integrate activity across sensory modalities and cortical regions. In our model in the previous chapter we highlighted the role of the fronto-insular cortex in the representational brain. It is possible that the claustrum is also important with linking information from the frontal and temporal poles. However, relatively little is known about the function of this structure.

HOW DO THE REPRESENTATIONAL BRAIN CONTROL SYSTEMS WORK?

We suggested in Chapter 11 that the representational brain is controlled by a dorsal control system linked to action and language and a ventral control system linked to emotional encoding. We view these systems as being more than just the attentional systems described above. Attention does not necessarily imply directed effort. What we are suggesting is that these control systems have become linked to a new system in humans that is associated with human functions, prospection, theory of mind, and language. Neuropsychiatric disorders tell us something about these new linkages.

Dysfunction in the dorsal control system is associated with schizophrenia, while dysfunction of the ventral control system is associated with mood disorders. It makes sense to us that representation should include information about action, language, and affect. However, we also recognize that much work is required to establish these connections. It ought to be possible to demonstrate that there is a link between the dorsal control system and language. There is some evidence that schizophrenic patients have aberrant linkages between the anterior cingulate and temporal regions projecting to speech areas during a word fluency task, but much remains to be done (Boksman et al., 2005). It also ought to be possible to study the relationship between the ventral control system and representation. To date studies have focused more on reward than representation of social behaviors.

Another suggestion that is more intuition than fact is the mechanism of symptom production arising from dysfunction in these systems. We suggested in

Chapter 11 that dysfunction of the dorsal control system leads to mislabeling of initiation, resulting in delusions of passivity, and release of language regions, leading to hallucinations. Studies of the coordination of these brain regions during these symptoms could provide some evidence for this suggestion. Similarly, studies of the coordination of the ventral brain regions might establish a similar release of the amygdala during mania. Simple activation studies will not provide much further information than we already have.

IS THE REPRESENTATIONAL BRAIN UNIQUE TO HUMANS?

We do not know for sure if the representational brain is unique to humans. As we discussed in Chapter 3, the human brain does not look a lot different than the chimpanzee brain, but there are some subtle differences, and it is interesting that these differences do correlate with unique human functions. The frontal and temporal poles associated with self-monitoring are particularly well developed in humans. Clearly, the language regions are also well developed in humans. The middle temporal gyrus seems to be prominent only in humans. When these features are combined with the ample cognitive and imaging literature reviewed in Chapters 8 and 9, a good case can be made that the representational brain is unique to humans. Animals are capable of living in very complex social systems, but their experiential life is not the same.

We know from brain imaging studies that medial brain regions seem to be associated with the social brain, and temporal and prefrontal regions are associated with language. But how does it work? We have much to learn about this process. As we suggested in Chapter 11, a good bet might be to think about Von Economo neurons, as they are present in higher mammals with complex social relationships and communication patterns and are particularly plentiful in humans. They also seem to be present in key areas associated with the representational brain: dorsal and anterior cingulate, fronto-insular cortex. What is not known is where they project to and what they do. The answers to these questions might tell us a lot about the human brain. One thing that is especially intriguing is the developmental consequences of synchronizing previously unsynchronized regions.

VON ECONOMO NEURONS AND BRAIN DEVELOPMENT

The Von Economo neurons may synchronize brain regions. Synchronizing the dorsal and ventral attentional systems with the medial and polar frontal cortex could allow complex social relationships to be coded and stored. The distribution of the projections of these neurons in chimpanzees compared to humans might confirm this possibility.

It is interesting that Von Economo neurons largely develop after birth, when the cognitive systems for language, theory of mind, and complex social relationships are developing (Allman et al., 2005; 2010). It is reasonable to suggest that Von Economo neurons are in an ideal position to allow the medial prefrontal cortex and temporal poles to interact with language areas and affective processing regions in a configuration much different from non-human primates. However, it is likely that differences in the number of Von Economo neurons are not the only differences that humans have from non-human primates. In Chapter 3 we highlighted the many differences between the human and non-human brain. No doubt many of these unique features also participate in the development of human capabilities.

SOME LIMITATIONS OF CURRENT BRAIN IMAGING

Brain imaging techniques have contributed much to our understanding of the representational brain, but there are some limitations. For example, there is fairly reliable midline activation during stimulus-independent thought, but the same regions are activated during theory of mind tasks or even during recall tasks. Surely there must be unique activation during these tasks that is not captured by these studies. Part of the answer may be to more carefully design studies that parse out these different functions. Another approach may be to develop better imaging techniques.

Low-frequency fluctuations of the blood oxygen level-dependent (BOLD) signal used in many default network studies offer a new window on brain networks. It is likely that they reflect high-frequency synchronization between regions, but there are many potential confounds, and it is not entirely clear at this point whether they are just reflecting synchronized networks. One of the problems with the BOLD technique is the time lag between the blood flow response and signal transduction in the brain. This is particularly problematic in regions such as the claustrum, which may depend in part on gap junction signaling. Some techniques done at higher field strengths show some promise to improve temporal resolution, but they are at an early stage of development (Li and Song, 2003).

A FINAL THOUGHT

One thing that occurred to us is that some readers may think that if neuropsychiatric disorders are related to the dysfunction of unique aspects of the human brain, then maybe the unfortunate people who suffer from these disorders are less human in some way. This is certainly not the case, just like the people who suffer from disorders of the hips and knees are no more ape-like than the rest of us. The human experience includes all of these conditions and more. In fact, we think that examining the relationship between these conditions and the human brain will make us all aware that people with these conditions share something with us. The people who suffer from schizophrenia, bipolar disorders, autism, and frontotemporal dementia have a human illness.

References

Abi-Dargham, A., Gil, R., Krystal, J., Baldwin, R.M., Seibyl, J.P., Bowers, M., van Dyck, C.H., Charney, D.S., Innis, R.B., and Laruelle, M. (1998). Increased striatal dopamine transmission in schizophrenia: Confirmation in a second cohort. *American Journal of Psychiatry,* **155**, 761–767.

Aboitiz, F., and García, R. (1997). The evolutionary origin of the language areas in the human brain. A neuroanatomical perspective. *Brain Research Reviews*, **25**, 381–396.

Abraham, A., Werning, M., Rakoczy, H., von Cramon, D.Y., and Schubotz, R.I. (2008). Minds, persons, and space: An fMRI investigation into the relational complexity of higher-order intentionality. *Consciousness and Cognition*, **17**, 438–450.

Abrams, R., and Taylor, M.A. (1979). Laboratory studies in the validation of psychiatric diagnoses. In J.H. Gruzelier and P. Flor-Henry (Eds.), *Hemispheric Asymmetries of Function in Psychopathology* (pp. 363–372). Amsterdam, Elsevier.

Addis, D.R., Wong, A.T., and Schacter, D.L. (2007). Remembering the past and imagining the future: Common and distinct neural substrates during event construction and elaboration. *Neuropsychologia*, **45**, 1363–1377.

Adler, C.M., Holland, S.K., Schmithorst, V., Wilke, M., Weiss, K.L., Pan, H., and Strakowski, S.M. (2004). Abnormal frontal white matter tracts in bipolar disorder: A diffusion tensor imaging study. *Bipolar Disorders*, **6**, 197–203.

Adolphs, R. (2003). Cognitive neuroscience of human social behaviour. *Nature Reviews Neuroscience*, **4**, 165–178.

Aggleton, J.P. (Ed.). (1992). *The Amygdala: Neurobiological Aspects of Emotion, Memory, and Mental Dysfunction*. New York, Wiley-Liss Inc.

Akbarian, S., Bunney, W.E., Potkin, S.G., Wigal, S.B., Hagman, J.O., Sandman, C.A., and Jones, E.G. (1993a). Altered distribution of nicotinamide-adenine dinucleotide phosphate-diaphorase cells in frontal lobe of schizophrenics implies disturbances of cortical development. *Archives of General Psychiatry,* **50**, 169–177.

Akbarian, S., Kim, J.J., Potkin, S.G., Hagman, J.O., Tafazzoli, A., Bunney, W.E., and Jones, E.G. (1995). Gene expression for glutamic acid decarboxylase is reduced without loss of neurons in prefrontal cortex of schizophrenics. *Archives of General Psychiatry,* **52**, 258–266.

Akbarian, S., Vinuela, A., Kim. J.J., Potkin, S.G., Bunney, W.E., and Jones, E.G. (1993b). Distorted distribution of nicotinamide-adenine dinucleotide phosphate-diaphorase neurons in temporal lobe of schizophrenics implies anomalous cortical development. *Archives of General Psychiatry,* **50**, 178–187.

Akiskal, H.S. (1981). Subaffective disorders: Dysthymic, cyclothymic and bipolar II disorders in the 'borderline' realm. *Psychiatric Clinics of North America*, **4**, 25–46.

Alberici, A., Gobbo, C., Panzacchi, A., Nicosia, F., Ghidoni, R., Benussi, L., Hock, C., Papassotiropoulos, A., Liberini, P., Growdon, J.H., Frisoni, G.B., Villa, A., Zanetti, O., Cappa, S., Fazio, F., and Binetti, G. (2004). Frontotemporal dementia: Impact of P301L tau mutation on a healthy carrier. *Journal of Neurology, Neurosurgery and Psychiatry*, **75**, 1607–1610.

Aleman, A., Hijman, R., de Haan, E.H.F., and Kahn, R.S. (1999). Memory impairment in schizophrenia: A meta-analysis. *American Journal of Psychiatry,* **156**, 1358–1366.

Alexander, A.L., Lee, J.E., Lazar, M., Boudos, R., DuBray, M.B., Oakes, T.R., Miller, J.N, Lu, J., Jeong, E.-K., McMahon, W.M., Bigler, E.D., and Lainhart, J.E. (2007). Diffusion tensor imaging of the corpus callosum in autism. *NeuroImage*, **34**, 61–73.

Alexander, G.E., Prohovnik, I., Sackeim, H.A., Stern, Y., and Mayeux, R. (1995). Cortical perfusion and gray matter weight in frontal lobe dementia. *Journal of Neuropsychiatry and Clinical Neurosciences*, **7**, 188–196.

Alexander, G.E., Crutchner, M.D., and De Long, M.R. (1990). Basal ganglia-thalamocortical circuits: Parallel substrates for motor, oculometer, "prefrontal" and "limbic" functions. *Progress in Brain Research,* **85**, 119–146.

Ali, F., and Meier, R. (2008). Positive selection of ASPM is correlated with cerebral cortex evolution across primates but not with whole-brain size. *Molecular Biology and Evolution,* **25,** 2247–2250.

Allman, J.M. (1982). Reconstructing the evolution of the brain in primates through the use of comparative neurophysiological data. In E. Armstrong and D. Falk (Eds.), *Primate Brain Evolution Methods and Concepts* (pp. 13–28). New York, Plenum.

Allman, J.M. (1990). Evolution of neocortex. In E.G. Jones and A. Peters (Eds.), *Cerebral Cortex. Volume B: Comparative Structure and Evolution of Cerebral Cortex* (pp. 269–283). New York, Plenum Press.

Allman, J.M. (1999). *Evolving Brains.* (Scientific American Library). New York, W.H. Freeman.

Allman, J.M. (2000). *Evolving Brains* (Scientific American Library Paperback). New York, W.H. Freeman.

Allman, J., Hakeem, A., and Watson, K. (2002). Two phylogenetic specializations in the human brain. *The Neuroscientist*, **8**, 335–346.

Allman, J.M., Hakeem, A., Erwin, J.M., Nimchinsky, E., and Hof, P. (2001). The anterior cingulate cortex: The evolution of an interface between emotion and cognition. *Annals of the New York Academy of Sciences*, **935**, 107–117.

Allman, J.M., Tetreault N.A., Hakeem, A.Y., Manaye, K.F., Semendeferi, K., Erwin, J., Park, S., Goubert, V., and Hof, P. (2010). The von Economo Neurons in Frontoinsular and Anterior Cingulate Cortex in Great Apes and Humans. *Brain Structure and Function*, **214**: 495–517.

Allman, J.M., Watson, K.K., Tetreault, N.A., and Hakeem, A.Y. (2005). Intuition and autism: A possible role for Von Economo neurons. *Trends in Cognitive Sciences*, **9**, 367–373.

Amodio, D.A., and Frith, C.D. (2006). Meeting of minds: The medial frontal cortex and social cognition. *Nature Reviews Neuroscience*, **7**, 268–277.

Anderson, J.E., Wible, C.G., McCarley, R.W., Jakab, M., Kasai, K., and Shenton, M.E. (2002). An MRI study of temporal lobe abnormalities and negative symptoms in chronic schizophrenia. *Schizophrenia Research,* **58**, 123–134.

Anderson, J.R., Finchman, J.M., Qin, Y., and Stocco, A. (2008). A central circuit of the mind. *Trends in Cognitive Sciences*, **12**, 136–143.

Andrés, A.M., Soldevila, M., Navarro, A., Kidd, K.K., Oliva, B., and Bertranpetit, J. (2004). Positive selection in MAOA gene is human exclusive: Determination of the putative amino acid change selected in the human lineage. *Human Genetics*, **115**, 377–386.

Andres, C. (2002). Molecular genetics and animal models in autistic disorder. *Brain Research Bulletin*, **57**, 109–119.

Angst, J., Sellaro, R., Stassen H.H., and Gamma, A. (2005). Diagnostic conversion from depression to bipolar disorders: Results of a long-term prospective study of hospital admissions. *Journal of Affective Disorders*, **84**, 149–157.

Angst, F., Stassen, H.H., Clayton, P.J., and Angst, J. (2002). Mortality of patients with mood disorders: Follow-up over 34–38 years. *Journal of Affective Disorders*, **68**, 167–181.

American Psychiatric Association. (2000). *Diagnostic and Statistical Manual of Mental Disorders*, Fourth Edition, Text Revision. Washington, D.C., American Psychiatric Association.

Andermann, A.A.J. (1997). Hughlings Jackson's deductive science of the nervous system: A product of his thought collective and formative years. *Neurology*, **48**, 471–481.

Andreasen, N.C., Rezai, K., Alliger, R., Swayze, V.W., Faum, M., Kircher, P., Cohen, G., and O'Leary, D.S. (1992). Hypofrontality in neuroleptic-naïve patients and in patients with chronic schizophrenia: Assessment with xenon 133 single-photon emission computed tomography and the Tower of London. *Archives of General Psychiatry,* **49**, 943–958.

Angst, J., and Marneros, A. (2001). Bipolarity from ancient to modern times: Conception, birth and rebirth. *Journal of Affective Disorders*, **67**, 3–19.

Arion, D., Unger, T., Lewis, D.A., Levitt, P., and Károly, M. (2007). Molecular evidence for increased expression of genes related to immune and chaperone function in the prefrontal cortex in schizophrenia. *Biological Psychiatry*, **62**, 711–721.

Arnone, D., Cavanagh, J., Gerber, D., Lawrie, S.M., Ebmeier, K.P., and McIntosh, A.M. (2009). Magnetic resonance imaging studies in bipolar disorder and schizophrenia: A meta-analysis. *British Journal of Psychiatry*, **195**, 194–201.

Arnone, D., McIntosh, A.M., Tan, G.M.Y., and Ebmeier, K.P. (2008). Meta-analysis of magnetic resonance imaging studies of the corpus callosum in schizophrenia. *Schizophrenia Research*, **101**, 124–132.

Artiges, E., Martinot, J.L., Verdys, M., Attar-Levy, D., Mazoyer, B., Tzourio, N., Giraud, M-J., and Paillère, M-L. (2000). Altered hemispheric functional dominance during word generation in negative schizophrenia. *Schizophrenia Bulletin*, **26**, 709–721.

Arts, B., Jabben, N., Krabbendam, L., and Os, J. van (2008). Meta-analyses of cognitive functioning in euthymic bipolar patients and their first-degree relatives. *Psychological Medicine*, **38**, 771–785.

Ashwood, P., Wills, S., and Van der Water, J. (2006). The immune response in autism: A new frontier for autism research. *Journal of Leukocyte Biology*, **80**, 1–15.

Asperger, H. (1944). Autistic psychopathy in childhood (U. Frith, Trans.). In U. Frith (Ed.), *Autism and Asperger Syndrome* (pp. 37–92). New York, Cambridge University Press, 1991.

Augustine, J.R. (1996). Circuitry and functional aspects of the insular lobe in primates including humans. *Brain Research Reviews*, **22**, 229–244.

Badre, D. (2008). Cognitive control, hierarchy, and the rostro-caudal organization of the frontal lobes. *Trends in Cognitive Sciences*, **12**, 193–200.

Baldessarini, R.J. (2000). A plea for integrity of the bipolar disorder concept. *Bipolar Disorders*, **2**, 3–7.

Badner, J.A., and Gershon, E.S. (2002). Meta-analysis of whole-genome linkage scans of bipolar disorder and schizophrenia. *Molecular Psychiatry*, **7**, 405–411.

Bailey, A., Le Couteur, A., Gottesman, I., Bolton, P., Simonoff, E., Yuzda, E., and Rutter, M. (1995). Autism as a strongly genetic disorder: Evidence from a British twin study. *Psychological Medicine,* **25**, 63–77.

Baird, G., Simonoff, E., Pickles, A., Chandler, S., Loucas, T., Meldrum, D., and Charman, T. (2006). Prevalence of disorders of the autism spectrum in a population cohort of children in South Thames: The Special Needs and Autism Project (SNAP). *Lancet*, **368**, 210–215.

Barbas, H., Ghashghaei, H., Dombrowski, S.M., and Rempel-Clower, N.L. (1999). Medial prefrontal cortices are unified by common connections with superior temporal cortices and distinguished by input from memory-related areas in the rhesus monkey. *Journal of Comparative Neurology*, **410**, 343–367.

Barkley, R.A. (2006). The relevance of the Still lectures to attention-deficit/hyperactivity disorder. *Journal of Attention Disorders*, **10**, 137–140.

Barkley, R.A., and Cox, D. (2007). A review of driving risks and impairments associated with attention-deficit/hyperactivity disorder and the effects of stimulant medication on driving performance. *Journal of Safety Research,* **38,** 113–128.

Barnea-Goraly, N., Kwon, H., Menon, V., Eliez, S., Lotspeich, L., and Reiss, A.L. (2004). White matter structure in autism; Preliminary evidence from diffusion tensor imaging. *Biological Psychiatry*, **55**, 323–326.

Barnett, J.H., and Smoller, J.W. (2009). The genetics of bipolar disorder. *Neuroscience,* **164**, 331–343.

Baron-Cohen, S., Leslie, A.M., and Frith, U. (1985). Does the autistic child have a "theory of mind"? *Cognition*, **21**, 37–46.

Baron-Cohen, S. (1995). *Mind Blindness*. Cambridge, MIT Press.

Barta, P.E., Pearlson, G.D., Powers, R.E., Richards, S.S., and Tune, L.E. (1990). Auditory hallucinations and smaller superior temporal gyral volume in schizophrenia. *American Journal of Psychiatry*, **147**, 1457–1462.

Bartels, A., and Zeki, S. (2004). The neural correlates of maternal and romantic love. *NeuroImage,* **21**, 1155–1166.

Bartha, R., Al-Semaan, Y.M., Williamson, P.C., Drost, D.J., Malla, A.K., Carr, T.J., Canaran, G., Densmore, M., and Neufeld, R.W.J. (1999). A short echo proton magnetic resonance spectroscopy study of the left temporal lobe in first-onset schizophrenic patients. *Biological Psychiatry*, **45**, 1403–1411.

Bartha, R., Williamson, P.C., Drost, D.J., Malla, A., Carr, T.J., Cortese, L., Canaran MacFabe, G., Rylett, R.J., and Neufeld, R.W.J. (1997). Measurement of glutamate and glutamine in the medial prefrontal cortex of never-treated schizophrenic patients and healthy controls using proton magnetic resonance spectroscopy. *Archives of General Psychiatry*, **54**, 959–965.

Barton, D.A., Esler, M.D., Dawood, T., Lambert, E.A., Haikerwal, D., Brenchley, C., Socratous, F., Hastings, J., Guo, L., Wiesner, G., Kaye, D.K., Bayles, R., Schlaich, M.P., and Lambert, G.W. (2008). Elevated brain serotonin turnover in patients with depression: Effect of genotype and therapy. *Archives of General Psychiatry*, **65**, 38–46.

Bauer, M.S., Altshuler, L., Evans, D.R., Beresford, T., Williford, W.O., and Hauger, R. (2005). Prevalence and distinct correlates of anxiety, substance, and combined comorbidity in a multi-site public sector sample with bipolar disorder. *Journal of Affective Disorders*, **85**, 301–315.

Bazin, N., Perruchet, P., Hardy-Bayle, M., and Feline, A. (2000). Context-dependent information processing in patients with schizophrenia. *Schizophrenia Research*, **45**, 93–101.

Bearden, C.E., Hoffman, K.M., and Cannon, T.D. (2001). The neuropsychology and neuroanatomy of bipolar disorder: A critical review. *Bipolar Disorders*, **3**, 106–150.

Bebbington, P., and Ramana, R. (1995). The epidemiology of bipolar affective disorder. *Social Psychiatry and Psychiatric Epidemiology*, **30**, 279–292.

Bello, S.C. (2007). Autism and environmental influences: Review and commentary. *Reviews on Environmental Health*, **22**, 139–156.

Ben Bashat, D., Kronfeld-Duenias, V., Zachor, D.A., Ekstein, P.M., Hendler, T., Tarrasch, R., Even, A., Levy, Y., and Ben Sira, L. (2007). Accelerated maturation of white matter in young children with autism: A high b value DWI study. *NeuroImage*, **37**, 40–47.

Benes, F.M., McSparren, J., Bird, E.D., Vincent, S.L., and SanGiovanni, J.P. (1991a). Deficits in small interneurons in prefrontal and cingulate cortices of schizophrenic and schizoaffective patients. *Archives of General Psychiatry*, **48**, 996–1001.

Benes, F.M., Sorenson, I., and Bird, E.D. (1991b). Reduced neuronal size in posterior hippocampus of schizophrenic patients. *Schizophrenia Research*, **17**, 597–608.

Benes, F.M., Sorensen, I., Vincent, S.L., Bird, E.D., and Sathi, M. (1992). Increased density of glutamate-immunoreactive vertical processes in superficial laminae in cingulate cortex of schizophrenic brain. *Cerebral Cortex*, **2**, 503–512.

Benes, F.M., Todtenkopf, M.S., Logiotatos, P., and Williams, M. (2000). Glutamate decarboxylase (65)-immunoreactive terminals in cingulate and prefrontal cortices of schizophrenia and bipolar brain. *Journal of Chemical Neuroanatomy*, **20**, 259–269.

Benes, F.M., Turtle, M., Khan, Y., and Farol, P. (1994). Myelination of a key relay zone in the hippocampal formation occurs in the human brain during childhood, adolescence, and adulthood. *Archives of General Psychiatry*, **51**, 477–484.

Bentall, R.P. (1990). The illusion of reality: A review and integration of psychological research on hallucinations. *Psychological Bulletin*, **107**, 82–95.

Berger, H. (1929). Uber das elektrenkephalogramm des Menschen. *Archiv fur Psychiatrie*, **87**, 527–570.

Berman, K.F., Torrey, E.F., Daniel, D.G., and Weinberger, D.R. (1992). Regional cerebral blood flow in monozygotic twins discordant and concordant for schizophrenia. *Archives of General Psychiatry*, **49**, 927–934.

Berthoz, S., Armony, L.J., Blair, R.J.R., and Dolan, R.J. (2002). An fMRI study of intentional and unintentional (embarrassing) violations of social norms. *Brain,* **125**, 1696–1708.

Bertolino, A., Breier, A., Callicott, J.H., Adler, C., Mattay, V.S., Shapiro, M., Frank, J.A., Pickar, D., and Weinberger, D.R. (2000a). The relationship between dorsolateral prefrontal neuronal N-acetylaspartate and evoked release of striatal dopamine in schizophrenia. *Neuropsychopharmacology*, **22**, 125–133.

Bertolino, A., Esposito, G., Callicott, J.H., Mattay, V.S., Van Horn, J.D., Frank, J.A., Berman, K.F., and Weinberger, D.R. (2000b). Specific relationship between prefrontal neuronal N-acetylaspartate and activation of the working memory cortical network in schizophrenia. *American Journal of Psychiatry*, **157**, 26–33.

Bertolino, A., Sawroz, S., Mattay, V.S., Barnett, A.S., Duyn, J.H., Moonen, C.T.W., Frank, J.H., Tedeschi, G., and Weinberger, D.R. (1996). Regionally specific pattern of neurochemical pathology in schizophrenia as assessed by multislice proton magnetic resonance spectroscopic imaging. *American Journal of Psychiatry*, **153**, 1554–1563.

Bertrand, M.C., Sutton, H., Achim, A.M., Malla, A.K., and LePage, M. (2007). Social cognitive impairments in first episode psychosis. *Schizophrenia Research*, **95**, 124–133.

Bezchlibnyk, Y., and Young, L.T. (2002). The neurobiology of bipolar disorder: Focus on signal transduction pathways and the regulation of gene expression. *Canadian Journal of Psychiatry*, **47**, 135–148.

Bianchin, M.M., Capella, H.M., Chaves, D.L., Steindel, M., Grisard, E.C., Ganev, G.G., da Silva, J.P., Jr., Neto, E.S., Poffo, M.A., Walz, R., Carlotti, C.G., Jr., and Sakamoto, A.C. (2004). Nasu-Hakola disease (polycystic lipomembranous osteodysplasia with sclerosing leukoencephalopathy—PLOSL): A dementia associated with bone cystic lesions. From clinical to genetic and molecular aspects. *Cellular and Molecular Neurobiology,* **24**, 1–24.

Bianco, I.H., and Wilson, S.W. (2008). The habenular nuclei: A conserved asymmetric relay station in the vertebrate brain. *Philosophical Transactions of the Royal Society,* **364**, 1005–1020.

Biederman, J., Monuteaux, M.C., Mick, E., Spencer, T., Wilens, T.E., Silva, J.M., Snyder, L.E., and Faraone, S.V. (2006). Young adult outcome of attention deficit hyperactivity disorder: a controlled 10-year follow-up study. *Psychological Medicine,* **36**, 167–179.

Bilder, R.M., Wu, H., Bogerts, B., Ashtari, M., Robinson, D., Woerner, M., Lieberman, J.A., and Degreef, G. (1999). Cerebral volume asymmetries in schizophrenia and mood disorders: A quantitative magnetic resonance imaging study. *International Journal of Psychophysiology*, **34**, 197–205.

Bird, C. M., Castelli, F., Malik, O., Frith U., and Husain M. (2004). The impact of extensive medial frontal lobe damage on 'theory of mind' and cognition. *Brain*, **127**, 914–28.

Blackwood, N.J., Bentall, R.P., Ffytche, D.H., Simmons, A., Murray, R.M., and Howard, R.J. (2004). Persecutory delusions and the determination of self-relevance: An fMRI investigation. *Psychological Medicine*, **34**, 591–596.

Blair, R.J.R., and Mithchell, D.G.V. (2009). Psychopathy, attention and emotion. *Psychological Medicine*, **39**, 543–555.

Blakemore, S-J., Oakley, D.A., and Frith, C.D. (2003). Delusions of alien control in the normal brain. *Neuropsychologia*, **41**, 1058–1067.

Blank, S.C., Scott, S.K., Murphy, K., Warburton, E., and Wise, R.J.S. (2002). Speech production: Wernicke, Broca and beyond. *Brain*, **125**, 1829–1838.

Bleuler, E. (1950). *Dementia Praecox; or the Group of Schizophrenias*. New York, International Universities Press.

Blouin, J-S., Bard, C., and Paillard, J. (2004). Contributions of the cerebellum to self-Initiated synchronized movements: A PET study. *Experimental Brain Research*, **155**, 63–68.

Bluhm, R.L., Miller, J., Lanius, R.A., Osuch, E.A., Boksman, K., Neufeld, R.W.J., Théberge, J., Schaefer, B., and Williamson, P. (2007). Spontaneous low-frequency fluctuations in the BOLD signal in schizophrenic patients: Anomalies in the default network. *Schizophrenia Research*, **33**, 1004–1012.

Blumberg, H.P., Stern, E., Martinez, D., Ricketts, S., de Asis, J., White, T., Epstein, J., McBride, P.A., Eidelberg, D., Kocsis, J.H., and Silbersweig, D.A. (2000). Increased anterior cingulate and caudate activity in bipolar mania. *Biological Psychiatry*, **48**, 1045–1052.

Blumberg, H.P., Stern, E., Ricketts, S., Martinez, D., de Asis, J., White, T., Epstein, J., Isenberg, N., McBride, P.A., Kemperman, I., Emmerich, S., Dhawan, V., Eidelberg, D., Kocsis, J.H., and Silbersweig, D.A. (1999). Rostral and orbital prefrontal cortex dysfunction in the manic state of bipolar disorder. *American Journal of Psychiatry*, **156**, 1986–1988.

Boccardi, M., Sabattoli, F., Laakso, M.P., Testa, C., Rossi, R., Beltramello, A., Soininen, H., and Frisoni, G.B. (2005). Frontotemporal dementia as a neural system disease. *Neurobiology of Aging*, **26**, 37–44.

Bogerts, B., Meertz, E., and Schonfeldt-Bausch, R. (1985). Basal ganglia and limbic system pathology in schizophrenia: A morphometric study of brain volume and shrinkage. *Archives of General Psychiatry*, **42**, 782–791.

Boivin, D.B. (2000). Influence of sleep-wake and circadian rhythm disturbances in psychiatric disorders. *Journal of Psychiatry and Neuroscience*, **25**, 446–458.

Boivin, D.B., Czeisler, C.A., Dijk, D.J., Duffy, J.F., Folkard, S., Minors, D.S., Totterdell, P., and Waterhouse, J.M. (1997). Complex interaction of the sleep-wake cycle and circadian phase modulates mood in healthy subjects. *Archives of General Psychiatry*, **54**, 145–152.

Boksman, K., Théberge, J., Neufeld, R.W.J., Williamson, P., Drost, D., Malla, A., Densmore, M., Takhar, J., Pavlosky, W., and Menon. R. (2005). A 4.0 Tesla fMRI study of brain connectivity during word fluency in first episode schizophrenia. *Schizophrenia Research*, **75**, 247–263.

Bond, J., Roberts, E., Mochida, G.H., Hampshire, D.J., Scott, S., Askham, J.M., Springel, K., Mahadevan, M., Crow, Y.J., Markham, A.F., Walsh, C.A., and Woods, C.G. (2002). ASPM is a major determinant of cerebral cortical size. *Nature Genetics*, **32**, 316–320.

Bora, E., Vahip, S., Gonul, A.S., Akdeniz, F., Alkan, M., Ogut, M., and Eryavuz, A. (2005). Evidence for theory of mind deficits in euthymic patients with bipolar disorder. *Acta Psychiatrica Scandinavica*, **112**, 110–116.

Bora, E., Yucel, M., and Pantelis, C. (2009). Theory of mind impairment in schizophrenia: Meta-analysis. *Schizophrenia Research*, **109**, 1–9.

Botvinick, M.M., Cohen, J.D., and Carter, C.S. (2004). Conflict monitoring and anterior cingulate cortex: An update. *Trends in Cognitive Sciences*, **8**, 539–546.

Bouhuys, A.L. (1991). Towards a model of mood responses to sleep deprivation in depressed patients. *Biological Psychiatry*, **29**, 600–612.

Bowen, D.M., Najlerahim, A., Procter, A.W., Francis, P.T., and Murphy, E. (1989). Circumscribed changes of the cerebral cortex in neuropsychiatric disorders of later life. *Proceedings of the National Academy of Sciences of the USA*, **86**, 9504–9508.

Boxer, A.L., and Miller, B.L. (2005). Clinical features of frontotemporal dementia. *Alzheimer Disease and Associated Disorders*, **19**, S3–S6.

Bradley, C. (1937). The behavior of children receiving Benzedrine. *American Journal of Psychiatry*, **94**, 577–585.

Bradshaw, G.A., Schore, A.N., Brown, J.L., Poole, J.H., and Moss, C.J. (2005). Elephant breakdown. Social trauma: Early disruption of attachment can affect the physiology, behavior and culture of animals and humans over generations. *Nature*, **433**, 807.

Braff, D.L., and Geyer, M.A. (1990). Sensorimotor gating and schizophrenia: human and animal model studies. *Archives of General Psychiatry*, **47**, 181–188.

Brans, R.G.H., van Haren, N.E.M., van Baal, C.M., Schnack, H.G., Kahn, R.S., and Hulshoff, H.E. (2008). Heritability of changes in brain volume over time in twin pairs discordant for schizophrenia. *Archives of General Psychiatry*, **65**, 1259–1268.

Brébion, G., Amador, X., David, A., Malaspina, D., Sharif, Z., and Gorman, J.M. (2000). Positive symptomatology and source-monitoring failure in schizophrenia: an analysis of symptom specific effects. *Psychiatry Research*, **95**, 119–131.

Breier, A., Su, T.P., Saunders, R., Carson, R.E., Kolachana, B.S., De Bartolomeis, A., Weinberger, D.R., Weisenfeld, N., Malholtra, A.K. Eckelman, W.C., and Pickar, D.

(1997). Schizophrenia is associated with elevated amphetamine-induced synaptic dopamine concentrations: Evidence from a novel positron emission tomography method. *Proceedings of the National Academy of Sciences of the USA*, **94**, 2569–2574.

Bremmer, M.A., Beekman, A.T., Deeg, D.J., Penninx, B.W., Dik, M.G., Hack, C.E., and Hoogendijk, W.J. (2008). Inflammatory markers in late-life depression: Results from a population-based study. *Journal of Affective Disorders*, **106**, 249–255.

Bremner, J.D., Innis, R.D., Salomon, R.M., Staib, L.H., Ng, C.K., Miller, H.L., Bronen, R.A., Krystal. J.H., Duncan, J., Rich, D., Price, L.H., Malison, R., Dey, H., Soufer, R., and Charney, D.S. (1997). Positron emission tomography measurement of cerebral metabolic correlates of tryptophan depletion-induced depressive relapse. *Archives of General Psychiatry*, **54**, 364–374.

Broe, M., Hodges, J.R., Schofield, E., Shephard, C.E., Kril, J.J., and Halliday, G.M. (2003). Staging disease severity in pathologically confirmed cases of frontotemporal dementia. *Neurology*, **60**, 1005–1011.

Brothers, L. (1990). The social brain: A project for investigating primate behavior and neurophysiology in a new domain. *Concepts in Neuroscience*, **1**, 27–51.

Brown, A.B., Biederman, J., Valera, E.M., Doyle, A.E., Bush, G., Spencer, T., Monuteaux, M.C., Mick, E., Whitfield-Gabrieli, S., Makris, N., LaViolette, P.S., Oscar-Berman, M., Faraone, S.V., and Siedman, L.J. (2010). Effect of dopamine transporter gene (SLC6A3) variation on dorsal anterior cingulate function in attention-deficit/hyperactivity disorder. *American Journal of Medical Genetics Part B: Neuropsychiatric Genetics*, **153B**, 365–375.

Brown, A.S., Hooton, J., Schaefer, C.A., Zhang, H., Petkova, E., Babulas, V., Perrin, M., Gorman, J.M., and Susser, E.R. (2004). Elevated maternal interleukin-8 levels and risk of schizophrenia in adult offspring. *American Journal of Psychiatry,* **161,** 889–895.

Brown, T.E. (2009). *ADHD Comorbidities: Handbook for ADHD Complications in Children and Adults.* Washington, D.C., American Psychiatric Publishing, Inc.

Broyd, S.J., Demanuele, C., Debener, S., Helps, S.K., James, C.J., and Sonuga-Barke, E.J.S. (2009). Default-mode brain dysfunction in mental disorders: A systematic review. *Neuroscience and Biobehavioral Reviews*, **33**, 279–296.

Brüne, M. (2005). 'Theory of mind' in schizophrenia: A review of the literature. *Schizophrenia Bulletin*, **31**, 21–42.

Brüne, M. (2003). Social cognition and behaviour in schizophrenia. In M. Brune, H. Ribbert, and W. Schiefenhövel (Eds.), *The Social Brain: Evolution and Pathology* (pp. 277–313). Chichester, West Sussex, England, John Wiley and Sons.

Brunet-Gouet, E., and Decety, J. (2006). Social brain dysfunction in schizophrenia: A review of neuroimaging studies. *Psychiatry Research: Neuroimaging*, **148**, 75–92.

Bucan, M., Abrahams, B.S., Wang, K., Glessner, J.T., Herman, E.I., Sonnenblick, L.I., Alvarez Retuerto, A.I., Imielinski, M., Hadley, D., Bradfield, J.P., Kim, C., Gidaya, N.B., Lindquist, I., Hutman, T., Sigman, M., Kustanovich, V., Lajonchere, C.M., Singleton, A., Kim, J., Wassink, T.H., McMahon, W.M., Owley, T., Sweeney, J.A., Coon, H., Nurnberger, J.I., Jr., Li, M., Cantor, R.M., Minshew, N.J., Sutcliffe, J.S., Cook, E.H., Dawson, G., Buxbaum, J.D., Grant, S.F.A., Schellenberg, G.D., Geschwind, D.H., and Hakonarson, H. (2009). Genome-wide analyses of exonic copy number variants in a family-based study point to novel autism susceptibility genes. *PLoS Genetics,* **5,** 1–12.

Büchel, C., Raedler, T., Sommer, M., Sach, M., Weiller, C., and Koch, M.A. (2004). White matter asymmetry in the human brain: A diffusion tensor MRI study. *Cerebral Cortex*, **14**, 945–951.

Buchsbaum, M.S., and Hazlett, E.A. (1998). Positron emission tomography studies of abnormal glucose metabolism in schizophrenia. *Schizophrenia Bulletin*, **24**, 343–364.

Buchsbaum, M.S., Tang, C.Y., Peled, S., Gudbjartsson, H., Lu, D., Hazlett, E.A., Downhill, J., Haznedar, M., Fallon, J.H., and Atlas, S.W. (1998). MRI white matter diffusion anisotropy and PET metabolic rate in schizophrenia. *NeuroReport*, **9**, 425–430.

Buckley, P.F., Moore, C., Long, H., Larkin, C., Thompson, P., Mulvany-Redmond, O., Stack, J.P., Ennis, J.T., and Waddington, J.L. (1994). ^{1}H-magnetic resonance spectroscopy of the left temporal and frontal lobes in schizophrenia: Clinical, neurodevelopmental and cognitive correlates. *Biological Psychiatry*, **36**, 792–800.

Buckner, R.L., Andrews-Hanna, J.R., and Schacter, D.L. (2008). The brain's default network: Anatomy, function, and relevance to disease. *Annals of the New York Academy of Sciences*, **1124**, 1–38.

Buckner, R.L., and Carroll, D.C. (2007). Self-projection and the brain. *Trends in Cognitive Sciences*, **11**, 49–57.

Budhani, S., Marsh, A.A., Pine, D.S., and Blair, R.J.R. (2007). Neural correlates of response reversal: Considering acquisition. *NeuroImage*, **34**, 1754–1765.

Buitelaar, J.K., and Willemsen-Swinkels, S.H.N. (2000). Medication treatment in subjects with autistic spectrum disorders. *European Child and Adolescent Psychiatry*, **9**, I/85–I/97.

Buka, S.L., and Fan, A.P. (1999). Association of prenatal and perinatal complications with subsequent bipolar disorder and schizophrenia. *Schizophrenia Research*, **39**, 113–119.

Bulik, C.M., Slof-Op't Landt, M.C.T., van Furth, E.F., and Sullivan, P.F. (2007). The genetics of anorexia nervosa. *Annual Review of Nutrition,* **27**, 263–275.

Bullmore, E., Brammer, M., Harvey, I., Murray, R., and Ron, M. (1995). Cerebral hemispheric asymmetry revisited: Effects of handedness, gender and schizophrenia measured by radius of gyration in magnetic resonance images. *Psychological Medicine*, **25**, 349–363.

Bullmore, E.T., Frangou, S., and Murray, R.M. (1997). The dysplastic net hypothesis: an integration of developmental and dysconnectivity theories of schizophrenia. *Schizophrenia Research*, **28**, 143–156.

Bunney, W.E., and Davis, J.M. (1965). Norepinephrine in depressive reactions: A review. *Archives of General Psychiatry*, **13**, 483–494.

Burgess, P.W., Dumontheil, I., and Gilbert, S.J. (2007). The gateway hypothesis of prefrontal cortex (area 10) function. *Trends in Cognitive Sciences*, **11**, 290–298.

Burki, F., and Kaessmann, H. (2004). Birth and adaptive evolution of a hominoid gene that supports high neurotransmitter flux. *Nature Genetics*, **36**, 1061–1063.

Burns, J., Job, D., Bastin, M.E., Whalley, H., MacGillivray, T., Johnstone, E.C., and Lawrie, S.M. (2003). Structural disconnectivity in schizophrenia: a diffusion tensor magnetic resonance imaging study. *British Journal of Psychiatry*, **182**, 439–443.

Burns, J.K. (2004). An evolutionary theory of schizophrenia: Cortical connectivity, metarepresentation, and the social brain. *Behavioral and Brain Sciences*, **27**, 831–885.

Burns, J.K. (2006). Psychosis: A costly by-product of social brain evolution in *Homo sapiens*. *Progress in Neuro-psychopharmacology and Biological Psychiatry*, **30**, 797–814.

Bush, E.C., and Allman, J.M. (2004). The scaling of frontal cortex in primates and carnivores. *Proceedings of the National Academy of Sciences of the USA*, **101**, 3962–3966.

Bush, G., Frazier, J.A., Rauch, S.L., Seidman, L.J., Whalen, P.J., Jenike, M.A., Rosen, B.R., and Biederman J. (1999). Anterior cingulate cortex dysfunction in attention-deficit/hyperactivity disorder revealed by fMRI and the counting Stroop. *Biological Psychiatry,* **45**, 1542–1552.

Bush, G., Luu, P., and Posner, M.I. (2000). Cognitive and emotional influences in anterior cingulate cortex. *Trends in Cognitive Sciences*, **4**, 215–222.

Butler, P.D., Abeles, I.Y., Weiskopf, N.G., Tambini, A., Jalbrzikowski, M., Legatt, M.E., Zemon, V., Loughead, J., Gur, R.C., and Javitt, D.C. (2009). Sensory contributions to impaired emotion processing in schizophrenia. *Schizophrenia Bulletin,* **35,** 1095–1107.

Buxhoeveden, D.P., and Casanova, M.F. (2002). The minicolumn and the evolution of the brain. *Brain, Behaviour and Evolution*, **60**, 125–151.

Byne, W., Hazlett, E.A., Buchsbaum, M.S., and Kemether, E. (2009). The thalamus and schizophrenia: Current status of research. *Acta Neuropathologica,* **117**, 347–368.

Cabeza, R., and Nyberg, L. (2000). Neural basis of learning and memory: Functional neuroimaging evidence. *Current Opinion in Neurology,* **13**, 415–421.

Cáceres, M., Lachuer, J., Zapala, M.A., Redmond, J.C., Kudo, L., Geschwind, D.H., Lockhart, D.J., Preuss, T.M., and Barlow, C. (2003). Elevated gene expression levels distinguish human from non-human primate brains. *Proceedings of the National Academy of Science of the USA*, **100**, 13030–13035.

Cáceres, M., Suwyn, C., Maddox, M., Thomas, J.W., and Preuss, T.D. (2007). Increased cortical expression of two synaptogenic thrombospondins in human brain evolution. *Cerebral Cortex*, **17**, 2312–2321.

Cahn, W., Hulshoff, H.E., Lems, E.B.T.E., van Haren, N.E.M., Schnack, H.G., van der Linden, J.A., Schothorst, P.F., van Engeland, H., and Kahn, R.S. (2002). Brain volume changes in first-episode schizophrenia: A 1-year follow-up study. *Archives of General Psychiatry*, **59**, 1002–1010.

Cahn, W., van Haren, N.E.M., Hulshoff Pol, H.E., Schnack, H.G., Caspers, E., Laponder, D.A.J., and Kahn, R.S. (2006). Brain volume changes in the first year of illness and 5-year outcome of schizophrenia. *British Journal of Psychiatry*, **189**, 381–382.

Calabrese, G., Deicken, R.F., Fein, P., Merrin, E.L., Schoenfeld, F., and Weiner, M.W. (1992). ^{31}Phosphorus magnetic resonance spectroscopy of the temporal lobes in schizophrenia. *Biological Psychiatry,* **32**, 26–32.

Calhoun, V.D., Kiehl, K.A., Liddle, P.F., and Pearlson, G.D. (2004). Aberrant localization of synchronous hemodynamic activity in auditory cortex reliably characterizes schizophrenia. *Biological Psychiatry*, **55**, 842–849.

Call, J., and Tomasella, M. (2008). Does the chimpanzee have a theory of mind? 30 years later. *Trends in Cognitive Sciences*, **12**, 187–192.

Callicott, J.H., Bertolino, A., Egan, M.F., Mattay, V.S., Langheim, F.J.P., and Weinberger, D.R. (2000). Selective relationship between prefrontal N-acetylaspartate measures and negative symptoms. *American Journal of Psychiatry*, **157**, 1646–1651.

Campbell, D.B., Sutcliffe, J.S., Ebert, P.J., Militerni, R., Bravaccio, C., Trillo, S., Elia, M., Schneider, C., Melmed, R., Sacco, R., Persico, A.M., and Levitt, P. (2006). A genetic variant that disrupts *MET* transcription is associated with autism. *Proceedings of the National Academy of Sciences of the USA*, **103**, 16834–16839.

Campbell, S., Marriott, M., Nahmias, C., and MacQueen, G.M. (2004). Lower hippocampal volume in patients suffering from depression: A meta-analysis. *American Journal of Psychiatry*, **161**, 598–607.

Cannon, D.M., Carson, R.E., Nugent, A.C., Eckelman, W.C., Kiesewetter, D.O., Williams, J., Rollis, D., Drevets, M., Gandhi, S., Solorio, G., and Drevets, W.C. (2006). Reduced muscarinic type 2 receptor binding in subjects with bipolar disorder. *Archives of General Psychiatry*, **63**, 741–747.

Cannon, D.M., Ichise, M., Rollis, D., Klaver, J.M., Gander, S.K., Charney, D.S., Manji, H.K., and Drevets, W.C. (2007). Elevated serotonin transporter binding in major depressive disorder assessed using positron emission tomography and [^{11}C] DASB; comparison with bipolar disorder. *Biological Psychiatry*, **62**, 870–877.

Cannon, T.D., van Erp, T.G.M., Huttunen, M., lonnqvist, J., Salonen, O., Valanne, L., Poutanen, V-P., Standertskjold-Nordenstam, C-G., Gur, R.E., and Yan, M. (1998). Regional gray matter, white matter, and cerebrospinal fluid distributions in schizophrenic patients, their siblings, and controls. *Archives of General Psychiatry*, **55**, 1084–1091.

Cardno, A.G., and Gottesman, I.I. (2000). Twin studies of schizophrenia: From bow-and-arrow concordances to Star Wars Mx and functional genomics. *American Journal of Medical Genetics*, **97**, 12–17.

Carlsson, A. (1988). The current status of the dopamine hypothesis of schizophrenia. *Neuropsychopharmacology*, **1**, 179–186.

Carroll, S.B. (2003). Genetics and the making of *Homo sapiens*. *Nature*, **422**, 849–857.

Carter, J.R., and Neufeld, R.W.J. (1999). Cognitive processing of multidimensional stimuli in schizophrenia: Formal modeling of judgment speed and content. *Journal of Abnormal Psychology*, **108**, 633–654.

Carter, C.S., Perlstein, W., Ganguli, R., Brar, J., Mintun, M., and Cohen, J.D. (1998). Functional hypofrontality and working memory dysfunction in schizophrenia. *American Journal of Psychiatry*, **155**, 1285–1287.

Casanova, M.F., van Kooten, I.A.J., Switala, A.E., Engeland, H., Heinsen, H., Steinbusch, H.W.M., Hof, P.R., Trippe, J., Stone, J., and Schmitz, C. (2006). Minicolumnar abnormalities in autism. *Acta Neuropathologica*, **112**, 287–303.

Castelli, F., Frith, C., Happé, F., and Frith, U. (2002). Autism, Asperger syndrome, and brain mechanisms for the attribution of mental states to animated shapes. *Brain*, **125**, 1839–1849.

Cecil, K.M., Lenkinski, R.E., Gur, R.E., and Gur, R.C. (1999). Proton magnetic resonance spectroscopy in the frontal and temporal lobes of neuroleptic naive patients with schizophrenia. *Neuropsychopharmacology*, **20**, 131–140.

Chae, T.H., and Walsh, C.A. (2007). Genes that control the size of the cerebral cortex. *Novartis Foundation Symposium,* **288,** 79–90.

Chai, X., Förster, E., Zhao, S., Bock, H.H., and Frotscher, M. (2009). Reelin acts as a stop signal for radially migrating neurons by inducing phosphorylation of n-cofilin at the leading edge. *Communicative & Integrative Biology,* **2,** 375–377.

Chalfonte, B.L., and Johnson, M.K. (1996). Feature memory and binding in young and older adults. *Memory and Cognition*, **24**, 403–416.

Chalmers, D.J. (1996). *The Conscious Mind: In Search of a Fundamental Theory*. New York, Oxford University Press.

Chandana, S.R., Behen, M.E., Juhász, C., Muzik, O., Rothermel, R.D., Manger, T.J., Chakraborty, P.K., Chugani, H.T., and Chugani, D.C. (2005). Significance of abnormalities in developmental trajectory and asymmetry of cortical serotonin synthesis in autism. *International Journal of Developmental Neuroscience*, **23**, 171–182.

Chapple, B., Grech, A., Sham, P., Toulopoulo, T., Walshe, M., Schulze, K., Morgan, K., Murray, R.M., and McDonald, C. (2004). Normal cerebral asymmetry in familial and non-familial schizophrenic probands and their unaffected relatives. *Schizophrenia Research*, **67**, 33–40.

Christoff, K., Ream, J.M., Geddes, L.P.T., and Gabrieli, J.D.E. (2003). Evaluating self-generated information: Anterior prefrontal contributions to human cognition. *Behavioral Neuroscience*, **117**, 1161–1168.

Christoph, G.R., Leonzio, R.J., and Wilcox, K.S. (1986). Stimulation of the lateral habenula inhibits dopamine-containing neurons in the substantia nigra and ventral tegmental area of the rat. *Journal of Neuroscience,* **6**, 613–619.

Christopherson, K.S., Ullian, E.M., Stokes, C.C.A., Mullowney, C.E., Hell, J.W., Agah, A., Lawler, J., Mosher, D.F., Bornstein, P., and Barres, B.A. (2005). Thrombospondins are astrocyte-secreted proteins that promote CNS synaptogenesis. *Cell,* **120**, 421–433.

Chubb, J.E., Bradshaw, N.J., Soares, D.C., Porteous, D.J., and Millar, J.K. (2008). The DISC locus in psychiatric illness. *Molecular Psychiatry,* **13**, 36–64.

Chugani, D.C., Muzik, O., Behen, M., Rothermel, R., Janisse, J.J., Lee, J., and Chugani, H.T. (1999). Developmental changes in brain serotonin synthesis capacity in autistic and nonautistic children. *Annals of Neurology*, **45**, 287–295.

Chow, T.W., Miller, B.L., Hayashi, V.N., and Geschwind, D.H. (1999). Inheritance of frontotemporal dementia. *Archives of Neurology*, **56**, 817–822.

Chowdari, K.V., Mirnics, K., Semwal, P., Wood, J., Lawrence, E., Bhatia, T., Deshpande, S.N., Thelma, B.K., Ferrell, R.E., Middleton. F.A., Devlin, B., Levitt, P., Lewis, D.A., and Nimgaonkar, V.L. (2002). Association and linkage analysis of *RGS4* polymorphisms in schizophrenia. *Human Molecular Genetics*, **11**, 1373–1380.

Chugani, D.C., Sundram, B., Behen, M., Lee, M.-L., and Moore, G.J. (1999). Evidence of altered energy metabolism in autistic children. *Progress in Neuro-psychopharmacology and Biological Psychiatry*, **23**, 635–641.

Churchland, P.S. (2002). Self-representation in nervous systems. *Science*, **296**, 308–310.

Ciompi, L. (1980). The natural history of schizophrenia in the long term. *British Journal of Psychiatry*, **136**, 413–420.

Clark, A.G., Glanowski, G., Nielson, R., Thomas, P.D., Kejariwal, A., Todd, M.A., Tannenbaum, D.M, Civello, D., Lu, F., Murphy, B., Ferriera, S., Wang, G., Zheng, X., White, T.J., Sninsky, J., Adams, M.D., and Cargill, M. (2003). Inferring nonneutral evolution from human-chimp-mouse orthologous gene trios. *Science*, **302**, 1960–1963.

Clark, L., Bechara, A., Damasio, H., Aitken, M.R.F., Sahakian, B.J., and Robbins, T.W. (2008). Differential effects of insular and ventromedial prefrontal cortex lesions on risky decision-making. *Brain,* **131**, 1311–1322.

Clark, L., and Goodwin, G.M. (2004). State- and trait-related deficits in sustained attention in bipolar disorder. *European Archives of Psychiatry and Clinical Neuroscience*, **254**, 61–68.

Cleeremans, A. (2003). *The Unity of Consciousness: Binding, Integration, and Dissociation,* New York, Oxford University Press.

Cody, H., Pelphrey, K., and Piven, J. (2002). Structural and functional magnetic resonance imaging of autism. *International Journal of Developmental Neuroscience*, **20**, 421–438.

Cole, M.W., and Schneider, W. (2007). The cognitive control network: Integrated cortical regions with dissociable functions. *NeuroImage*, **37**, 343–360.

Cole, M.W., Yeung, N., Freiwald, W.A., and Botvinick, M. (2009). Cingulate cortex: Diverging data from humans and monkeys. *Trends in Neurosciences*, **32**, 566–574.

Colombo, M., and Graziano, M. (1994). Effects of auditory and visual interference on auditory-visual delayed matching to sample in monkeys. *Behavioral Neuroscience*, **108**, 636–639.

Constantinidis, C., Williams, G.V., and Goldman-Rakic, P.S. (2002). A role for inhibition in shaping the temporal flow of information in prefrontal cortex. *Nature Neuroscience*, **5**, 175–180.

Copolov, D.L., Seal, M.L., Maruff, P., Ulusoy, R., Wong, M.T.H., Tochon-Danguy, H.J., and Egan, G.F. (2003). Cortical activation associated with the experience of auditory hallucinations and perception of human speech in schizophrenia: A PET correlation study. *Psychiatry Research: Neuroimaging*, **122**, 139–152.

Corbetta, M., and Shulman, G.L. (2002). Controls of goal-directed and stimulus-driven attention in the brain. *Nature Reviews Neuroscience*, **3**, 201–215.

Cornblatt, B.A., and Keilp, J.G. (1994). Impaired attention, genetics, and the pathophysiology of schizophrenia. *Schizophrenia Bulletin*, **20**, 31–46.

Coryell, W., Leon, A.C., Turvey, C., Akiskal, H.S., Mueller, T., and Endicott, J. (2001). The significance of psychotic features in manic episodes: A report from the NIMH collaborative study. *Journal of Affective Disorders*, **67**, 79–88.

Coryell, W., Scheftner, W., Keller, M., Endicott, J., Maser, J., and Klerman, G.L. (1993). The enduring psychosocial consequences of mania and depression. *American Journal of Psychiatry*, **150**, 720–727.

Courchesne, E., Karns, C.M., Davis, H.R., Ziccardi, R., Carper, R.A., Tigue, Z.D., Chisum, H.J., Moses, P., Pierce, K., Lord, C., Lincoln, A.J., Pizzo, S., Schreibman, L., Haas, R.H., Akshoomoff, N.A., and Courchesne, R.Y. (2001). Unusual brain growth patterns in early life in patients with autistic disorder. *Neurology*, **57**, 245–254.

Craddock, N., and Owen, M.J. (2010). The Kraepelinian dichotomy: going, going…but still not gone. *British Journal of Psychiatry*, **196**, 92–95.

Craig, A.D. (2003). A new view of pain as a homeostatic emotion. *Trends in Neurosciences,* **26**, 303–307.

Craig, A.D. (2005). Forebrain emotional asymmetry: A neuroanatomical basis? *Trends in Cognitive Sciences*, **9**, 566–571.

Craig, A.D. (2009). How do you feel—now? The anterior insula and human awareness. *Nature Reviews Neuroscience,* **10**, 59–70.

Craik, F.I.M., Moroz, T.M., Moscovitch, M., Stuss, D.T., Winocur, G., Tulving, E., and Kapur, S. (1999). In search of the self: A positron emission tomography study. *Psychological Science*, **10**, 26–34.

Crawford, J.R., Obonsawin, M.C., and Bremner, M. (1993). Frontal lobe impairment in schizophrenia: Relationship to intellectual functioning. *Psychological Medicine*, **23**, 787–790.

Crespi, B., and Badcock, C. (2008). Psychosis and autism as diametrical disorders of the social brain. *Behavioral and Brain Sciences*, **31**, 241–320.

Crespi, B., Summers, K., and Dorus, S. (2007). Adaptive evolution of genes underlying schizophrenia. *Proceedings of the Royal Society B,* **274,** 2801–2810.

Crick, F. (1984). Function of the thalamic reticular complex: The searchlight hypothesis. *Proceedings of the National Academy of Sciences of the USA*, **81**, 4586–4590.

Crick, F.C., and Koch, C. (2005). What is the function of the claustrum? *Philosophical Transactions of the Royal Society B*, **360**, 1271–1279.

Critchley, H.D., Corfield, D.R., Chandler, M.P., Mathias, C.J., and Dolan, R.J. (2001). Cerebral correlates of autonomic cardiovascular arousal: A functional neuroimaging investigation in humans, *Journal of Physiology*, **523**, 259–270.

Critchley, H.D., Daly, E.M., Bullmore, E.T., Williams, S.C.R., Van Amelsvoort, T., Robertson, D.M., Rowe, A., Phillips, M., McAlonam, G., Howlin, P., and Murphy, D.G.M. (2000). The functional neuroanatomy of social behaviour: Changes in cerebral blood flow when people with autistic disorder process facial expressions. *Brain*, **123**, 2203–2312.

Critchley, H.D., Mathias, J., and Dolan, R.J. (2001). Neural activity in the human brain relating to uncertainty and arousal during anticipation. *Neuron,* **29**, 537–545.

Crow, T.J. (1990a). The continuum of psychosis and its genetic origins: The sixty-fifth Maudsley lecture. *British Journal of Psychiatry*, **156**, 788–797.

Crow, T.J. (1990b). Temporal lobe asymmetries as the key to the etiology of schizophrenia. *Schizophrenia Bulletin*, **16**, 433–443.

Crow, T.J. (1995). A Darwinian approach to the origins of psychosis. *British Journal of Psychiatry*, **167**, 12–25.

Crow, T.J. (1997a). Schizophrenia as failure of hemispheric dominance for language. *Trends in Neuroscience*, **20**, 339–343.

Crow, T.J. (1997b). Is schizophrenia the price that *Homo sapiens* pays for language? *Schizophrenia Research*, **28**, 127–141.

Crow, T.J. (1998). Schizophrenia as a transcallosal misconnection syndrome. *Schizophrenia Research*, **30**, 111–114.

Cullen, T.J., Walker, M.A., Eastwood, S.L., Esiri, M.M., Harrison, P.J., and Crow, T.J. (2006). Anomalies of asymmetry of pyramidal cell density and structure in dorsolateral prefrontal cortex in schizophrenia. *British Journal of Psychiatry*, **188**, 26–31.

Cullheim, S., and Thams, S. (2007). The microglial networks of the brain and their role in neuronal network plasticity after lesion. *Brain Research Reviews,* **55,** 89–96.

Dalgleish, T. (2004). The emotional brain. *Nature Reviews Neuroscience*, **5**, 582–589.

Damasio, A. (1999). *The Feeling of What Happens: Body and Emotion in the Making of Consciousness.* New York, Harcourt Brace and Company.

Damasio, A.R., and Van Hoesen, G.W. (1983). Focal lesions of the limbic frontal lobe. In K.M. Heilman and P. Satz (Eds.), *Neuropsychology of Human Emotion* (pp. 85–110). New York, Guilford Press.

Damasio, H., Tranel, D., Grabowski, T., Adolphs, R., and Damasio, A. (2004). Neural systems behind word and concept retrieval. *Cognition*, **92**, 179–229.

Danion, J.M., Rizzo, L., and Bruant, A. (1999). Functional mechanisms underlying impaired recognition memory and conscious awareness in patients with schizophrenia. *Archives of General Psychiatry*, **56**, 639–644.

Dantzer, R., Bluthe, R., Castanon, N., Kelly, K., Konsman, J.P., Laye, S., Lestage, J., and Parnet, P. (2007). Cytokines, sickness behavior and depression. In R. Ader (Ed.), *Psychoneuroimmunology* (4th ed., pp. 281–318). Amsterdam, Elsevier.

Dao-Castellana, M.H., Paillèere-Martinot, M.L., Hantraye, P., Attar-Lévy, D., Rémy, P., Crouzel, C., Artiges, E., Féline, A., Syrota, A., and Martinot, J.L. (1997). Presynaptic dopaminergic function in the striatum of schizophrenic patients. *Schizophrenia Research*, **23**, 167–174.

Daprati, E., Franck, N., Georgieff, N., Proust, J., Pacherie, E., Dalery, J., and Jeannerod, M. (1997). Looking for agent: An investigation into consciousness of action and self-consciousness in schizophrenic patients. *Cognition*, **65**, 71–86.

Dapretto, M., Davies, M.S., Pfeifer, J.H., Scott, M.A., Sigman, M., Bookheimer, S.Y., and Iacoboni, M. (2006). Understanding emotions in others: Mirror neuron dysfunction in children with autism spectrum disorders. *Nature Neuroscience*, **9**, 28–30.

Darwin, C. (1886). *The Principal Works of Charles Darwin: The Origin of the Species, Descent of Man.* New York, J.B. Alden. Davidson, L.L., and Heinrichs, R.W. (2002). Quantification of frontal and temporal lobe brain-imaging findings in schizophrenia: A meta-analysis. *Psychiatry Research: Neuroimaging*, **122**, 69–87.

Davidson, L.L., and Heinrichs, R.W. (2003). Quantification of frontal and temporal lobe brain-imaging findings in schizophrenia: A meta-analysis. *Psychiatry Research: Neuroimaging*, **122**, 69–87.

Davis, K.L., Kahn, R.S., Ko, G., and Davidson, M. (1991). Dopamine in schizophrenia: A review and reconceptualization. *American Journal of Psychiatry*, **148**, 1474–1486.

Davis, K.L., Stewart, D.G., Friedman, J.I., Buchsbaum, M., Harvey, P.D., Hof, P.R., Buxbaum, J., and Haroutunian, V. (2003). White matter changes in schizophrenia: evidence for myelin-related dysfunction. *Archives of General Psychiatry*, **60**, 443–456.

Davis, M., and Whalen, P.J. (2001). The amygdala: Vigilance and emotion. *Molecular Psychiatry*, **6**, 13–34.

Deakin, J.F.W., Slater, P., Simpson, M.D.C., Gilchrist, A.C., Skan, W.J., Royston, M.C., Reynolds, G.P., and Cross, A.J. (1989). Frontal cortical and left temporal glutamatergic dysfunction in schizophrenia. *Journal of Neurochemistry*, **52**, 1781–1786.

Dehaene, S., Kerszberg, M., and Changeux, J.-P. (1998). A neuronal model of a global workspace in effortful cognitive tasks. *Proceedings of the National Academy of Sciences of the USA*, **95**, 14529–14534.

Dehaene-Lambertz, G., Hertz-Pannier, L., and Dubois, J. (2006). Nature and nurture in language acquisition: Anatomical and functional brain-imaging studies in infants. *Trends in Neurosciences*, **29**, 367–373.

Deicken, R.F., Calabrese, G., Merris, E.L., Meyerhoff, D.J., Dillon, W.P., Weiner, M.W., and Fein, G. (1994). ^{31}Phosphorus magnetic resonance spectroscopy of the frontal and parietal lobes in chronic schizophrenia. *Biological Psychiatry*, **36**, 503–510.

Deicken, R.F., Pegues, M., and Amend, D. (1999). Reduced hippocampal N-acetylaspartate without volume loss in schizophrenia. *Schizophrenia Research*, **37**, 217–223.

Deicken, R.F., Zhou, L., Schuff, N., Fein, G., and Weiner, M.W. (1998). Hippocampal neuronal dysfunction in schizophrenia as measured by proton magnetic resonance spectroscopy. *Biological Psychiatry*, **43**, 483–488.

del Rio, M.R., and DeFelipe, J. (1997). Colocalization of parvalbumin and calbindin D-28k in neurons including chandelier cells of the human temporal neocortex. *Journal of Chemical Neuroanatomy*, **12**, 165–173.

Delamillieure, P., Constans, J-M., Fernandez, J., Brazo, P., Benali, K., Courthéoux, P., Thibaut, F., Petit, M., and Dollfus, S. (2002). Proton magnetic resonance spectroscopy (^{1}H MRS) in schizophrenia: Investigation of the right and left hippocampus, thalamus, and prefrontal cortex. *Schizophrenia Bulletin*, **28**, 329–339.

Delamillieure, P., Fernandez, J., Coustans, J-M., Brazo, P., Benalo, K., Abadie, P., Vasse, T., Thibaut, F., Courtleoux, P., Petit, M., and Dollfus, S. (2000). Proton magnetic resonance spectroscopy of the medial prefrontal cortex in patients with deficit schizophrenia: Preliminary report. *American Journal of Psychiatry*, **157**, 641–643.

DeLisi, L.E. (2000). Critical overview of current approaches to genetic mechanisms in schizophrenia research. *Brain Research Reviews*, **31**, 187–192.

DeLisi, L.E. (2008). The concept of progressive brain change in schizophrenia: Implications for understanding schizophrenia. *Schizophrenia Bulletin*, **34**, 312–321.

DeLisi, L.E., Sakuma, M., Kushner, M., Finer, D.L., Hoff, A.L., and Crow, T.J. (1997). Anomalous cerebral asymmetry and language processing in schizophrenia. *Schizophrenia Bulletin*, **23**, 255–271.

Delisi, L.E., Tew, W., Xie, S., Hoff, A.L., Sakuma, M., Kushner, M., Lee, G., Shedlack, K., Smith, A.M., and Grimson, R. (1995). A prospective follow-up study of brain morphology and cognition in first-episode schizophrenic patients: preliminary findings. *Biological Psychiatry*, **38**, 349–360.

De Luca, M., Beckmann, C.F., De Stefano, N., Matthews, P.M., and Smith, S.M. (2006). fMRI resting state networks define distinct modes of long-distance interactions in the human brain. *NeuroImage*, **29**, 1359–1367.

den Ouden, H.E.M., Frith, U., and Blakemore, S.-J. (2005). Thinking about intentions. *NeuroImage*, **28**, 787–796.

de Quervain, D. J.-F., Fischbacher, U., Treyer, V., Schellhammer, M., Schnyder, U., Buck, A., and Fehr, E. (2004). The neural basis of altruistic punishment. *Science,* **305**, 1254–1258.

Desco, M., Gispert, J.D., Reig, S., Sanz, J., Pascau, J., Sarramea, F., Benito, C., Santos, A., Palomo, T., and Molina, V. (2003). Cerebral metabolic patterns in chronic and recent-onset schizophrenia. *Psychiatry Research*, **122**, 125–135.

Deutch, A.Y. (1993). Prefrontal cortical dopamine systems and the elaboration of functional corticostriatal circuits: Implications for schizophrenia and Parkinson's disease. *Journal of Neural Transmission*, **91**, 197–221.

Devinsky, O., and Luciano, D. (1993). The contributions of the anterior cingulate cortex to human behaviour. In B.A. Vogt and M. Gabriel (Eds.), *Neurobiology of the Cortex and Limbic Thalamus* (pp. 527–556). Boston, Birkhauser.

Devinsky, O., Morrell, M.J., and Vogt, B.A. (1995). Contributions of the anterior cingulate cortex to behaviour. *Brain*, **118**, 279–306.

DeVito, T.J., Drost, D.J., Neufeld, R.W.J., Rajakumar, N., Pavlosky, W., Williamson, P., and Nicolson, R. (2007). Evidence for cortical dysfunction in autism: A proton magnetic resonance spectroscopic imaging study. *Biological Psychiatry*, **61**, 465–473.

Dewey, S.L., Smith, G.S., Logan, J., Alexoff, D., Ding, Y.S., King, P., Pappas, N., Brodie, J., and Ashley, C.R. (1995). Serotonergic modulation of striatal dopamine measured with positron emission tomography (PET) and in vivo microdialysis. *Journal of Neuroscience*, **15**, 821–829.

Diehl-Schmid, J., Grimmer, T., Drzezga, A., Bornschein, S., Riemenschneider, M., Förstl, H., Schwaiger, M., and Kurz, A. (2007). Decline of cerebral glucose metabolism in frontotemporal dementia: A longitudinal 18F-FDG-PET-study. *Neurobiology of Aging*, **28**, 42–50.

Di Martino, D., Shehzad, Z., Kelly, C., Roy, A.K., Gee, D.G., Uddin, L.Q., Gotimer, K., Klein, D.F., Castellanos, F.X., and Milham, M.P. (2009). Relationship between cingulo-insular functional connectivity and autistic traits in neurotypical adults. *American Journal of Psychiatry*, **166**, 891–899.

Doja, A., and Roberts, W. (2006). Immunizations and autism: A review of the literature. *Canadian Journal of Neurological Sciences*, **33**, 341–346.

Dorph-Petersen, K.-A., Caric, D., Saghafi, R., Zhang, W., Sampson, A.R., and Lewis, D.A. (2009). Volume and neuron number of the lateral geniculate nucleus in schizophrenia and mood disorders. *Acta Neuropathologica*, **177**, 369–384.

Dorph-Petersen, K.-A., Pierri, J.N., Wu, Q., Sampson, A.R., and Lewis, D.A. (2007). Primary visual cortex volume and total neuron number are reduced in schizophrenia. *Journal of Comparative Neurology,* **501,** 290–301.

Dosenbach, N.U.F., Visscher, K.M, Palmer, E.D., Miezin, F.M., Wenger, K.K., Kang, H.C., Burgund, E.D., Grimes, A.L., Schlaggar, B.L., and Petersen, S.E. (2006). A core system for the implementation of task sets. *Neuron*, **50**, 799–812.

Drevets, W.C. (2000). Neuroimaging studies of mood disorders. *Biological Psychiatry*, **48,** 813–829.

Drevets, W.C. (2007). Orbitofrontal cortex function and structure in depression. *Annals of the New York Academy of Sciences*, **1121**, 499–527.

Drevets, W.C. (1999). Prefrontal cortical-amygdalar metabolism in major depression. *Annals of the New York Academy of Sciences*, **877**, 614–637.

Drevets, W.C. (2003). Neuroimaging abnormalities in the amygdala in mood disorders. *Annals of the New York Academy of Sciences*, **985**, 420–444.

Drevets, W.C., Gautier, C., Price, J.C., Kupfer, D.J., Kinahan, P.E., Grace, A.A., Price, J.L., and Mathis, C.A. (2001). Amphetamine-induced dopamine release in human ventral striatum correlates with euphoria. *Biological Psychiatry*, **49**, 81–96.

Drevets, W.C., Price, J.L., Bardgett, M.E., Reich, T., Todd, R.D., and Raichle, M.E. (2002). Glucose metabolism in the amygdala in depression: Relationship to diagnostic subtype and plasma cortisol levels. *Pharmacology, Biochemistry and Behaviour*, **71**, 431–447.

Drevets, W.C., Price, J.L., Simpson, J.R., Todd, R.D., Reich, T., Vannier, M., and Raichle, M.E. (1997). Subgenual prefrontal abnormalities in mood disorders. *Nature*, **386**, 824–827.

Duan, X., Chang, J.H., Ge, S., Faulkner, R.L., Kim, J.Y., Kitabatake, Y., Liu, X-B., Yang, C-H., Jordan, J.D., Ma, D.K., Liu, C.Y., Ganesan, S., Cheng, H-J., Ming, G-I., Lu, B., and Song, H. (2007). Disrupted-in-schizophrenia 1 regulates integration of newly generated neurons in the adult brain. *Cell,* **130**, 1146–1158.

Dunbar, R.I.M., and Shultz, S. (2007). Understanding primate brain evolution. *Philosophical Transactions of the Royal Society*, **362**, 649–658.

Duncan, J., and Owen, A.M. (2000). Common regions of the human frontal lobe recruited by diverse cognitive demands. *Trends in Neurosciences*, **23**, 475–483.

Dworzynski, K., Happé, F., Bolton, P., and Ronald, A. (2009). Relationship between symptom domains in autism spectrum disorders: A population-based twin study. *Journal of Autism Developmental Disorders,* **39**, 1197–1210.

Dye, S.M., Spence, S.A., Bench, C.J., Hirsch, S.R., Stefan, M.D., Sharma, T., and Grasby, P.M. (1999). No evidence for left superior temporal dysfunction in asymptomatic schizophrenia and bipolar disorder: PET study of verbal fluency. *British Journal of Psychiatry*, **175**, 367–374.

Egan, M.F., Goldberg, T.E., Kolachana, B.S., Callicott, J.H., Mazzanti, C.M., Straub, R.E., Goldman, D., and Weinberger, D.R. (2001). Effect of COMT Val$^{108/158}$ Met genotype on frontal lobe function and risk for schizophrenia. *Proceedings of the National Academy of Sciences of the USA*, **98**, 6917–6922.

Eisenberg, L. (1981). Leo Kanner, M.D. 1894–1981. *American Journal of Psychiatry*, **138**, 1122–1125.

Ekman, P. (1984). Expression and nature of emotion. In K. Scherer and P. Ekman (Eds.), *Approaches to Emotion* (pp. 319–343). Hillsdale, NJ, Erlbaum.

Elkashef, A.M., Doudet, D., Bryant, T., Cohen, R.M., Li, S.H., and Wyatt, R.J. (2000). 6-(18)F-DOPA PET study in patients with schizophrenia: positron emission tomography. *Psychiatry Research*, **100**, 1–11.

Elkis, H., Friedman, L., Wise, A., and Meltzer, H.Y. (1995). Meta-analysis of studies of ventricular enlargement and cortical sulcal prominence in mood disorders: Comparisons with controls or patients with schizophrenia. *Archives of General Psychiatry*, **52**, 735–746.

Elliott, R., Dolan, R.J., and Frith, C.D. (2000). Dissociable functions in the medial and lateral orbitofrontal cortex: Evidence from human neuroimaging studies. *Cerebral Cortex*, **10**, 308–317.

Elliott, R., Newman, J.L., Longe, O.A., and Deakin, J.F. (2003). Differential response patterns in the striatum and orbitofrontal cortex to financial reward in humans: A parametric functional magnetic resonance imaging study. *Journal of Neuroscience*, **23**, 303–307.

Ellison-Wright, I., and Bullmore, E. (2009). Meta-analysis of diffusion tensor imaging studies in schizophrenia. *Schizophrenia Research*, **108**, 3–10.

Enard, W., Khaitovich, P., Klose, J., Zöllner, S., Heissig, F., Giavalisco, P., Nieselt-Struwe, K., Muchmore, E., Varki, A., Ravid, R., Doxiadis, G.M., Bontrop, R.E., and Pääbo, S. (2002). Intra- and interspecific variation in primate gene expression patterns. *Science*, **296**, 340–343.

Enard, W., Przeworski, M., Fisher, S.E., Lai, C.S., Wiebe, V., Kitano, T., Monaco, A.P., and Pääbo, S. (2002). Molecular evolution of FOXP2, a gene involved in speech and language. *Nature*, **418**, 869–872.

Ende, G., Braus, D.F., Walter, S., Weber-Fahr, W., Soher, B., Maudsley, A.A., and Henn, F.A. (2001). Effects of age, medication, and illness duration on the N-acetylaspartate signal of the anterior cingulate region in schizophrenia. *Schizophrenia Research*, **41**, 389–395.

Epstein, J., Stern, E., and Silbersweig, D. (1999). Mesolimbic activity associated with psychosis in schizophrenia: Symptom-specific PET studies. *Annals of the New York Academy of Sciences*, **877**, 562–574.

Evans, C.L., McGuire, P.K., and David, A.S. (2000). Is auditory imagery defective in patients with auditory hallucinations? *Psychological Medicine*, **30**, 137–148.

Evans, P.D., Gilbert, S.L., Mekel-Bobrov, N., Vallender, E.J., Anderson, J.R., Vaez-Azizi, L.M., Tishkoff, S.A., Hudson, R.R., and Lahn, B.T. (2005). Microcephalin, a gene regulating brain size, continues to evolve adaptively in humans. *Science,* **309**, 1717–1720.

Faedda, G.L., Baldessarini, R.J., Suppes, T., Tondo, L., Becker, I., and Lipschitz, D. (1995). Pediatric-onset bipolar disorder: A neglected clinical and public health problem. *Harvard Review of Psychiatry*, **3**, 171–195.

Fair, D.A., Cohen, A.L., Dosenbach, N.U.F., Church, J.A., Miezin, F.M., Barch, D.M., Raichle, M.E., Petersen, S.E., and Schlaggar, B.L. (2008). The maturing architecture of the brain's default network. *Proceedings of the National Academy of Sciences of the USA*, **105**, 4028–4032.

Fair, D.A., Dosenbach, N.U.F., Church, J.A., Cohen, A.L., Brahmbhatt, S., Miezin, F.M., Barch, D.M., Raichle, M.E., Petersen, S.E., and Schlaggar, B.L. (2007). Development of distinct control networks through segregation and integration. *Proceedings of the National Academy of Sciences of the USA*, **104**, 13507–13512.

Falkai, P., and Bogerts, B. (1986). Cell loss in the hippocampus of schizophrenics. *European Archives of Psychiatry and Neurological Sciences*, **236**, 154–161.

Falkai, P., and Bogerts, B. (1993). Cytoarchitectonic and developmental studies in schizophrenia. In R. Kerwin (Ed.), *Neurobiology and Psychiatry* (pp. 43–70). Cambridge, U.K., Cambridge University Press.

Fannon, D., Simmons, A., Tennakoon, L., O'Céallaigh, S., Sumich, A., Doku, V., Shew, C., and Sharma, T. (2003). Selective deficit of hippocampal N-acetylaspartate in antipsychotic-naïve patients with schizophrenia. *Biological Psychiatry*, **54**, 587–598.

Faraone, S.V., Perlis, R.H., Doyle, A.E., Smoller, J.W., Goralnick, J.J., Holmgren, M.A., and Sklar, P. (2005). Molecular genetics of attention-deficit/hyperactivity disorder. *Biological Psychiatry,* **57**, 1313–1323.

Faraone, S.V., Sergeant, J., Gillberg, C., and Biederman, J. (2003). The worldwide prevalence of ADHD: Is it an American condition? *World Psychiatry*, **2**, 104–113.

Farrer, C., Franck, N., Georgieff, N., Frith, C.D., Decety, J., and Jeannerod, M. (2003). Modulating the experience of agency: A positron emission tomography study. *Neuroimage*, **18**, 324–333.

Farrer, C., Franck, N., Frith, C.D., Decety, J., Georgieff, N., d'Amato, T., and Jeannerod, M. (2004). Neural correlates of action attribution in schizophrenia. *Psychiatry Research: Neuroimaging*, **131**, 31–44.

Farrow, S.J. (2006). Sir George Frederick Still (1868–1941). *Rheumatology,* **45,** 777–778.

Feinberg, I. (1982/1983). Schizophrenia: Caused by a fault in programmed synaptic elimination during adolescence? *Journal of Schizophrenia Research*, **17**, 319–334.

Feinberg, I., and Guazzelli, M. (1999). Schizophrenia: A disorder of the corollary discharge systems that integrate the motor systems of thought with the sensory systems of consciousness. *British Journal of Psychiatry*, **174**, 196–204.

Flaum, M., O'Leary, D.S., Swayze, V.W., Miller, D.D., Arndt, S., and Andreasen, N.C. (1995). Symptom dimensions and brain morphology in schizophrenia and related psychotic disorders. *Journal of Psychiatry Research*, **29**, 261–276.

Flechsig, P.E. (1921). Die myelogenetische Gliederung der Leitungsbahnen des Linsenkerns beim Menschen. *Berichte über die Verhandlungen der Königlich Sächsischen Gesellschaft der Wissenschaften zu Leipzig: Mathematisch-Physische Klasse*, **73**, 295–302.

Flor-Henry, P. (1969). Psychosis and temporal lobe epilepsy: A controlled investigation. *Epilepsia*, **10**, 363–395.

Fombonne, E. (2009). Epidemiology of pervasive developmental disorders. *Pediatric Research,* **65**, 591–598.

Fossati, P., Hevenor, S.J., Graham, S.J., Grady, C., Keightley, M., Craik F., and Mayberg, H. (2003). In search of the emotional self: An fMRI study using positive and negative emotional words. *American Journal of Psychiatry*, **160**, 1938–1945.

Fox, M.D., Corbetta, M., Snyder, A.Z., Vincent, J.L., and Raichle, M.E. (2006). Spontaneous neuronal activity distinguishes human dorsal and ventral attention systems. *Proceedings of the National Academy of Sciences of the USA*, **103**, 10046–10051.

Fox, M.D., and Raichle, M.E. (2007). Spontaneous fluctuations in brain activity observed with functional magnetic resonance imaging. *Nature Reviews Neuroscience*, **8**, 700–711.

Fox, M.D., Snyder, A.Z., Vincent, J.L., Corbetta, M., Van Essen, D.C., and Raichle, M.E. (2005). The human brain is intrinsically organized into dynamic, anticorrelated functional networks. *Proceedings of the National Academy of Sciences of the USA,* **102**, 9673–9678.

Foxe, J.J., Murray, M.M., and Javitt, D.C. (2005). Filling-in in schizophrenia: A high-density electrical mapping and source-analysis investigation of illusory contour processing. *Cerebral Cortex,* **15,** 1914–1927.

Franceschi, M., Anchisi, D., Pelati, O., Zuffi, M., Matarrese, M., Moresco, R.M., Fazio, F., and Perani, D. (2005). Glucose metabolism and serotonin receptors in the frontotemporal lobe degeneration. *Annals of Neurology*, **57**, 216–225.

Franck, N., Farrer, C., Georgieff, N., Marie-Cardine, M., Daléry, J., d'Amato, T., and Jeannerod, M. (2001). Defective recognition of one's own actions in patients with schizophrenia. *American Journal of Psychiatry*, **158**, 454–459.

Franke, B., Neale, B.M., and Faraone, S.V. (2009). Genome-wide association studies in ADHD. *Human Genetics,* **126**, 13–50.

Fransson, P. (2005). Spontaneous low-frequency BOLD signal fluctuations: An fMRI investigation of resting-state default mode of brain function hypothesis. *Human Brain Mapping,* **26**, 15–29.

Fransson, P., Skiöld, B., Horsch, S., Nordell, A., Blennow, M., Lagercrantz, H., and Åden, U. (2007). Resting-state networks in the infant brain. *Proceedings of the National Academy of Sciences of the USA*, **104**, 15531–15536.

French, C.C., and Beaumont, J.G. (1984). A critical review of EEG coherence studies of hemisphere function. *International Journal of Psychophysiology*, **1**, 241–254.

Friedman, D., and Squires-Wheeler, E. (1994). Event-related potentials (ERPs) as indicators of risk for schizophrenia. *Schizophrenia Bulletin*, **20**, 63–74.

Friedman, E.M., Hayney, M.S., Love. G.D., Urry, H.L., Rosenkranz, M.A., Davidson, R.J., Singer, B.H., and Ryff, C.D. (2005). Social relationships, sleep quality, and interleukin-6 in aging women. *Proceedings of the National Academy of Sciences of the USA,* **102,** 18757–18762.

Friedman, J.I., Tang, C., Buchsbaum, M., Schmeidler, J., Flanagan, L., Golembo, S., Kanellopoulo, I., Ng, J., Hof, P.R., Harvey, P.D., Tsopelas, N.D., Stewart, D., and Davis, K.L. (2008). Diffusion tensor imaging findings in first-episode and chronic schizophrenic patients. *American Journal of Psychiatry*, **165**, 1024–1032.

Friedman, S.D., Shaw, D.W., Artru, A.A., Richards, T.L., Gardner, J., Dawson, G., Posse, S., and Dager, S.R. (2003). Regional brain chemical alterations in young children with autism spectrum disorder. *Neurology*, **60**, 100–107.

Foster, N.L. (2003). Validating FDG-PET as a biomarker for frontotemporal dementia. *Experimental Neurology*, **184**, S2–S8.

Franceschi, M., Anchisi, D., Pelati, O., Zuffi, M., Matarrese, M., Moresco, R.M., Fazio, F., and Perani, D. (2005). Glucose metabolism and serotonin receptors in the frontotemporal lobe degeneration. *Annals of Neurology*, **57**, 216–225.

Friederici, A.D. (2009). Pathways to language: Fiber tracts in the human brain. *Trends in Cognitive Sciences*, **13**, 175–181.

Friedland, R.P., Koss, A., Lerner, A., Hedera, P., Ellis, W., Dronkers, N., Ober, B.A., and Jagust, W.J. (1993). Functional imaging, the frontal lobes and dementia. *Dementia*, **4**, 192–203.

Frith, C.D. (1987). The positive and negative symptoms of schizophrenia reflect impairments in the perception and initiation of action. *Psychological Medicine*, **17**, 631–648.

Frith, C.D. (1992). *The Cognitive Neuropsychology of Schizophrenia*. Hove, East Essex, U.K., Lawrence Erlbaum Associates Ltd.

Frith, C. (1995). Functional imaging and cognitive abnormalities. *Lancet*, **346**, 615–620.

Frith, C.D. (2007). The social brain? *Philosophical Transactions of the Royal Society B*, **362**, 671–678.

Frith, C.D., Blakemore, S.-J., and Wolpert, D.M. (2000). Explaining the symptoms of schizophrenia: Abnormalities in the awareness of action. *Brain Research Reviews*, **31**, 357–363.

Frith, C., and Dolan, R. (1996). The role of the prefrontal cortex in higher cognitive functions. *Cognitive Brain Research,* **5**, 175–181.

Fritz, J., Mishkin, M., and Saunders, R.C. (2005). In search of an auditory engram. *Proceedings of the National Academy of Sciences of the USA*, **102**, 9359–9364.

Frodl, T.S., Koutsouleris, N., Bottlender, R., Born, C., Jäger, M., Scupin, I., Reiser, M., Möller, H.-J., and Meisenzahl, E.M. (2008). Depression-related variation in brain morphology over 3 years. *Archives of General Psychiatry*, **65**, 1156–1165.

Fujimoto, T., Nakano, T., Takano, T., Hokazono, Y., Asakura, T., and Tsuji, T. (1992). Study of chronic schizophrenics using ^{31}P magnetic resonance chemical shift imaging. *Acta Psychiatrica Scandinavica*, **86**, 455–462.

Fujiwara, H., Namiki, C., Hirao, K., Miyata, J., Shimizu, M., Fukuyama, H., Sawamoto, N., Hayashi, T., and Murai, T. (2007). Anterior and posterior cingulum abnormalities and their association with psychopathology in schizophrenia: A diffusion tensor imaging study. *Schizophrenia Research*, **95**, 215–222.

Fukuzako, H., Fukuzako, T., Hashiguchi, T., Kodaura, S., Takigawa, M., and Fujimoto, T. (1999a). Changes in levels of phosphorous metabolites in temporal lobes of drug-naive schizophrenic patients. *American Journal of Psychiatry*, **156**, 1205–1208.

Fukuzako, H., Kodama, S., Fukuzako, T., Yamada, K., Doi, W., Sato, D., and Takigawa, M. (1999b). Subtype-associated metabolite differences in the temporal lobe in schizophrenia detected by proton magnetic resonance spectroscopy. *Psychiatry Research: Neuroimaging*, **92**, 45–56.

Fukuzako, H., Takeuchi, K., Hozazano, Y., Fugako, T., Yamada, K., Hashiguchi, T., Obo, Y., Ueyama, K., Takigawa, M., and Fujimoto, T. (1995). Proton magnetic resonance spectroscopy of the left medial temporal and frontal lobes in chronic schizophrenia: preliminary report. *Psychiatry Research: Neuroimaging*, **61**, 193–200.

Fuller, R., Nopoulos, P., Arndt, S., O'Leary, D., Beng-Choon, H., and Andreasen, N.C. (2002). Longitudinal assessment of premorbid cognitive functioning in patients with schizophrenia through examination of standardized scholastic test performance. *American Journal of Psychiatry*, **159**, 1183–1189.

Funnell, E. (2001). Evidence for scripts in semantic dementia: Implications for theories of semantic memory. *Cognitive Neuropsychology*, **18**, 323–341.

Fuster, J.M. (Ed.). (1989). *The Prefrontal Cortex: Anatomy, Physiology, and Neuropsychology of the Frontal Lobes*, 2nd ed. New York, Raven Press.

Gagneux, P., and Varki, A. (2001). Genetic differences between humans and great apes. *Molecular Phylogenetics and Evolution*, **18**, 2–13.

Gallagher, H.L., and Frith, C.D. (2003). Functional imaging of 'theory of mind.' *Trends in Cognitive Sciences*, **7**, 77–83.

Gallese, V. (2007). Before and below 'theory of mind': Embodied simulation and the neural correlates of social cognition. *Philosophical Transactions of the Royal Society*, **362**, 659–669.

Gallup, G.G. (1970). Chimpanzees: Self-recognition. *Science*, **167**, 86–87.

Gao, W., Zhu, H., Giovanello, K.S., Smith, J.K., Shen, D., Gilmore, J.H., and Lin, W. (2009). Evidence on the emergence of the brain's default network from 2-week-old to 2-year-old healthy pediatric subjects. *Proceedings of the National Academy of Sciences of the USA*, **106**, 6790–6795.

Garrity, A.G., Pearlson, G.D., McKiernan, K.A., Lloyd, D., Kiehl, K.A., and Calhoun, V.D. (2007). Aberrant 'default mode' functional connectivity in schizophrenia. *American Journal of Psychiatry*, **164**, 450–457.

Garver, D.L., Nair, T.R., Christensen, J.D., Holcomb, J.A., and Kingsbury, S.J. (2000). Brain and ventricle instability during psychotic episodes of the schizophrenias. *Schizophrenia Research*, **44**, 11–22.

Gentile, J.P., Atiq, R., and Gillig, P.M. (2006). Adult ADHD: Diagnosis, differential diagnosis, and medication management. *Psychiatry,* **3**, 24–30.

George, M.S., Ketter, T.A., Parekh, P.I., Gill, D.S., Marangell, L., Pazzaglia, P.J., Herscovitch, P., and Post, R.M. (1997). Depressed subjects have decreased rCBF activation during facial emotional recognition. *CNS Spectrums*, **2**, 45–55.

Georgieff, N., and Jeannerod, M. (1998). Beyond consciousness of external reality: A 'who' system for consciousness of action and self-consciousness. *Consciousness and Cognition*, **7**, 465–477.

Gerber, D.J., Hall, D., Miyakawa, T., Demars, S., Gogos, J.A., Karayiorgou, M., and Tonegawa, S. (2003). Evidence for association of schizophrenia with genetic variation in the 8p21.3 gene, *PPP3CC,* encoding the calcineurin gamma subunit. *Proceedings of the National Academy of Sciences of the USA*, **100**, 8993–8998.

Geschwind, D.H., and Levitt, P. (2007). Autism spectrum disorders: Developmental disconnection syndromes. *Current Opinion in Neurobiology*, **17**, 103–111.

Gilbert, S.J., Spengler, S., Simons, J.S., Steele, J.D., Lawrie, S.M., Frith, C.D., and Burgess, P.W. (2006). Functional specialization within rostral prefrontal cortex (area 10): A meta-analysis. *Journal of Cognitive Neuroscience*, **18**, 932–948.

Gillberg, C.L. (1992). The Emanuel Miller memorial lecture 1991. Autism and autistic-like conditions: Subclasses among disorders of empathy. *Journal of Child Psychology and Psychiatry,* **33,** 813–842.

Gillberg, C., Santosh, P., and Brown, T. (2009). ADHD with autism spectrum disorders. In T. Brown (Ed.), *ADHD Comorbidities: Handbook for ADHD Complications in Children and Adults* (pp. 265–278). Washington, D.C., American Psychiatric Publishing, Inc.

Gillihan, S.J., and Farah, M.J. (2005). Is self special? A critical review of evidence from experimental psychology and cognitive neuroscience. *Psychological Bulletin*, **131**, 76–97.

Glahn, D.C., Winkler, A.M., Kochunov, P., Almasy, L., Duggirala, R., Carless, M.A., Curran, J.C., Olvera, R.L., Laird, A.R., Smith, S.M., Beckmann, C.F., Fox, P.T., and

Blangero, J. (2010). Genetic control over the resting brain. *Proceedings of the National Academy of Sciences of the USA*, **107**, 1223–1228.

Glessner, J.T., Wang, K., Cai, G., Korvatska, O., Kim, C.E., Wood, S., Zhang, H., Estes, A., Brune, C.W., Bradfield, J.P., Imielinski, M., Frackelton, E.C., Reichert, J., Crawford, E.L., Munson, J., Sleiman, P.M.A., Chiavacci, R., Annaiah, K., Thomas, K., Hou, C., Glaberson, W., Flory, J., Otieno, F., Garris, M., Soorya, L., Klei, L., Piven, J., Meyer, K.J., Anagnostou, E., Sakuai, T., Game, R.M., Rudd, D.S., Zurawiecki, D., McDougle, C.J., Davis, L.K., Miller, J., Posey, D.J., Michaels, S., Kolevzon, A., Silverman, J.M., Bernier, R., Levy, S.E., Schultz, R.T., Dawson, G., Owley, T., McMahon, W.M., Wassink, T.H., Sweeney, J.A., Nurnberger, J.I., Coon, H., Sutcliffe, J.S., Minshew, N.J., Grant, S.F.A., Bucan, M., Cook, E.H., Buxbaum, J.D., Devlin, B., Schellenberg, G.D., and Hakonarson, H. (2009). Autism genome-wide copy number variation reveals ubiquitin and neuronal genes. *Nature*, **459**, 569–573.

Gluck, M.R., Thomas, R.G., Davis, K.L., and Haroutunian, V. (2002). Implications for altered glutamate and GABA metabolism in dorsolateral prefrontal cortex of aged schizophrenic patients. *American Journal of Psychiatry*, **159**, 1165–1173.

Gogtay, N., Giedd, J.N., Lusk, L., Hayashi, K.M., Greenstein, D., Vaituzis, A.C., Nugent, T.F., Herman, D.H., Clasen, L.S., Toga, A.W., Rapoport, J.L., and Thompson, P.M. (2004). Dynamic mapping of human cortical development during childhood through early adulthood. *Proceedings of the National Academy of Sciences of the USA*, **101**, 8174–8179.

Gold, J.M., Carpenter, C., Randolf, C., Goldberg, T.E., and Weinberger, D.R. (1997). Auditory working memory and Wisconsin Card Sorting Test performance in schizophrenia. *Archives of General Psychiatry*, **54**, 159–165.

Goldberg, J.F., Harrow, M., and Grossman, L.S. (1995). Course and outcome in bipolar affective disorder: A longitudinal follow-up study. *American Journal of Psychiatry*, **152**, 379–384.

Goldberg, T.E., Saint-Cyr, J.A., and Weinberger, D.R. (1990). Assessment of procedural learning and problem solving in schizophrenic patients by Tower of Hanoi type tasks. *Journal of Neuropsychiatry and Clinical Neuroscience*, **2**, 165–173.

Goldberg, T.E., Torrey, E.F., Berman, K.F., and Weinberger, D.R. (1994). Relations between neuropsychological performance and brain morphology and physiological measures in monozygotic twins discordant for schizophrenia. *Psychiatry Research: Neuroimaging*, **55**, 51–61.

Goldman-Rakic, P.S. (1987). Circuitry of primate prefrontal cortex and regulation of behavior by representational memory. In F. Plum (Ed.), *Handbook of Physiology: The Nervous System, Higher Functions of the Brain, Section I, Volume V, Part 1* (pp. 373–417). Bethesda, MD: American Physiological Society.

Goldman-Rakic, P.S. (1994). Working memory dysfunction in schizophrenia. *Journal of Neuropsychiatry and Clinical Neuroscience*, **6**, 348–357.

Goldman-Rakic, P.S., Selemon, L.D., and Schwartz, M.L. (1984). Dual pathways connecting the dorsolateral prefrontal cortex with the hippocampal formation and parahippocampal cortex in the rhesus monkey. *Neuroscience*, **12**, 719–743.

Goldner, E.M., Hsu, .L, Waraich, P., and Somers, J.M. (2002). Prevalence and incidence studies of schizophrenic disorders: A systematic review of the literature. *Canadian Journal of Psychiatry*, **47**, 833–843.

Gonzalez, N., Moody, T.W., Igarashi, H., Ito, T., and Jensen, R.T. (2008). Bombesin-related peptides and their receptors: Recent advances in their role in physiology and disease states. *Current Opinion in Endocrinology, Diabetes & Obesity*, **15**, 58–64.

Goodwin, F.K., and Jamison, K.R. (2007). *Manic-Depressive Illness: Bipolar Disorders and Recurrent Depression*, 2nd ed. New York, Oxford University Press.

Gottfried, J.A., Deichmann, R., Winston, J.S., and Dolan, R.J. (2002). Functional heterogeneity in human olfactory cortex: An event-related functional magnetic resonance imaging study. *Journal of Neuroscience*, **22**, 10819–10828.

Graybiel, A.M. (1997). The basal ganglia and cognitive pattern generators. *Schizophrenia Bulletin*, **23**, 459–469.

Grace, A.A. (1993). Cortical regulation of subcortical systems and its possible relevance to schizophrenia. *Journal of Neural Transmission*, **1**, 111–134.

Graff-Radford, N.R., and Woodruff, B.K. (2007). Frontotemporal dementia. *Seminars in Neurology*, **27**, 48–57.

Gray, J.A. (1995). The contents of consciousness: A neuropsychological conjecture. *Behavioral and Brain Sciences*, **18**, 659–722.

Gray, J.A. (2004). *Consciousness: Creeping Up on the Hard Problem*. New York, Oxford University Press.

Graybiel, A.M. (1995). Building action repertoires: Memory and learning functions of the basal ganglia. *Current Opinion in Biology*, **5**, 733–741.

Greene, J.D., Sommerville, R.B., Nystrom, L.E., Darley, J.M., and Cohen, J.D. (2001). An fMRI investigation of emotional engagement in moral judgement. *Science*, **293**, 2105–2108.

Gregory, C., Lough, S., Stone, V., Erzinclioglu, S., Martin, L., Baron-Cohen, S., and Hodges, J.R. (2002). Theory of mind in patients with frontal variant frontotemporal dementia and Alzheimer's disease: Theoretical and practical implications. *Brain*, **125**, 752–764.

Greicius, M.D., Flores, B.H., Menon, V., Glover, G.H., Solvason, H.B., Kenna, H., Reiss, A.L., and Schatzberg, A.F. (2007). Resting-state functional connectivity in major depression: Abnormally increased contribution from subgenual cingulate cortex and thalamus. *Biological Psychiatry*, **62**, 429–437.

Greicius, M.D., Krasnow, B., Reiss, A.L., and Menon, V. (2003). Functional connectivity in the resting brain: A network analysis of the default mode hypothesis. *Proceedings of the National Academy of Sciences of the USA,* **100**, 253–258.

Greicius, M.D., Srivastava, G., Reiss, A.L., and Menon, V. (2004). Default-mode network activity distinguishes Alzheimer's disease from healthy aging: Evidence from functional MRI. *Proceedings of the National Academy of Sciences of the USA*, **101**, 4637–4642.

Grether, D.M., Plott, C.R., Rowe, D.B., Sereno, M., and Allman, J.M. (2007). Mental processes and strategic equilibration: An fMRI study of selling strategies in second price auctions. *Experimental Economics,* **10**, 105–122.

Grice, D.E., and Buxbaum, J.D. (2006). The genetics of autism spectrum disorders. *NeuroMolecular Medicine*, **8**, 451–460.

Grimmer, T., Diehl, J., Drezga, A., Förstl, H., and Kurz, A. (2004). Region-specific decline of cerebral glucose metabolism in patients with frontotemporal dementia: A prospective ^{18}F-FDG-PET study. *Dementia and Geriatric Cognitive Disorders*, **18**, 32–36.

Guilmatre, A., Dubourg, C., Mosca, A-L., Legallic, S., Goldenberg, A., Drouin-Garraud, V., Layet, V., Rosier, A., Briault, S., Bonnet-Brilhault, F., Laumonnier, F., Odent, S., Le Vacon, G., Joly-Helas, G., David, V., Bendavid, C., Pinoit, J-M., Henry, C., Impallomeni, C., Germano, E., Tortorella, G., Di Rosa, G., Barthelemy, C., Andres, C., Faivre, L., Frébourg, T., Veber, P.S., and Campion, D. (2009). Recurrent rearrangements in synaptic and neurodevelopmental genes and shared biologic pathways in schizophrenia, autism, and mental retardation. *Archives of General Psychiatry,* **66**, 947–956.

Gruzelier, J.H. (1984). Hemispheric imbalances in schizophrenia. *International Journal of Psychophysiology*, **1**, 227–240.

Gruzelier, J.H. (1999). Functional neurophysiological asymmetry in schizophrenia: A review and reorientation. *Schizophrenia Bulletin*, **25**, 91–120.

Gruzelier, J.H., and Flor-Henry, P. (Eds.) (1979). *Hemispheric Asymmetries of Function in Psychopathology*. Amsterdam, Elsevier.

Gruzelier, J., Seymour, K., Wilson, L., Jolley, A., and Hirsch, S. (1988). Impairments on neuropsychologic tests of temporohippocampal and frontohippoampal functions and word fluency in remitting schizophrenia and affective disorders. *Archives of General Psychiatry*, **45**, 623–629.

Gur, R.E., Cowell P., Turetsky, B.I., Gallacher, F., Cannon, T., Bilker, W., and Gur, R.C. (1998). A follow-up magnetic resonance imaging study of schizophrenia: Relationship of neuroanatomical changes to clinical and neurobehavioural measures. *Archives of General Psychiatry*, **55**, 145–152.

Gur, R.E., Jaggi, J.L., Shtasel D.L., Ragland, J.D., and Gur, R.C. (1994). Cerebral blood flow in schizophrenia: Effects of memory processing on regional activation. *Biological Psychiatry*, **35**, 3–15.

Gur, R.E., Turetsky, B.I., Bilker, W.B., and Gur, R.C. (1999). Reduced gray matter volume in schizophrenia. *Archives of General Psychiatry*, **56**, 905–911.

Gusnard, D.A., Akbudak, E., Shulman, G.L., and Raichle, M.E. (2001). Medial prefrontal cortex and self-referential mental activity: Relation to a default mode of brain function. *Proceedings of the National Academy of Sciences of the USA*, **98**, 4259–4264.

Hacia, J.G. (2001). Genome of the apes. *Trends in Genetics*, **17**, 637–645.

Häfner, H., and an der Heiden, W. (1997). Epidemiology of schizophrenia. *Canadian Journal of Psychiatry*, **42**, 139–151.

Haldane, M., and Frangou, S. (2004). New insights help define the pathophysiology of bipolar affective disorder: Neuroimaging and neuropathology findings. *Progress in Neuro-Psychopharmacology and Biological Psychiatry*, **28**, 943–960.

Hall, M.-H., Rijsdijk, F., Kalidindi, S., Schulze, K., Kravariti, E., Kane, F., Sham, P., Bramon, E., and Murray, R.M. (2007). Genetic overlap between bipolar illness and event-related potentials. *Psychological Medicine*, **37**, 667–678.

Halmi, K.A. (2009). Anorexia nervosa: An increasing problem in children and adolescents. *Dialogues in Clinical Neuroscience,* **11,** 100–103.

Hanley, J., Rickles, W.R., Crandall, P.H., and Walter, R.D. (1972). Automatic recognition of EEG correlates of behavior in a chronic schizophrenic patient. *American Journal of Psychiatry*, **128**, 74–78.

Happé, F., Ronald, A., and Plomin, R. (2006). Time to give up on a single explanation for autism. *Nature Neuroscience*, **9**, 1218–1220.

Harciarek, M., and Jodzio, K. (2005). Neuropsychological differences between frontotemporal dementia and Alzheimer's disease: A review. *Neuropsychology Review*, **15**, 131–145.

Harrison, N.A., Brydon, L., Walker, C., Gray, M., Steptoe, A., and Critchley, H.D. (2009a). Inflammation causes mood changes through alterations in subgenual cingulate activity and mesolimbic connectivity. *Biological Psychiatry*, **66**, 407–414.

Harrison, N.A., Brydon, L., Walker, C., Gray, M., Steptoe, A., Dolan, R.J., and Critchley, H.D. (2009b). Neural origins of human sickness in interoceptive responses to inflammation. *Biological Psychiatry*, **66**, 415–422.

Harrison, N.A., Gray, M.A., and Critchley, H.D. (2009). Dynamic pupillary exchange engages brain regions encoding social salience. *Social Neuroscience,* **4**, 233–243.

Harrison, P.J. (1999). The neuropathology of schizophrenia: A critical review of the data and their interpretation. *Brain*, **122**, 593–624.

Harrison, P.J., and Owen, M.J. (2003). Genes for schizophrenia? Recent findings and their pathophysiological implications. *Lancet*, **361**, 417–419.

Harrison, P.J., and Weinberger, D.R. (2005). Schizophrenia genes, gene expression, and neuropathology: On the matter of their convergence. *Molecular Psychiatry*, **10**, 40–68.

Hart, B.L. (1988). Biological basis of the behavior of sick animals. *Neuroscience and Biobehavioral Reviews*, **12**, 123–137.

Hartmann, T. (2003). *The Edison Gene*. Rochester, Park Press.

Hashimoto, R., Numakawa, T., Ohnishi, T., Kumamaru, E., Yagasaki, Y., Ishimoto, T., Mori, T., Nemoto, K., Adachi, N., Izumi, A., Chiba, S., Noguchi, H., Suzuki, T., Iwata, N., Ozaki, N., Taguchi, T., Kamiya, A., Kosuga, A., Tatsumi, M., Kamijima, K., Weinberger, D.R., Sawa, A., and Kunugi, H. (2006). Impact of the DISC1 Ser704Cys polymorphism on risk for major depression, brain morphology and ERK signaling. *Human Molecular Genetics,* **15,** 3024–3033.

Hashimoto, T., Tayama, M., Miyazaki, M., Yoneda, Y., Yoshimoto, T., Harada, M., Miyoshi, H., Tanouchi, M., and Kuroda, Y. (1997). Differences in brain metabolites between patients with autism and mental retardation as detected by in vivo localized proton magnetic resonance spectroscopy. *Journal of Child Neurology*, **12**, 91–96.

Hasler, G., van der Veen, J.W., Tumonis, T., Meyers, N., Shen, J., and Drevets, W.C. (2007). Reduced prefrontal glutamate/glutamine and -aminobutyric acid levels in major depression determined using proton magnetic resonance spectroscopy. *Archives of General Psychiatry*, **64**, 193–200.

Haun, D.B.M., Rapold, C.J., Call, J., Janzen, G., and Levinson, S.C. (2006). Cognitive cladistics and cultural override in Hominid spatial cognition. *Proceedings of the National Academy of Sciences of the USA*, **103**, 17568–17573.

Hauser, M.D., Chomsky, N., and Fitch, W.T. (2002). The faculty of language: What is it, who has it, and how did it evolve? *Science*, **298**, 1569–1579.

Hazlett, H.C., Poe, M., Gerig, G., Smith, R.G., Provenzale, J., Ross, A., Gilmore, J., and Piven, J. (2005). Magnetic resonance imaging and head circumference study of brain size in autism: Birth through age 2 years. *Archives of General Psychiatry*, **62**, 1366–1376.

Haznedar, M.M., Roversi, F., Pallanti, S., Baldini-Rossi, N., Schnur, D.B., LiCalzi, E.M., Tang, C., Hof, P.R., Hollander, E., and Buchsbaum, M.S. (2005). Fronto-thalamo-striatal gray and white matter volumes and anisotropy of their connections in bipolar spectrum illnesses. *Biological Psychiatry*, **57**, 733–742.

Heath, R.G. (1954). *Studies in Schizophrenia: A Multidisciplinary Approach to Mind-Body Relationships*. Cambridge, Harvard University Press.

Heckers, S., Goff, D., Schacter, D.L., Savage, C.R., Fischman, A.J., Alpert, N.M., and Rauch, S.L. (1999). Functional imaging of memory retrieval in deficit vs nondeficit schizophrenia. *Archives of General Psychiatry*, **56**, 1117–1123.

Heimberg, C., Kosmoroski, R.A., Lawson, W.B., Cardwell, D., and Karson, C.N. (1998). Regional proton magnetic resonance spectroscopy in schizophrenia and exploration of drug effect. *Psychiatry Research: Neuroimaging*, **83**, 105–115.

Heimer, L. (2000). Basal forebrain in the context of schizophrenia. *Brain Research Reviews*, **31**, 205–235.

Heinrichs, R.W., and Zakzanis, K.K. (1998). Neurocognitive deficit in schizophrenia: a quantitative review of the evidence. *Neuropsychology*, **12**, 426–445.

Hemsley, D.R. (1987). An experimental psychological model for schizophrenia. In H. Häfner, W.F. Gattaz, and W. Janzarik (Eds.), *Search for the Causes of Schizophrenia* (pp. 179–188). New York, Springer-Verlag.

Hennah, W., Thompson, P., McQuillin, A., Bass, N., Loukola, A., Anjorin, A., Blackwood, D., Curtis, D., Deary, I.J., Harris, S.E., Isomtesä, E.T., Lawrence, J., Lönnqvist, J.,

Muir, W., Palotie, A., Partonen, T., Paunio, T., Pylkkö, E., Robinson, M., Soronen, P., Suominen, K., Suvisaari, J., Thirumalai, S., St. Clair, D., Gurling, H., Peltonen, L., and Porteous, D. (2009). DISC1 association, heterogeneity and interplay in schizophrenia and bipolar disorder. *Molecular Psychiatry*, **14**, 865–873.

Herbert, M.R. (2005). Larger brains in autism: The challenge of pervasive abnormality. *The Neuroscientist*, **11**, 417–440.

Herbert, M.R., Ziegler, D.A., Makris, N., Filipek, P.A., Kemper, T.L., Normandin, J.J., Sanders, H.A., Kennedy, D.N., and Caviness, V.S. (2004). Localization of white matter volume increase in autism and developmental language disorder. *Annals of Neurology*, **55**, 530–540.

Herold, R., Feldmann, A., Simon, M., Tényi, T., Kövér, F., Nagy, F., Varga, E., and Fekete, S. (2009). Regional gray matter reduction and theory of mind deficit in the early phase of schizophrenia: A voxel-based morphometric study. *Acta Psychiatrica Scandinavica*, **119**, 199–208.

Hickok, G., and Poeppel, D. (2004). Dorsal and ventral streams: A framework for understanding aspects of the functional anatomy of language. *Cognition*, **92**, 67–99.

Hickok, G., and Poeppel, D. (2007). The cortical organization of speech processing. *Nature Reviews Neuroscience*, **8**, 393–402.

Hietala, J., Syvälahti, E., Vilkman, H., Vuorio, K., Räakköläinen, V., Bergman, J., Haaparanta, M., Solin, O., Kuoppamäki, M., Eronen, E., Ruotsalainen, U., and Salokangas, R.G. (1999). Depressive symptoms and presynaptic dopamine function in neuroleptic-naïve schizophrenia. *Schizophrenia Research*, **35**, 41–50.

Hietala, J., Syvälahti, E., Vuorio, K., Räkköläinen, V., Bergman, J., Haaparanta, M., Solin, O., Kuoppamäki, M., Kirvelä, O., Ruotsalainen, U., and Salokangas, R.G. (1995). Presynaptic dopamine function in striatum of neuroleptic-naïve schizophrenic patients. *Lancet*, **346**, 1130–1131.

Higdon, R., Foster, N.L., Koeppe, R.A., DeCarli, C.S., Jagust, W.J., Clark, C.M., Barbas, N.R., Arnold, S.E., Turner, R.S., Heidebrink, J.L., and Minoshima, S. (2004). A comparison of classification methods for differentiating fronto-temporal dementia from Alzheimer's disease using FDG-PET imaging. *Statistics in Medicine*, **23**, 315–326.

Hill, S.K., Schuepbach, D., Herbener, E.S., Keshavan, M.S., and Sweeney, J.A. (2004). Pretreatment and longitudinal studies of neuropsychological deficits in antipsychotic-naïve patients with schizophrenia. *Schizophrenia Research*, **68**, 49–63.

Hisaoko, S., Harada, M., Nishitani, H., and Mori, K. (2001). Regional magnetic resonance spectroscopy of the brain in autistic individuals. *Neuroradiology*, **43**, 496–498.

Ho, B-C., Andreasen, N.C., Nopoulos, P., Arndt, S., Magnotta, V., and Flaum, M. (2003). Progressive structural brain abnormalities and their relationship to clinical outcome: A longitudinal magnetic resonance imaging study early in schizophrenia. *Archives of General Psychiatry*, **60**, 585–594.

Hodges, J.R., Davies, R., Xuereb, J., Kril, J., and Halliday, G. (2003). Survival in frontotemporal dementia. *Neurology*, **61**, 349–354.

Hodges, J.R., and Graham, K.S. (2001). Episodic memory: Insights from semantic dementia. *Philosophical Transactions of the Royal Society London* B, **356**, 1423–1434.

Hoffman, R.E., Anderson, A.W., Varanko, M., Gore, J.C., and Hampson, M. (2008). Time course of regional brain activation associated with onset of auditory/verbal hallucinations. *British Journal of Psychiatry*, **193**, 424–425.

Hogarty, G.E., Goldberg, S.C., and Schooler, N.R. (1974). Drug and sociotherapy in the aftercare of schizophrenic patients III. Adjustment of nonrelapsed patients. *Archives of General Psychiatry*, **31**, 609–618.

Holinger, D.P., Galaburda, A.M., and Harrison, P.J. (2000). Cerebral asymmetry. In P. J. Harrison and G. W. Roberts (Eds.), *The Neuropathology of Schizophrenia: Progress and Interpretation* (pp. 151–171). New York, Oxford.

Holtzheimer, P.E., and Mayberg, H.S. (2009). The cingulate cortex as organizing principle in neuropsychiatric disease. In B.A. Vogt (Ed.), *Cingulate Neurobiology and Disease* (pp. 237–244). New York, Oxford.

Holzman, P.S. (1987). Recent studies of psychophysiology in schizophrenia. *Schizophrenia Bulletin*, **13**, 49–75.

Horie, M., Honda, T., Suzuki, Y., Kobayashi, Y, Daito, T., Oshida, T, Ikuta, K., Jern, P. Gojobori, T., Coffin, J., and Tomonaga, K. (2010). Endogenous non-retroviral RNA virus elements in mammalian genomes, *Nature*, 463, 84–88.

Horn, H., Federspiel, A., Wirth, M., Müller, T.J., Wiest, R., Wang, J.-J., and Strik, W. (2009). Structural and metabolic changes in language areas linked to formal thought disorder. *British Journal of Psychiatry*, **194**, 130–138.

Horovitz, S.G., Braun, A.R., Carr, W.S., Picchioni, D., Balkin, T.J., Fukunaga, M., and Duyn, J.H. (2009). Decoupling of the brain's default mode network during sleep. *Proceedings of the National Academy of Sciences of the USA*, **106**, 11376–11381.

Horton, H.L., and Levitt, P. (1988). A unique membrane protein is expressed on early developing limbic system axons and cortical targets. *Journal of Neuroscience*, **8**, 4653–4661.

Houdé, O., Rossi, S., Lubin, A., and Joliot, M. (2010). Mapping numerical processing, reading and executive functions in the developing brain: An fMRI meta-analysis of 52 studies including 842 children. *Developmental Science* (in press).

Houenou, J., Wessa, M., Douand, G., Leboyer, M., Chanraud, S., Perrin, M., Poupon, C., Martinot, J.L., and Paillere-Martinot, M.-L. (2007). Increased white matter connectivity in euthymic bipolar patients: Diffusion tensor tractography between the subgenual cingulate and amygdalo-hippocampal complex. *Molecular Psychiatry*, **12**, 1001–1010.

Hsiao, M.-C., Lin, K.-J., Liu, C.-Y., Tzen, K.-Y., and Yen, T.-C. (2003). Dopamine transporter change in drug-naïve schizophrenia: an imaging study with ^{99m}Tc-TRODAT-1. *Schizophrenia Research*, **65**, 39–46.

Huber, G., Gross, G., Schüttler, R., and Linz, M. (1980). Longitudinal studies of schizophrenic patients. *Schizophrenia Bulletin*, **6**, 592–605.

Hudson, J.I., Lipinski, J.F. Keck, P.E., Aizley, H.G., Lukas, S.E., Rothschild, A.J., Waternaux, C.M., and Kupfer, D.J. (1992). Polysomnographic characteristics of young manic patients: Comparison with unipolar depressed patients and normal control subjects. *Archives of General Psychiatry*, **49**, 378–383.

Hunt, N., Sayer, H., and Silverstone, T. (1992). Season and manic relapse. *Acta Psychiatrica Scandinavica*, **85**, 123–126.

Hunter, M.D., Eickhoff, S.B., Miller, T.W.R., Farrow, T.F.D., Wilkinson, I.D., and Woodruff, P.W.R. (2006). Neural activity in speech-sensitive auditory cortex during silence. *Proceedings of the National Academy of Sciences of the USA,* **103**, 189–194.

Huttenlocher, P.R., and Dabholkar, A.S. (1997). Regional differences in synaptogenesis in the human cerebral cortex. *Journal of Comparative Neurology*, **387**, 167–178.

Ibach, B., Poljansky, S., Marienhagen, J., Sommer, M., Männer, P., and Hajak, G. (2004). Contrasting metabolic impairment in frontotemporal degeneration and early Alzheimer's disease. *NeuroImage*, **23**, 739–743.

Imamoto, K., and Leblond, C.P. (1978). Radioautographic investigation of gliogenesis in the corpus callosum of young rats. II. Origin of microglial cells. *Journal of Comparative Neurology*, **180**, 139–163.

Ingraham, L.J., and Kety, S.S. (2000). Adoption studies of schizophrenia. *American Journal of Medical Genetics*, **97**, 18–22.

Ingvar, D.H., and Franzen, G. (1974). Abnormalities of cerebral blood flow distribution in patients with chronic schizophrenia. *Acta Psychiatrica Scandinavica*, **50**, 425–462.

International Schizophrenia Consortium, (2008). Rare chromosomal deletions and duplications increase risk of schizophrenia. *Nature*, **455**, 237–241.

Ishii, K., Sakamoto, S., Sasaki, M., Kitagaki, H., Yamaji, S., Hashimoto, M., Imamura, T., Shimomura, T., Hirono, N., and Mori, E. (1998). Cerebral glucose metabolism in patients with frontotemporal dementia. *Journal of Nuclear Medicine*, **39**, 1875–1878.

Ishimaru, M., Kurumaji, A., and Toru, M. (1994). Increases in strychnine-insensitive glycine binding sites in cerebral cortex of chronic schizophrenics: evidence for glutamate hypothesis. *Biological Psychiatry*, **35**, 84–95.

Jabbi, M., Bastiaansen, J., and Keysers, C. (2008). A common anterior insular representation of disgust observation, experience and imagination shows divergent functional connectivity pathways. *PLOS ONE* 8:e2939.

Jackson, J.H. (1932a). Remarks on evolution and dissolution of the nervous system. In J. Taylor (Ed.), *Selected Writings of John Hughlings Jackson*, Volume 2 (pp. 76–91). London, Hodder and Stoughton.

Jackson, J.H. (1932b). Remarks on dissolution of the nervous system as exemplified by certain post-epileptic conditions. In J. Taylor (Ed.), *Selected Writings of John Hughlings Jackson,* Volume 2 (pp. 3–28). London, Hodder and Stoughton.

Jackson, J.H. (1932c). Evolution and dissolution of the nervous system. In J. Taylor (Ed.), *Selected Writings of John Hughlings Jackson,* Volume 2 (pp. 45–75). London, Hodder and Stoughton.

Jacob, H., and Beckmann, H. (1986). Prenatal developmental disturbances in the limbic allocortex in schizophrenics. *Journal of Neural Transmission*, **65**, 303–326.

Jacobsen, L.K., Giedd, J.N., Castellanos, F.X., Vaituzis, A.C., Hamburger, S.D., Kumra, M.S.S., Lenane, M.C., and Rapaport, J.L. (1998). Progressive reduction of temporal lobe structures in childhood-onset schizophrenia. *American Journal of Psychiatry*, **155**, 678–685.

James, A.C.D., Javaloyes, A., James, S., and Smith, D.M. (2002). Evidence for non-progressive changes in adolescent-onset schizophrenia: Follow-up magnetic resonance imaging study. *British Journal of Psychiatry*, **180**, 339–344.

Jarskog, L.F., Glantz, L.A., Gilmore, J.H., and Lieberman, J.A. (2005). Apoptotic mechanisms in the pathophysiology of schizophrenia. *Progress in Neuro-psychopharmacology and Biological Psychiatry*, **29**, 846–858.

Javitt, D.C. (2009). Sensory processing in schizophrenia: Neither simple nor intact. *Schizophrenia Bulletin,* **35,** 1059–1064.

Jaynes, J. (1977). *The Origin of Consciousness in the Breakdown of the Bicameral Mind.* Boston, Houghton Mifflin Co.

Jedema, H.P., Gianaros, P.J., Greer, P.J., Kerr, D.D., Liu, S., Higley, J.D., Suomi, S.J., Olsen, A.S., Porter, J.N., Lopresti, B.J., Hariri, A.R., and Bradberry, C.W. (2010). Cognitive impact of genetic variation of the serotonin transporter in primates is associated with differences in brain morphology rather than serotonin neurotransmission. *Molecular Psychiatry*, **15**, 512–522.

Jeong, Y., Cho, S.S., Park, J.M., Kang, S.J., Lee, J.S., Kang, E., Na, D.L., Kim, S.A. (2005). ^{18}F-FDG PET findings in frontotemporal dementia: An SPM analysis of 29 patients. *Journal of Nuclear Medicine*, **46**, 233–239.

Jentsch, J.D., Taylor, J.R., and Roth, R.H. (1998). Subchronic phencyclidine administration increases mesolimbic dopamine system responsivity and augments stress- and amphetamine-induced hyperlocomotion. *Neuropsychopharmacology*, **19**, 105–113.

Jentsch, J.D., and Roth, R.H. (1999). The neuropsychopharmacology of phencyclidine: From NMDA receptor hypofunction to the dopamine hypothesis of schizophrenia. *Neuropsychopharmacology*, **20**, 201–225.

Jeste, D.V., Del Carmen, R., Lohr, J.B., and Wyatt, R.J. (1985). Did schizophrenia exist before the eighteenth century? *Comprehensive Psychiatry*, **26**, 493–503.

Jocham, G., Klein, T.A., Neumann, J., von Cramon, D.Y., Reuter, M., and Ullsperger, M. (2009). Dopamine DRD2 polymorphism alters reversal learning and associated neural activity. *Journal of Neuroscience*, **29**, 3695–3704.

Johnson, J.K., Diehl, J., Mendez, M.F., Neuhaus, J., Shapira, J.S., Forman, M., Chute, D.J., Roberson, E.D., Pace-Savitsky, C., Neumann, M., Chow, T., Rosen, H.J., Forstl, H., Kurz, A., and Miller, B. L. (2005). Frontotemporal lobar degeneration: Demographic characteristics of 353 patients. *Archives of Neurology*, **62**, 925–930.

Johnson, S.C., Baxter, L.C., Wilder, L.S., Pipe, J.G., Heiserman, J.E., and Prigatano, G.P. (2002). Neural correlates of self-reflection. *Brain*, **125**, 1808–1814.

Jones, E.G. (2001). The thalamic matrix and thalamocortical synchrony. *Trends in Neurosciences*, **24**, 595–601.

Jones, P., and Cannon, M. (1998). The new epidemiology of schizophrenia. *Psychiatric Clinics of North America*, **21**, 1–25.

Jurgens, U. (1995). Neural control of vocal production in non-human and human primates. In E. Zimmermann, J. D. Newman, and U. Jurgens (Eds.), *Current Topics in Primate Vocal Communication* (pp. 199–206). New York, Plenum Press.

Just, M.A., Cherkassky, V.L., Keller, T.A., Kana, B.K., and Minshew, N.J. (2007). Functional and anatomical cortical underconnectivity in autism: Evidence from an fMRI study of an executive function task and corpus callosum morphometry. *Cerebral Cortex*, **17**, 951–961.

Just, M.A., Cherkassky, V.L., Keller, T.A., and Minshew, N.J. (2004). Cortical activation and synchronization during sentence comprehension in high-functioning autism: Evidence of underconnectivity. *Brain*, **127**, 1811–1821.

Kana, R.K., Keller, T.A., Cherkassky, V.L., Minshew, N.J., and Just, M.A. (2006). Sentence comprehension in autism: Thinking in pictures with decreased functional connectivity. *Brain*, **129**, 2484–2493.

Kandel, E.R. (2006). *In Search of Memory: The Emergence of a New Science of Mind*. New York, Norton.

Kandel, E.R., Schwartz, J.H., and Jessell, T.M. (2000). *Principles of Neural Science*, 4th ed. New York, McGraw-Hill.

Kanner, L. (1965). Infantile autism and the schizophrenias. *Behavioral Science*, **10**, 412–442.

Kanner, L. (1943). Autistic disturbances of affective contact. *Nervous Child*, **2**, 217–250.

Kantrowitz, J.T., Butler, P.D., Schecter, I., Silipo, G., and Javitt, D.C. (2009). Seeing the world dimly: The impact of early visual deficits on visual experience in schizophrenia. *Schizophrenia Bulletin,* **35,** 1085–1094.

Kaplan, H.S., Hooper, P.L., and Gurven, M. (2009). The evolutionary and ecological roots of human social organization. *Philosophical Transactions of the Royal Society B,* **364**, 3289–3299.

Kapur, S., and Remington, G. (1996). Serotonin-dopamine interaction and its relevance to schizophrenia. *American Journal of Psychiatry*, **153**, 466–476.

Karama, S., Lecours, A.R., Leroux, J-M., Bourgouin, P., Beaudoin, G., Joubert, S., and Beauregard, M. (2002). Areas of brain activation in males and females during viewing of erotic film excerpts. *Human Brain Mapping,* **16**, 1–13.

Karmiloff-Smith, A. (1992). *Beyond Modularity: A Developmental Perspective on Cognitive Science*. Cambridge, MIT Press.

Kasai, K., Shenton, M.E., Salisbury, D.F., Hirayasu, Y., Lee, C-U., Ciszewski, A.A., Yurgelun-Todd, D., Kikinis, R., Jolesz, F.A., and McCarley, R.W. (2003). Progressive decrease of left superior temporal gyrus gray matter volume in patients with first-episode schizophrenia. *American Journal of Psychiatry*, **160**, 156–164.

Kasari, C., and Rotheram-Fuller, E. (2005). Current trends in psychological research on children with high-functioning autism and Asperger disorder. *Current Opinion in Psychiatry*, **18**, 497–501.

Kato, C., Petronis, A., Okazaki, Y., Tochigi, M., Umekage, T., and Sasaki, T. (2002). Molecular genetic studies of schizophrenia: Challenges and insights. *Neuroscience Research*, **43**, 295–304.

Kato, T., Shiori, T., Murashita, J., Hamakawa, H., Inubushi, T., and Takahashi, S. (1995). Lateralized abnormality of high-energy phosphate and bilateral reduction of phosphomonoesterase measured by phosphorus-31 magnetic resonance spectroscopy of the frontal lobes in schizophrenia. *Psychiatry Research: Neuroimaging*, **61**, 151–160.

Kawasaki, Y., Maeda, Y., Suzuki, M., Urata, K., Higashima, M., Kiba, K., Yamaguchi, N., Matsuda, H., and Hisada, K. (1993). SPECT analysis of regional cerebral blood flow changes in patients with schizophrenia during the Wisconsin Card Sorting Test. *Schizophrenia Research*, **10**, 109–116.

Kaye, W.H., Fudge, J.L., and Paulus, M. (2009). New insights into symptoms and neuro-circuit function of anorexia nervosa. *Nature Reviews Neuroscience*, **10,** 573–584.

Keane, J., Calder, A.J., Hodges, J.R., and Young, A.W. (2002). Face and emotion processing in frontal variant frontotemporal dementia. *Neuropsychologia*, **40**, 655–665.

Keefe, R.S.E. (2000). Working memory dysfunction and its relevance in schizophrenia. In T. Sharma, and P.D. Harvey (Eds.), *Cognitive Functioning in Schizophrenia* (pp. 16–49). New York, Oxford University Press.

Kegeles, L.S., Shungu, D.C., Anjilvel, S., Chan, S., Ellis, S.P., Xanthopoulos, E., Malaspina, D., Gorman, J.M., Mann, J.J., Laruelle, M., and Kaufman, C.A. (2000b). Hippocampal pathology in schizophrenia: Magnetic resonance imaging and spectroscopy studies. *Psychiatry Research: Neuroimaging*, **98**, 163–175.

Kelemen, O., Nagy, O. Mátyássy, A., Bitter, I., Benedek, G., Vidnyánsky, Z., and Kéri, S. (2007). How well do patients with schizophrenia track moving targets? *Neuropsychology*, **21**, 319–325.

Keller, T.A., Kana, R.K., and Just, M.A. (2007). A developmental study of the structural integrity of white matter in autism. *NeuroReport*, **18**, 23–27.

Kelley, W.M., Macrae, C.N., Wyland, C.L., Caglar, S., Inati, S., and Heatherton, T.F. (2002). Finding the self? An event-related fMRI study. *Journal of Cognitive Neuroscience*, **14**, 785–794.

Kemper, T.L., and Bauman, M. (1998). Neuropathology of infantile autism. *Journal of Neuropathology and Experimental Neurology*, **57**, 645–652.

Kempton, M.J., Geddes, J.R., Ettinger, U., Williams, S.C.R., and Grasby, P.M. (2008). Meta-analysis, database, and meta-regression of 98 structural imaging studies in bipolar disorder. *Archives of General Psychiatry*, **65**, 1017–1032.

Kendler, K.S., McGuire, M., Gruenberg, A.M., O'Hare, A., Spellman, M., and Walsh, D. (1993). The Roscommon Family Study. I. Methods, diagnosis of probands, and risk of schizophrenia in relatives. *Archives of General Psychiatry*, **50**, 527–540.

Kennedy, D.P., Redcay, E., and Courchesne, E. (2006). Failing to de-activate: Resting functional abnormalities in autism. *Proceedings of the National Academy of Sciences of the USA*, **103**, 8275–8280.

Kéri, S., Kelemen, O., Benedek, G., and Janka, Z. (2004). Vernier threshold in patients with schizophrenia and in their unaffected siblings. *Neuropsychology*, **18**, 537–542.

Kéri, S., Kelemen, O., and Benedek, G. (2009). Attentional modulation of perceptual organization in schizophrenia. *Cognitive Neuropsychiatry*, **14**, 77–86.

Kertesz, A., and Kalvach, P. (1996). Arnold Pick and German neuropsychiatry in Prague. *Archives of Neurology*, **53**, 935–938.

Keshavan, M.S., Haas, G.L., Kahn, C.E., Aguilar, E., Dick, E.L., Schooler, N.R., Sweeney, J.A., and Pettegrew, J.W. (1998). Superior temporal gyrus and the course of early schizophrenia: progressive, static or reversible? *Journal of Psychiatry Research*, **32**, 161–167.

Keski-Rahkonen, A., Hoek, H.W., Susser, E.S., Linna, M.S., Sihvola, E., Raevuori, A., Bulik, C.M., Kaprio, J., and Rissanen, A. (2007). Epidemiology and course of anorexia nervosa in the community. *American Journal of Psychiatry,* **164**, 1259–1265.

Kessler, R.C., Berglund, P., Demler, O., Jin, R., Merikangas, K.R., and Walters, E.E. (2005a). Lifetime prevalence and age-of-onset distributions of DSM-IV disorders in the National Comorbidity Survey Replication. *Archives of General Psychiatry*, **62**, 593–602.

Kessler, R.C., Chiu, W.T., Demler, O., and Walters, E.E. (2005b). Prevalence, severity, and comorbidity of 12-month DSM-IV disorders in the National Comorbidity Survey Replication. *Archives of General Psychiatry*, **62**, 617–627.

Khaitovich, P., Muetzel, B., She, X., Lachmann, M., Hellman, I., Dietzsch, J., Steigele, S., Do, H.-H., Weiss, G., Enard, W., Heissig, F., Arendt, T., Nieselt-Struwe, K., Eichler, E.E., and Pääblo, S. (2004). Regional patterns of gene expression in human and chimpanzee brains. *Genome Research*, **14**, 1462–1472.

Killackey, H.P. (1995). Evolution of the human brain: A neuroanatomical perspective. In M.S. Gazzaniga (Ed.), *The Cognitive Neurosciences* (pp. 1243–1253). Cambridge, MIT Press.

Kilpinen, H., Ylisaukko-oja, T., Hennah, W., Palo, O.M., Varilo, T., Vanhala, R., Nieminen-von Wendt, T., von Wendt, L., Paunio, T., and Peltonen, L. (2008). Association of DISC1 with autism and Asperger syndrome. *Molecular Psychiatry*, **13**, 187–196.

Kinney, H.C., Brody, B.A., Kloman, A.S., and Gilles, F.H. (1988). Sequence of central nervous system myelination in human infancy II. Patterns of myelination in autopsied infants. *Journal of Neuropathology and Experimental Neurology*, **47**, 217–234.

Kircher, T.T.J., Senior, C., Phillips, M.L., Rabe-Hesketh, S., Benson, P.J., Bullmore, E.T., Brammer, M., Simmons, A., Bartels, M., and David, A.S. (2000). Recognizing one's own face. *Cognition*, **78**, B1–B15.

Kirkpatrick, B., Xu, L., Cascella, N., Ozeki, Y., Sawa, A., and Roberts, R.C. (2006). DISC1 immunoreactivity at the light and ultrastructural level in the human neocortex. *Journal of Comparative Neurology*, **497**, 436–450.

Kirov, G., Rujescu, D., Ingason, A., Collier, D.A., O'Donovan, M.C., and Owen, M.J. (2009). Neurexin 1 (NRXN1) deletions in schizophrenia. *Schizophrenia Bulletin,* **35,** 851–854.

Klerman, G.L. (1981). The spectrum of mania. *Comprehensive Psychiatry*, **22**, 11–20.

Knibb, J.A., Kipps, C.M., and Hodges, J.R. (2006). Frontotemporal dementia. *Current Opinion in Neurology*, **19**, 565–571.

Knight, R.T., Staines, W.R., Swick, D., and Chao, L.L. (1999). Prefrontal cortex regulates inhibition and excitation in distributed neural networks. *Acta Psychologica*, **101**, 159–178.

Knutson, B., Fong, G.W., Bennett, S.M., Adams, C.M., and Hommer, D. (2003). A region of mesial prefrontal cortex tracks monetarily rewarding outcomes: Characterization with rapid event-related fMRI. *NeuroImage,* **18**, 263–272.

Knutson, B., Taylor, J., Kaufman, M., Peterson, R., and Glover, G. (2005). Distributed neural representation of expected value. *Journal of Neuroscience*, **25**, 4806–4812.

Kolb, B., and Whishaw, I.Q. (1983). Performance of schizophrenic patients on tests sensitive to left or right frontal temporal parietal function in neurologic patients. *Journal of Nervous and Mental Disease*, **171**, 435–443.

Kolevzon, A., Gross, R., and Reichenberg, A. (2007). Prenatal and perinatal factors for autism: A review and integration of findings. *Archives of Pediatric and Adolescent Medicine*, **161**, 326–333.

Konick, L.C., and Friedman, L. (2001). Meta-analysis of thalamic size in schizophrenia. *Biological Psychiatry*, **49**, 28–38.

Koo, M.S., Levitt, J.J., Salisbury, D.F., Nakamura, M., Shenton, M.E., and McCarley, R.W. (2008). A cross-sectional and longitudinal magnetic resonance imaging study of cingulate gyrus gray matter volume abnormalities in first-episode schizophrenia and first-episode affective psychosis. *Archives of General Psychiatry*, **65**, 746–760.

Konopka, G., Bomar, J.M., Winden, K., Coppola, G., Jonsson, Z.O., Gao, F., Peng, S., Preuss, T.M., Wohlschlegel, J.A., and Geschwind, D.H. (2010). Human-specific transcriptional regulation of CNS development genes by FOXP2. *Nature*, **462**, 213–218.

Kort, E.J., Paneth, N., and Vande Woude, G.F. (2009). The decline in U.S. cancer mortality in people born since 1925. *Cancer Research,* **69,** 6500–6505.

Koshino, H., Carpenter, P.A., Minshew, N.J., Cherkassky, V.L., Keller, T.A., and Just, M.A. (2005). Functional connectivity in an fMRI working memory task in high-functioning autism. *NeuroImage*, **24**, 810–821.

Kovelman, J.A., and Scheibel, A.B. (1984). A neurohistological correlate of schizophrenia. *Biological Psychiatry*, **19**, 1601–1621.

Kowalska, D.M., Ku mierek, P., Kosmal, A., and Mishkin, M. (2001). Neither perirhinal/entorhinal nor hippocampal lesions impair short-term auditory recognition memory in dogs. *Neuroscience*, **104**, 965–978.

Kraepelin, E. (1919). *Dementia Praecox and Paraphrenia* (R.M. Barclay, Trans., G.M. Robertson, Ed.), special edition, 1989. Birmingham, AL, The Classics of Medicine Library.

Kraepelin, E. (1921). *Manic-Depressive Insanity and Paranoia* (R.M. Barclay, Trans., G.M. Robertson. Ed.), special edition, 1989. Birmingham, AL, The Classics of Medicine Library.

Kreutzberg, G.W. (1996). Microglia: A sensor for pathological events in the CNS. *Trends in Neuroscience*, **19**, 312–318.

Krystal, J.H., Belger, A., Abi-Saab, W., Moghaddam, B., Charney, D.S., Anand, A., Madonick, S., and D'Souza, D.C. (2000). Glutamatergic contributions to cognitive dysfunction in schizophrenia. In T. Sharma and P. Harvey (Eds.), *Cognition in Schizophrenia: Impairments, Importance, and Treatment Strategies* (pp. 126–153). New York, Oxford.

Krystal, J.H., Karper, L.P., Seibyl, J.P., Freeman, G.K., Delaney, R., Bremner, J.D., Heninger, G.R., Bowers, M.B., and Charney, D.S. (1994). Subanesthetic effects of the noncompetitive NMDA antagonist, ketamine in humans: Psychomimetic, perceptual, cognitive, and neuroendocrine responses. *Archives of General Psychiatry*, **51**, 199–214.

Kubicki, M., Westin, C-F., Nestor, P.G., Wible, C.G., Frumin, M., Maier, S.E., Kikinis, R., Jolesz, F.A., McCarley, R.W., and Shenten, M.E. (2003). Cingulate fasciculus integrity disruption in schizophrenia: A magnetic resonance diffusion tensor imaging study. *Biological Psychiatry*, **54**, 1171–1180.

Laasko, A., Vilkman, H., Alakare, B., Haaparanta, M., Bergman, J., Solin, O., Peurasaari, J., Räkköläinen, V., Syvälahti, E., and Hietala, J. (2000). Striatal dopamine transporter binding in neuroleptic-naïve patients with schizophrenia studied with positron emission tomography. *American Journal of Psychiatry*, **157**, 269–271.

Laberge, D.L. (1995). *Attentional Processing: The Brain's Art of Mindfulness.* Cambridge, Harvard University Press.

Lahera, G., Montes, J.M., Benito, A., Valdivia, M., Medina, E., Mirapeix, I., and Sáiz-Ruiz, J. (2008). Theory of mind deficit in bipolar disorder: Is it related to a previous history of psychotic symptoms? *Psychiatry Research*, **161**, 309–317.

Lahti, A.C., Holcomb, H.H., Medoff, D.R., Weiler, M.A., Tamminga, C.A., and Carpenter, W.T. (2001). Abnormal patterns of regional cerebral blood flow in schizophrenia with primary negative symptoms during an effortful auditory recognition task. *American Journal of Psychiatry*, **158**, 1797–1808.

Lahti, A.C., Koffel, B., Laporte, D., and Tamminga, C.A. (1995b) Subanesthetic doses of ketamine stimulate psychosis in schizophrenia. *Neuropsychopharmacology*, **13**, 9–19.

Lahti, A.C., Weiler, M.A., Holcomb, H.H., Tamminga, C.A., Tamminga, C.A., Carpenter, W.T., and McMahon, R. (2006). Correlations between rCBF and symptoms in two independent cohorts of drug-free patients with schizophrenia. *Neuropsychopharmacology*, **31**, 221–230.

Lai, C.S.L., Fisher, S.E., Hurst, J.A., Vargha-Khadem, F., and Monaco, A.P. (2001). A fork-domain gene is mutated in a severe speech and language disorder. *Nature*, **413**, 519–523.

Lainhart, J.E. (2006). Advances in autism neuroimaging research for the clinician and geneticist. *American Journal of Medical Genetics C (Seminars in Medical Genetics)*, **142**, 33–39.

Landrigan, P. (2010). What causes autism? Exploring the environmental contribution. *Current Opinion in Pediatrics*, **22**, 1–7.

Lane, H.Y., Chang, Y.-C., Liu, Y.-C., Chiu, C.C., and Tsai, G.E. (2005). Sarcosine or D-serine add-on treatment for acute exacerbation of schizophrenia: A randomized, double-blind, placebo-controlled study. *Archives of General Psychiatry*, **62**, 1196–1204.

Lane, R.D., and Nadel, L. (Eds.) (2000). *Cognitive Neuroscience of Emotion.* New York, Oxford University Press.

Lanius, R.A., Williamson, P.C., Densmore, M., Boksman, K., Gupta, M., Neufeld, R.W.J., Gati, J.S., and Menon, R. (2001). Neural correlates of traumatic memories in post-traumatic stress disorder: A functional MRI investigation. *American Journal of Psychiatry*, **158**, 1920–1922.

Lanius, R., Williamson, P.C., Densmore, M., Boksman, K., Neufeld, R.W.J., Gati, J., and Menon, R.S. (2004). The nature of traumatic memories: A functional MRI connectivity analysis. *American Journal of Psychiatry*, **161**, 36–44.

Laruelle, M. (1998). Imaging dopamine transmission in schizophrenia: A review and meta-analysis. *Quarterly Journal of Nuclear Medicine*, **42**, 211–221.

Laruelle, M., Abi-Dargham, A., Van Dyck, C.H., Gil, R., DeSouza, C.D., Erdos, J., McCance, E., Rosenblatt, W., Fingado, C., Zoghbi, S.S., Baldwin, R.M., Seibyl, J.P., Krystal, J.H., Charney, D.S., and Innis, R.B. (1996). Single photon emission computerized tomography imaging of amphetamine-induced dopamine release in drug-free schizophrenic subjects. *Proceedings of the National Academy of Sciences of the USA*, **93**, 9235–9240.

Lasky-Su, J.A., Faroane, S.V., Glatt, S.J., and Tsuang, M.T. (2005). Meta-analysis of the association between two polymorphisms in the serotonin transporter gene and affective disorders. *American Journal of Medical Genetics Part B (Neuropsychiatric Genetics)*, **133B**, 110–115.

Lavenu, I., Pasquier, F., Lebert, F., Petit, H., and Van der Linden, M. (1999). Perception of emotion in frontotemporal dementia and Alzheimer disease. *Alzheimer Disease and Associated Disorders*, **13**, 96–101.

Lawrie, S.M., and Abukmeil, S. (1998). Brain abnormality in schizophrenia: A systematic and quantitative review of volumetric magnetic resonance imaging studies. *British Journal of Psychiatry*, **172**, 110–120.

Lawrie, S.M., Whalley, H., Kestelman, J.N., Abukmeil, S.S., Byrne, M., Hodges, A., Rimmington, J.E., Best, J.J.K., and Johnstone, E.C. (1999). Magnetic resonance imaging of the brain in people at high risk of developing schizophrenia. *Lancet*, **353**, 30–33.

Lazarus, R.S. (1991). Cognition and motivation in emotion. *American Psychologist*, **46**, 352–367.

LeDoux, J. (1996). *The Emotional Brain: The Mysterious Underpinnings of Emotional Life*. New York, Simon and Schuster.

Lee, J.E., Bigler, E.D., Alexander, A.L., Lazar, M., DuBray, M.B., Chung, M.K., Johnson, M., Morgan, J., Miller, J.N., McMahon, W.M., Lu, J., Jeong, E.K., and Lainhart, J.E. (2007). Diffusion tensor imaging of white matter in the superior temporal gyrus and temporal stem in autism. *Neuroscience Letters*, **424**, 127–132.

Legrand, D., and Ruby, P. (2009). What is self-specific? Theoretical investigation and critical review of neuroimaging results. *Psychological Review*, **116**, 252–282.

Leigh, S.R. (2004). Brain growth, life history, and cognition in primate and human evolution. *American Journal of Primatology*, **62**, 139–164.

Leonhard, K. (1957). *The Classification of Endogenous Psychoses* (E. Robins, Ed., R. Berman, Trans.), 5th ed, 1979. New York, Irvington Publishers, Inc. Originally published as *Aufteilung der endogenen psychochosen*, 1957, Berlin, Akademie-Verlag.

Leonard, S., Gault, J., Hopkins, J., Logel, J., Vianzon, R., Short, M., Drebing, C., Berger, R., Venn, D., Sirota, P., Zerbe, G., Olincy, A., Ross, R.G., Adler, L., and Freedman, R. (2002). Association of promoter variants in the 7 nicotinic acetylcholine receptor subunit gene with inhibitory deficit found in schizophrenia. *Archives of General Psychiatry*, **59**, 1085–1096.

Leopold, D.A., Murayama, Y., and Logothetis, N.K. (2003). Very slow activity fluctuations in monkey visual cortex: Implications for functional brain imaging. *Cerebral Cortex*, **13**, 423–433.

Lesch, K.P., Meyer, J., Glatz, K., Flügge, G., Hinney, A., Hebebrand, J., Klauck, S.M., Poustka, F., Begel, D., Mössner, R., Riederer, P., and Heils, A. (1997). The 5-HT transporter gene-linked polymorphic region (5-HTTLPR) in evolutionary perspective: Alternative biallelic variation in rhesus monkeys. *Journal of Neural Transmission*, **104**, 1259–1266.

Levitan, C., Ward, P.B., and Catts, S.V. (1999). Superior temporal gyral volumes and laterality correlates of auditory hallucinations in schizophrenia. *Biological Psychiatry*, **46**, 955–962.

Levitt, J.G., O'Neill, J., Blanton, R.E., Smalley, S., Fardale, D., McCracken, J.T., Guthrie, D., Toga, A.W., and Alger, J.R. (2003). Proton magnetic resonance spectroscopic imaging of the brain in childhood autism. *Biological Psychiatry*, **54**, 1355–1366.

Lewis, C.M., Levinson, D.F., Wise, L.H., DeLisi, L.E., Straub, R.E., Hovatta, I., Williams, N.M., Schwab, S.G., Pulver, A.E. Faraone, S.V., Brzustowicz, L.M., Kaufmann, C.A., Garver, D.L., Gurling, H.M.D., Lindholm, E., Coon, H., Moises, H.W., Byerley, W., Shaw, S.H., Mesen, A., Sherrington, R., O'Neill, F.A., Walsh, D., Kendler, K.S., Ekelund, J., Paunio, T., Lönnqvist, J., Peltonen, L., O'Donovan M.C., Owen, M.J., Wildenauer, D.B., Maier, W., Nestadt, G., Blouin, J.-L., Antonarakis, D.B., Mowry, B.J., Silverman, J.M., Crowe, R.C., Cloninger, C.R., Tsuang, M.T., Malaspina, D., Harkavy-Friedman, J.M., Svrakic, D.M., Bassett, A.S., Holcomb, J., Kalsi, G., McQuillin, A., Brynjolfson, J., Sigmundsson, T., Petursson, H., Jazin, E., Zoëga, T., and Helgason, T. (2003). Genome scan meta-analysis of schizophrenia and bipolar disorder, Part II: Schizophrenia. *American Journal of Human Genetics*, **73**, 34–48.

Lewis, D.A. (1997). Development of the prefrontal cortex during adolescence: Insights into vulnerable neural circuits in schizophrenia. *Neuropsychopharmacology*, **16**: 385–398.

Lewis, D.A., and González-Burgos, G. (2006). Pathophysiologically based treatment interventions in schizophrenia. *Nature Medicine*, **12**, 1016–1022.

Lewis, D.A., and González-Burgos, G. (2008). Neuroplasticity of neocortical circuits in schizophrenia. *Neuropsychopharmacology Reviews*, **33**, 141–165.

Lewis, D.A., Hashimoto, T., and Volk, D.W. (2005). Cortical inhibitory neurons and schizophrenia. *Nature Review Neuroscience*, **6**, 312–324.

Lewis, D.A., Melchitzky, D.S., and González-Burgos, G. (2002). Specificity in functional architecture of primate prefrontal cortex. *Journal of Neurocytology,* **31**, 265–276.

Lewis, S.W., Ford, R.A., Syed, G.M., Revely, A.M., and Toone, B.K. (1992). A controlled study of 99mTc-HMPAO single-photon emission imaging in chronic schizophrenia. *Psychological Medicine*, **22**, 27–35.

Li, T., and Song, A.W. (2003). Fast functional brain signal changes detected by diffusion weighted fMRI. *Magnetic Resonance Imaging*, **21**, 829–833.

Li, X., Chauhan, A., Sheikh, A.M., Patil, S., Chauhan, V., Li, X-M., Ji, L., Brown, T., and Malik, M. (2009). Elevated immune response in the brain of autistic patients. *Journal of Neuroimmunology,* **207,** 111–116.

Liang, M., Zhou, Y., Jiang, T, Liu, Z., Tian, L., Liu, H., and Hao, Y. (2006). Widespread functional disconnectivity in schizophrenia with resting-state functional magnetic resonance imaging. *NeuroReport*, **17**, 209–213.

Lichtenstein, P., Yip, B.H., Björk, C., Pawitan, Y., Cannon, T.D., Sullivan, P.F., and Hultman, C.M. (2009). Common genetic determinants of schizophrenia and bipolar disorder in Swedish families: A population-based study. *Lancet*, **373**, 234–239.

Liddle, P.F., Friston, K.J., Frith, C.D., Hirsch, S.R., Jones T., and Frackowiak, R.S.J. (1992). Patterns of cerebral blood flow in schizophrenia. *British Journal of Psychiatry*, **160**, 179–186.

Lieberman, J., Chakos, M., Wu, H., Alvir, J., Hoffman, E., Robinson, D., and Bilder, R. (2001). Longitudinal study of brain morphology in first episode schizophrenia. *Biological Psychiatry*, **49**, 487–499.

Lieberman, P. (1985). On the evolution of human syntactic ability. Its pre-adaptive bases-motor control and speech. *Journal of Human Evolution*, **14**, 657–668.

Lim, K.O., and Helpern, J.A. (2002). Neuropsychiatric applications of DTI: A review. *NMR in Biomedicine*, **15**, 587–593.

Lindström, L.H., Gefvert, O., Hagberg, G., Lundberg, T., Bergström, M., Hartvig, P., and Långström, B. (1999). Increased dopamine synthesis rate in medial prefrontal cortex and striatum in schizophrenia indicated by L-($-^{11}$C) dopa and PET. *Biological Psychiatry*, **46**, 681–688.

Llinás, R.R., and Pare, D. (1991). Of dreaming and wakefulness. *Neuroscience*, **44**, 521–535.

Llinás, R., Ribary, U., Joliot, M., and Wang, X-J. (1994). Content and context in temporal thalamocortical binding. In G. Buzáki, R. Llinás, W. Singer, A. Berthoz, and Y. Christen (Eds.), *Temporal Coding in the Brain* (pp. 251–272), Berlin, Springer-Verlag.

Ludwig, H., and Bode, L. (2000). Borna disease virus: New aspects on infection, disease, diagnosis and epidemiology. *Scientific and Technical Review of the Office International des Epizooties*, **19**, 259–288.

Machón, R.A., Mednick, S.A., and Huttunen, M.O. (1997). Adult major affective disorder after prenatal exposure to an influenza epidemic. *Archives of General Psychiatry*, **54**, 322–328.

MacQueen, G.M., Campbell, S., McEwen, B.S., Macdonald, K., Amano, S., Joffe, R.T., Nahmias, C., and Young, T. (2003). Course of illness, hippocampal function, and hippocampal volume in major depression. *Proceedings of the National Academy of Sciences USA*, **100**, 1387–1392.

MacLean, P.D. (1978). Challenges of the Papez heritage. In K.E. Livingston and O. Hornykiewcz (Eds.), *Limbic Mechanisms: The Continuing Evolution of the Limbic System Concept* (pp. 1–15). New York, Plenum.

Maddock, R.J. (1999). The retrosplenial cortex and emotion: New insights from functional neuroimaging of the human brain. *Trends in Neurosciences*, **22**, 310–316.

Maguire, E.A., and Mummery, C.J. (1999). Differential modulation of a common memory retrieval network revealed by positron emission tomography. *Hippocampus,* **9**, 54–61.

Mahmood, T., and Silverstone, T. (2001). Serotonin and bipolar disorder. *Journal of Affective Disorders*, **66**, 1–11.

Maier, M., Ron, M.A., Barker, G.J., and Tofts, P.S. (1995). Proton magnetic resonance spectroscopy: An in vivo method of estimating hippocampal neuronal depletion in schizophrenia. *Psychological Medicine*, **25**, 1201–1209.

Makris, N., Biederman, J., Valera, E.M., Bush, G., Kaiser, J., Kennedy, D.N., Caviness, V.S., Faraone, S.V., and Seidman, L.J. (2007). Cortical thinning of the attention and executive function networks in adults with attention-deficit/hyperactivity disorder. *Cerebral Cortex,* **17,** 1364–1375.

Makris, N., Goldstein, J.M., Kennedy, D., Hodge, S.M., Caviness, V.S., Faraone, S.V., Tsuang, M.T., and Seidman, L.J. (2006). Decreased volume of left and total anterior insular lobule in schizophrenia. *Schizophrenia Research,* **83,** 155–171.

Malhi, G.S., Ivanovski, B., Szekeres, V., and Olley, A. (2004). Bipolar disorder: It's all in your mind? The neuropsychological profile of a biological disorder. *Canadian Journal of Psychiatry*, **49**, 813–819.

Manaye, K.F., Lei, D.-L., Tizabi, Y., Dávila-Garcia, M.I., Mouton, P.R., and Kelley, P.H. (2005). Selective neuronal loss in the paraventricular nucleus of the hypothalamus in patients suffering from major depression and bipolar disorder. *Journal of Neuropathology and Experimental Neurology*, **64**, 224–229.

Manji, H.K., Drevets, W.C., and Charney, D.S. (2001). The cellular neurobiology of depression. *Nature Medicine*, **5**, 541–547.

Manji, H.K., and Lenox, R.H. (2000). Signaling: Cellular insights into the pathophysiology of bipolar disorder. *Biological Psychiatry*, **48**, 518–530.

Mariani, C., Defendi, S., Mailland, E., and Pomati, S. (2006). Frontotemporal dementia. *Neurological Sciences*, **27**, S35–S36.

Marques-Bonet, T., Kidd, J.M., Ventura, M., Graves, T.A., Cheng, Z., Hillier, L.W., Jiang, Z., Baker, C., Malfavron-Borja, R., Fulton, L.A., Alkan, C., Aksay, G., Girirajan, S., Siswara, P., Chen, L., Cardone, M.F., Navarro, A., Mardis, E.R., Wilson, R.K., and Eichler, E.E. (2009). A burst of segmental duplications in the genome of the African great ape ancestor. *Nature*, **457**, 877–881.

Marshall, C.R., Noor, A., Vincent, J.B., Lionel, A.C., Feuk, L., Skaug, J., Shago, M., Moessner, R., Pinto, D., Ren, Y., Thiruvahindrapduram, B., Fiebig, A., Schreiber, S., Friedman, J., Ketelaars, C.E.J., Vos, V.J., Ficicioglu, C., Kirkpatrick, S., Nicolson, R., Sloman, L., Summers, A., Gibbons, C.A., Teebi, A., Chitayat, D., Weksberg, R., Thompson, A., Vardy, C., Crosbie, V., Luscombe, S., Baatjes, R., Zwaigenbaum, L., Roberts, W., Fernandez, B., Szatmari, P., and Scherer, S.W. (2008). Structural variation of chromosomes in autism spectrum disorder. *American Journal of Human Genetics,* **82,** 477–488.

Mataix-Cols, D., An, S.K., Lawrence, N.S., Caseras, X., Speckens, A., Giampietro, V., Brammer, M.J., and Phillips, M.L. (2008). Individual differences in disgust sensitivity modulate neural response to aversive disgusting stimuli. *European Journal of Neuroscience,* **27**, 3050–3058.

Martin, A., Wiggs, C.L., Ungerleider, L.G., and Haxby, J.V. (1996). Neural correlates of category-specific knowledge. *Nature*, **379**, 649–652.

Martin, L.A., Ashwood, P, Braunschweig, D., Cabanlit, M., Van de Water, J., and Amaral, D.G. (2008). Stereotypes and hyperactivity in rhesus monkeys exposed to IgG from mothers of children with autism. *Brain Behaviour and Immunity*, **22**, 804–805.

Marquès-Bonet, T., Cáceres, M., Bertranpetit, J., Preuss, T.M., Thomas, J.M., and Navarro, A. (2004). Chromosomal rearrangements and the genomic distribution of gene-expression divergence in humans band chimpanzees. *Trends in Genetics*, **20**, 524–529.

Mason, M.F., Norton, M.I,. Van Horn, J.D., Wegner, D.M., Grafton, S.T., and Macrae, C.N. (2007). Wandering minds: The default network and stimulus-independent thought. *Science*, **315**, 393–395.

Mata, I., Perez-Iglesias, R., Roiz-Santianez, R., Tordesillas-Gutierrez, D., Gonzalez-Mandly, A., Vazquez-Barquero, J.L., and Crespo-Facorro, B. (2009). A neuregulin 1 variant is associated with increased lateral ventricular volume in patients with first-episode schizophrenia. *Biological Psychiatry*, **65**, 535–540.

Mathalon, D.H., Sullivan, E.V., Lim, K.O., and Pfefferbaum, A. (2001). Progressive brain volume changes and the clinical course of schizophrenia in men: A longitudinal magnetic resonance imaging study. *Archives of General Psychiatry*, **58**, 148–157.

Matsumoto, M., and Hikosaka, O. (2007). Lateral habenula as a source of negative reward signals in dopamine neurons. *Nature,* **447**, 1111–1115.

Matsumoto, M., and Hikosaka, O. (2009). Two types of dopamine neuron distinctly convey positive and negative motivational signals. *Nature*, **459**, 837–841.

May, P.R.A., Tuma, A.H., and Dixon, W.J. (1981). Schizophrenia: A follow-up study of the results of five forms of treatment. *Archives of General Psychiatry*, **38**, 776–784.

Mayberg, H.S. (2003). Positron emission tomography imaging in depression: A neural systems perspective. *Neuroimaging Clinics of North America*, **13**, 805–815.

Mayberg, H.S., Liotti, M., Brannan, S.K., McGinnis, S., Mahurin, R.K., Jerabek, P.A., Silva, J.A., Tekell, J.L., Martin, C.C., Lancaster, J.L., and Fox, P.T. (1999). Reciprocal limbic-cortical function and negative mood: Converging PET findings in depression and normal sadness. *American Journal of Psychiatry*, **156**, 675–682.

Mayberg, H.S., Lozano, A.M., Voon, V., McNeeley, H.E., Seminowicz, D., Hamani, C., Schwalb, J.M., and Kennedy, S.H. (2005). Deep brain stimulation for treatment-resistant depression. *Neuron*, **45**, 651–660.

McGhie, A., and Chapman, J. (1961). Disorders of attention and perception in early schizophrenia. *British Journal of Medical Psychology*, **34**, 103–116.

McGowan, P., Sasaki, A., Alessio, A., Dymov, S., Labonte, B., Szyf, M., Turecki, G., and Meaney, M. (2009). Epigenetic regulation of the glucocorticoid receptor in human brain associated with childhood abuse. *Nature Neuroscience,* **12**, 342–348.

McGowan, S., Lawrence, A.D., Sales, T., Quested, D., and Grasby, P. (2004). Presynaptic dopaminergic dysfunction in schizophrenia: a positron emission tomographic [^{18}F] fluorodopa study. *Archives of General Psychiatry*, **61**, 134–142.

McGrath, J.J., and Murray, R.M. (1995). Risk factors for schizophrenia: From conception to birth. In S. Hirsch and D. Weinberger (Eds.), *Schizophrenia* (pp. 187–205). Oxford, Blackwell.

McGuire, P.K., Silbersweig, D.A., Wright, I., Murray, R.M., David, A.S., Frackowiak, R.S.J., and Frith, C.D. (1995). Abnormal monitoring of inner speech: A physiological basis for auditory hallucinations. *Lancet*, **346**, 596–600.

McQueen, M.B., Devlin, B., Faraone, S.V., Nimgaonkar, V.L., Sklar, P., Smoller, J., Jamra, R.A., Albus, M., Bacanu, S.-A., Baron, M., Barrett, T.B., Berrettini, W., Blacker, D., Byerley, W., Cichon, S., Coryell, W., Craddock, N., Daly, M.J., DePaulo, J.R., Edenberg, H.J., Foroud, T., Gill, M., Gilliam, C., Hamshere, M., Jones, I., Jones, L., Juo, S.-H., Kelsoe, J.R., Lambert, D., Lange, C., Lerer, B., Liu, J., Maier, W., MacKinnon, J.D., McInnis, M.G., McMahon, F.J., Murphy, D.L., Nöthen, M.M., Numberger, J.I., Pato, C.N., Pato, M.T., Potash, J.B., Propping, P., Pulver, A.E., Rice, J.P., Rietschel, M., Scheftner, W., Schumacher, J., Segurado, R., Van Steen, K., Xie, W., Zandi, P.P., and Laird, N.M. (2005). Combined analysis from eleven linkage studies of bipolar disorder provides strong evidence of susceptibility loci on chromosome 6q and 8q. *American Journal of Human Genetics*, **77**, 582–595.

McNeil, T.F., Cantor-Graae, E., and Weinberger, D.R. (2000). Relationship of obstetrical complications and differences in size of brain structures in monozygotic twin pairs discordant for schizophrenia. *American Journal of Psychiatry*, **157**, 203–212.

Meador-Woodruff, J.H., and Healy, D.J. (2000). Glutamate receptor expression in schizophrenic brain. *Brain Research Reviews*, **31**, 288–294.

Mega, M.S., Cummings, J.L., Salloway, S., and Malloy, P. (1997). The limbic system: An anatomic, phylogenetic, and clinical perspective. *Journal of Neuropsychiatry*, **9**, 315–330.

Mesulam, M-M. (1990). Large-scale neurocognitive networks and distributed processing for attention, language, and memory. *Annals of Neurology*, **28**, 597–613.

Mesulam, M-M. (2000). Behavioural neuroanatomy. In M.M. Mesulam (Ed.), *Principles of Behavioural and Cognitive Neurology* (pp. 1–120). New York, Oxford.

Metzinger, T. (Ed.) (2000). *Neural Correlates of Consciousness: Empirical and Conceptual Questions*. Cambridge, MIT Press.

Meyer-Lindenberg, A., Miletich, R.S., Kohn, P.D., Esposito, G., Carson, R.E., Quarantelli, M., Weinberger, D.R., and Berman, K.F. (2002). Reduced prefrontal activity predicts exaggerated striatal dopaminergic function in schizophrenia. *Nature Neuroscience*, **5**, 267–271.

Middleton, F.A., and Strick, P.L. (2001). A revised neuroanatomy of frontal-subcortical circuits. In D.G. Lichter and J.L. Cummings (Eds.), *Frontal-Subcortical Circuits in Psychiatric and Neurological Disorders* (pp. 44–58). New York, Guilford Press.

Miller, B.L., and Gearhart, R. (1999). Neuroimaging in the diagnosis of frontotemporal dementia. *Dementia and Geriatric Cognitive Disorders*, **10**, 71–74.

Miller, B.L., Seeley, W.W., Mychack, P., Rosen, H.J., Mena, I., and Boone, K. (2001). Neuroanatomy of the self: Evidence from patients with frontotemporal dementia. *Neurology*, **57**, 817–821.

Miller, E.K., and Cohen, J.D. (2001). An integrative theory of prefrontal cortex function. *Annual Reviews of Neuroscience*, **24**, 167–202.

Miller, J.N., and Ozonoff, S. (2000). The external validity of Asperger disorder: Lack of evidence from the domain of neuropsychology. *Journal of Abnormal Psychology*, **109**, 227–238.

Mimmack, M.L., Ryan, M., Baba, H., Navarro-Ruiz, J., Iritani, S., Faull, R.L.M., McKenna, P.J., Jones, P.B., Arai, H., Starkey, M., Emson, P.C., and Bahn, S. (2002). Gene expression analysis in schizophrenia: Reproducible up-regulation of several members of the apolipoprotein L family located in a high-susceptibility locus for schizophrenia on chromosome 22. *Proceedings of the National Academy of Sciences of the USA,* **99,** 4680–4685.

Minio-Paluello, I., Baron-Cohen, S., Avenanti, A., Walsh, V., and Aglioti, S.M. (2009). Absence of embodied empathy during pain observation in Asperger syndrome. *Biological Psychiatry,* **65**, 55–62.

Minshew, N.J., Goldstein, G., Dombrowski, S.M., Panchalingam, K., and Pettegrew, J.W. (1993). A preliminary ^{31}P MRS study of autism: Evidence for undersynthesis and increased degradation of brain metabolites. *Biological Psychiatry*, **33**, 762–773.

Minshew, N.J., Goldstein, G., and Siegel, D.J. (1997). Neuropsychological functioning in autism: Profile of a complex information processing disorder. *Journal of the International Neuropsychological Society*, **3**, 303–316.

Minshew, N.J., and Williams, D.L. (2007). The new neurobiology of autism: Cortex, connectivity, and neuronal organization. *Archives of Neurology*, **64**, 945–950.

Minzenberg, M.J., Laird, A.R., Thelen, S., Carter, C.S., and Glahn, D.C. (2009). Meta-analysis of 41 functional neuroimaging studies of executive function in schizophrenia. *Archives of General Psychiatry*, **66**, 811–822.

Missler, M., Zhang, W., Rohlmann, A., Kattenstroth, G., Hammer, R.E., Gottman, K., and Südhof, T.C. (2003). a-Neurexins couple Ca^{21} channels to synaptic vesicle exocytosis. *Nature,* **423**, 939–948.

Mitchell, J.P., Banaji, M.R., and Macrae, C.N. (2005a). General and specific contributions of the medial prefrontal cortex to knowledge about mental states. *NeuroImage,* **28**, 757–762.

Mitchell, J.P., Banaji, M.R., and Macrae, C.N. (2005b). The link between social cognition and self-referential thought in the medial prefrontal cortex. *Journal of Cognitive Neuroscience*, **17**, 1306–1315.

Mogenson, G.J., Jones, D.L., and Yim, C.Y. (1980). From motivation to action: Functional interface between limbic system and the motor system. *Progress in Neurobiology*, **14**, 69–97.

Moghaddam, B. (2002). Stress activation of glutamate neurotransmission in the prefrontal cortex: implications for dopamine-associated psychiatric disorders. *Biological Psychiatry*, **51**, 775–787.

Molina Rodriguez, V., Andreé, R.M., Castejón, M.J.P., Labrador, R.G., Navarrete, F.F., Delgado, J.L.C., and Vila, F.J.R. (1997). Cerebral perfusion correlates of negative symptomatology and parkinsonism in a sample of treatment-refractory schizophrenics: An exploratory 99mTc-HMPAO SPET study. *Schizophrenia Research*, **25**, 11–20.

Molloy, C.A., Morrow, A.L., Meinzen-Derr, J., Dawson, G., Bernier, R., Dunn, M., Hyman, S.L., McMahon, W.M., Goudie-Nice, J., Hepburn, S., Minshew, N., Rogers, S., Sigman, M., Spence, M.A., Tager-Flusberg, H., Volkmar, F.R., and Lord, C. (2006). Familial autoimmune thyroid disease as a risk factor for regression in children with autism spectrum disorder: A CPEA study. *Journal of Autism and Developmental Disorders*, **36**, 317–324.

Morcom, A.M., and Fletcher, P.C. (2007). Does the brain have a baseline? Why we should be resisting a rest. *NeuroImage,* **37**, 1073–1082.

Morrison, A.P., and Haddock, G. (1997). Cognitive factors in source monitoring and auditory hallucinations. *Psychological Medicine*, **27**, 669–679.

Morrison-Stewart, S.L., Williamson, P.C., Corning, W.C., Kutcher, S.P., Snow, W.G., and Merskey, H. (1992). Frontal and non-frontal lobe neuropsychological test performance and clinical symptoms of schizophrenia. *Psychological Medicine*, **22**, 353–359.

Moses-Kolko, E.L., Price, J.C., Thase, M.E., Meltzer, C.C., Kupfer, D.J., Mathis, C.A., Bogers, W.D., Berman, S.R., Houck, P.R., Schneider, T.N., and Drevets, W.C. (2007). Measurement of 5-HT_{1A} receptor binding in depressed adults before and after antidepressant drug treatment using positron emission tomography and [^{11}C] WAY-100635. *Synapse*, **61**, 523–530.

Mulligan, A., Anney, R.J.L., O'Regan, M., Chen, W., Butler, L., Fitzgerald, M., Buitelaar, J., Steinhausen, H-C., Rothenberger, A., Minderaa, R., Nijmeijer, J., Hoekstra, P.J.,

Oades, R.D., Roeyers, H., Buschgens, C., Christiansen, H., Franke, B., Gabriels, I., Hartman, C., Kuntsi, J., Marco, R., Meidad, S., Mueller, U., Psychogiou, L., Rommelse, N., Thompson, M., Uebel, H., Banaschewski, T., Ebstein, R., Eisenberg, J., Manor, I., Miranda, A., Mulas, F., Sergeant, J., Sonuga-Barke, E., Asherson, P., Faraone, S.V., and Gill, M. (2009). Autism symptoms in attention-deficit/hyperactivity disorder: A familial trait which correlates with conduct, oppositional defiant, language and motor disorders. *Journal of Autism and Developmental Disorders,* **39,** 197–209.

Murphy, D.G.M., Daly, E., Schmitz, N., Toal, F., Murphy, K., Curran, S., Erlandsson, K., Eersels, J., Kerwin, R., Ell, P., and Travis, M. (2006). Cortical serotonin 5-HT_{2A} receptor binding and social communication in adults with Asperger's syndrome: An in vivo SPECT study. *American Journal of Psychiatry*, **163**, 934–936.

Murray, C.J.L., and Lopez, A.D. (Ed.). (1996). *The Global Burden of Disease: A Comprehensive Assessment of Mortality, and Disability from Diseases, Injuries, and Risk Factors in 1990 and Projected to 2020.* Boston, Harvard University Press.

Murray, E.A. (2007). The amygdala, reward and emotion. *Trends in the Cognitive Sciences*, **11**, 489–497.

Nair, T.R., Christensen, J.D., Kingsbury, S.J., Kumar, N.G., Terry, W.M., and Garver, D.L. (1997). Progression of cerebroventricular enlargement and the subtyping of schizophrenia. *Psychiatry Research: Neuroimaging*, **74**, 141–150.

Nakamura, M., Salisbury, D.F., Hirayasu, Y., Bouix, S., Pohl, K.M., Yoshida, T., Koo, M.-S., Shenton, M.E., and McCarley R.W. (2007). Neocortical gray matter volume in first-episode schizophrenia and first-episode affective psychosis: A cross-sectional and longitudinal study. *Biological Psychiatry*, **62**, 773–783.

Narr, K.L., Sharma, T., Woods, R.P., Thompson, P.M., Sowell, E.R., Rex, D., Kim, S., Asuncion, D., Jang, S., Mazziotta, J., and Toga, A.W. (2003). Increases in regional subarachnoid CSF without apparent cortical gray matter deficits in schizophrenia: Modulating effects of sex and age. *American Journal of Psychiatry*, **160**, 2169–2180.

Nasrallah, H.A. (1985). The unintegrated right cerebral hemispheric consciousness as alien intruder: A possible mechanism for Schneiderian delusions in schizophrenia. *Comprehensive Psychiatry*, **26**, 273–282.

Nasrallah, H.A. (1986). Cerebral hemispheric asymmetries and interhemispheric integration in schizophrenia. In H.A. Nasrallah and D.R. Weinberger (Eds.), *Handbook of Schizophrenia, Vol. 1: The Neurology of Schizophrenia* (pp. 157–174). Amsterdam, Elsevier.

Nasrallah, H.A., Skinner, T.E., Schmalbrock, P., and Robitaille, P.M. (1994). In vivo proton magnetic resonance spectroscopy (H-1 MRS) of the hippocampal formation in schizophrenia: A pilot study. *British Journal of Psychiatry*, **165**, 481–485.

Neary, D., Snowden, J.S., Gustafson, L., Passant, U., Stuss, D., Black, S., Freedman, M., Kertesz, A., Robert, P.H., Albert, M., Boone, K., Miller, B.L., Cummings, J., and Benson, D.F. (1998). Frontotemporal lobar degeneration: A consensus on clinical diagnostic criteria. *Neurology*, **51**, 1546–1554.

Neary, D., Snowden, J.S., and Mann, D. (2005). Frontotemporal dementia. *Lancet*, **4**, 771–780.

Nelson, M.D., Saykin, A.J., Flashman, L.A., and Riordan, H.J. (1998). Hippocampal volume reduction in schizophrenia as assessed by magnetic resonance imaging: A meta-analytic study. *Archives of General Psychiatry*, **55**, 433–440.

Nestor, P.G., Shenton, M.E., McCarley, R.W., Haimson, J., Smith, R.S., O'Donnell, B., Kimble, M., Kikinis, R., and Jolesz, F.A. (1993). Neuropsychological correlates of MRI temporal lobe abnormalities in schizophrenia. *American Journal of Psychiatry*, **150**, 1849–1855.

Neuchterlein, K.H., Dawson, M.E., and Green, M.F. (1994). Information processing abnormalities as neuropsychological vulnerability indicators for schizophrenia. *Acta Psychiatrica Scandinavica*, **90** (Suppl 384), 71–79.

Neumann, H., and Takahashi, K. (2007). Essential role of the microglial triggering receptor expressed on myeloid cells-2 (TREM2) for central nervous tissue immune homeostasis. *Journal of Neuroimmunology,* **184**, 92–99.

Neumärker, K.-J. (2003). Leo Kanner: His years in Berlin, 1906-24. The roots of autistic disorder. *History of Psychiatry*, **14**, 205–218.

Newman, J. (1997a). Putting the puzzle together. Part I: Towards a general theory of the neural correlates of consciousness. *Journal of Consciousness Studies*, **4**, 47–66.

Newman, J. (1997b). Putting the puzzle together. Part II: Towards a general theory of the neural correlates of consciousness. *Journal of Consciousness Studies*, **4**, 100–121.

Newman, J., and Grace, A.A. (1999). Binding across time: The selective gating of frontal and hippocampal systems modulating working memory and attentional states. *Consciousness and Cognition*, **8**, 196–212.

Newschaffer, C.J., Croen, L.A., Daniels, J., Giarelli, E., Grether, J.K., Levy, S.E., Mandell, D.S., Miller, L.A., Pinto-Martin, J., Reaven J., Reynolds, A.M., Rice, C.E., Schendel, D., and Windham, G.C. (2007). The epidemiology of autism spectrum disorders. *Annual Review of Public Health*, **28**, 235–258.

Nicholas, A.K., Swanson, E.A., Cox, J.J., Karbani, G., Malik, S., Springell, K., Hampshire, D., Ahmed, M., Bond, J., Di Benedetto, D., Fichera, M., Romano, C., Dobyns, W.B., and Woods, C.G. (2009). The molecular landscape of ASPM mutations in primary microcephaly. *Journal of Medical Genetics,* **46,** 249–253.

Nimchinsky, E.A., Gilissen, E., Allman, J.M., Perl, D.P., Erwin, J.M., and Hof, P.R. (1999). A neuronal morphologic type unique to humans and great apes. *Proceedings of the National Academy of Sciences of the USA*, **96**, 5268–5273.

Nimmerjahn, A., Kirchhoff, F., and Helmchen, F. (2005). Resting microglial cells are highly dynamic surveillants of brain parenchyma in vivo. *Science,* **308**, 1314–1318.

Norman, R.M.G., and Malla, A.K. (1993). Stressful life events and schizophrenia I: A review of the research. *British Journal of Psychiatry*, **162**, 161–166.

Northoff, G., Heinzel, A., de Greck, M., Bermpohl, F., Dobrowolny, H., and Panksepp, J. (2006). Self-referential processing in our brain: A meta-analysis of imaging studies on the self. *NeuroImage*, **31**, 440–457.

Nyberg, L., McIntosh, A.R., Cabeza, R., Habib, R., Houle, S., and Tulving, E. (1996). General and specific brain regions involved in encoding and retrieval of events: What, where and when. *Proceedings of the National Academy of Sciences of the USA*, **93**, 11280–11285.

Oberheim, N.A., Wang, X., Goldman, S., and Nedergaard, M. (2006). Astrocytic complexity distinguishes the human brain. *Trends in Neurosciences*, **29**, 547–553.

Oberman, L.M., and Ramachandran, V.S. (2007). The simulating social mind: The role of the mirror neuron system and simulation in the social and communicative deficits of autism spectrum disorders. *Psychological Bulletin*, **133**, 310–327.

O'Connor, M.-F., Irwin, M.R., and Wellisch, D.K. (2009). When grief heats up: Pro-inflammatory cytokines predict regional brain activation. *Neuroimage*, **47**, 891–896.

O'Callaghan, E., Redmond, O., Ennis, R., Stack, J., Kinsella, A., Ennis, J.T., Larkin, C., and Waddington, J.L. (1991). Initial investigation of the left temporoparietal region in schizophrenia by ^{31}P magnetic resonance spectroscopy. *Biological Psychiatry*, **29**, 1149–1152.

Ochsner, K.N. (2008). The social-emotional processing stream: Five core constructs and their translational potential for schizophrenia and beyond. *Biological Psychiatry*, **64**, 48–61.

O'Doherty, J., Critchley, H., Deichmann, R., and Dolan, R.J. (2003). Dissociating valence of outcome from behavioral control in human orbital and ventral prefrontal cortices. *Journal of Neuroscience*, **23**, 7931–7939.

O'Doherty, J., Kringelbach, M.L., Rolls, E.T., Hornak, J., and Andrew, C. (2001). Abstract reward and punishment representations in the human orbitofrontal cortex. *Nature Neuroscience*, **4**, 95–102.

O'Donnell, B.F., Vohs, J.L., Hetrick, W.P., Carroll, C.A., and Shekhar, A. (2004). Auditory event-related potential abnormalities in bipolar disorder and schizophrenia. *International Journal of Psychophysiology*, **53**, 45–55.

O'Donnell, P., and Grace, A.A. (1998). Dysfunction in multiple interrelated systems as the neurobiological bases of schizophrenic symptom clusters. *Schizophrenia Bulletin*, **24**, 267–283.

O'Donnell, P., Greene, J., Pabello, N., Lewis, B.L., and Grace, A.A. (1999). Modulation of cell firing in the nucleus accumbens. *Annals of the New York Academy of Sciences*, **877**, 157–175.

Olhmeier, M., Zhang, Y., Bode, L., Sieg, S., Feutl, S., Ludwig, H., Emrich, H., and Dietrich, D. (2008). Amantadine reduces mania in Borna disease virus-infected non-psychotic bipolar patients. *Pharmacopsychiatry*, **41**, 202–203.

Okuda, J., Fujii, T., Yamadori, A., Kawashima, R., Tsukiura, T., Fukatsu, R., Suzuki, K., Ito, M., and Fukuda, H. (1998). Participation of the prefrontal cortices in prospective memory: Evidence from a PET study in humans. *Neuroscience Letters,* **253**, 127–130.

O'Leary, D.D.M., Schlaggar, B.L., and Tuttle, R. (1994). Specification of neocortical areas and thalamocortical connections. *Annals of Neuroscience*, **17**, 419–439.

Olley, A.L., Malhi, G.S., Bachelor, J., Cahill, C.M., Mitchell, P.B., and Berk, M. (2005). Executive functioning and theory of mind in euthymic bipolar disorder. *Bipolar Disorders*, **7**, 43–52.

Olley, A., Malhi, G.S., Mitchell, P.B., Batchelor, J., Lagopoulis, J., and Austin, M.-P.V. (2005). When euthymia is just not good enough: The neuropsychology of bipolar disorder. *Journal of Nervous and Mental Diseases*, **193**, 323–330.

Olney, J.W., and Farber, N.B. (1995). Glutamate receptor dysfunction and schizophrenia. *Archives of General Psychiatry*, **52**, 998–1007.

Ongur, D., and Price, J.L. (2000). The organization of networks within the orbital and medial prefrontal cortex of rats, monkeys and humans. *Cerebral Cortex*, **10**, 206–219.

Oquendo, M.A., Hastings, R.S., Huang, Y.-Y., Simpson, N., Ogden, R.T., Hu, X.-Z., Goldman, D., Arango, V., Van Heertum., R.L., Mann, J.J., and Parsey, R.V. (2007). Brain serotonin transporter binding in depressed patients with bipolar disorder using positron emission tomography. *Archives of General Psychiatry*, **64**, 201–208.

Orzack, M.H., and Kornetsky, C. (1966). Attention dysfunction in chronic schizophrenia. *Archives of General Psychiatry*, **14**, 323–326.

Otsuka, H., Harada, M., Mora, K., Hisaoka, S., and Nishitani, H. (1999). Brain metabolites in the hippocampus-amygdala region and cerebellum in autism: An ^{1}H MR spectroscopy study. *Neuroradiology*, **41**, 517–519.

Owen, A.M., Evans, A.C., and Petrides, M. (1996). Evidence for a two-stage model of spatial working memory processing within the lateral frontal cortex: A positron emission tomography study. *Cerebral Cortex*, **6**, 31–38.

Owen, M.J., Craddock, N., and Jablensky, A. (2007). The genetic deconstruction of psychosis. *Schizophrenia Bulletin*, **33**, 905–911.

Owen, M.J., Williams, N.M., and O'Donovan, M.C. (2004). The molecular genetics of schizophrenia: New findings promise new insights. *Molecular Psychiatry*, **9**, 14–27.

Paillère-Martinot, M-L., Caclun, A., Artiges, E., Poline, J-B., Joliot, M., Mallet, L., Recasens, C., Attar-Lévy, D., and Martinot, J-L. (2001). Cerebral gray matter and white matter reductions and clinical correlates in patients with early onset schizophrenia. *Schizophrenia Research*, **50**, 19–26.

Pakkenberg, B. (1990). Pronounced reduction of total neuron number in mediodorsal thalamic nucleus and nucleus accumbens in schizophrenics. *Archives of General Psychiatry*, **47**, 1023–1028.

Pakkenberg, B. (1992). The volume of the mediodorsal thalamic nucleus in treated and untreated schizophrenics. *Schizophrenia Research*, **7**, 95–100.

Palmen, S.J.M.C., van Engeland, H., Hof, P.R., and Schmitz, C. (2004). Neuropathological findings in autism. *Brain,* **127**, 2572–2583.

Pandya, D.N. (1995). Anatomy of the auditory cortex. *Review of Neurology (Paris)*, **151**, 486–494.

Pantelis, C., Velakoulis, D., McGorry, P.D., Wood, S.J., Suckling, J., Phillips, L.J., Yung, A.R., Bullmore, E.T., Brewer, W., Soulsby, B., Desmond, P., and McGuire, P.K. (2003). Neuroanatomical abnormalities before and after onset of psychosis: A cross-sectional and longitudinal MRI comparison. *Lancet*, **361**, 281–288.

Papadopoulos, F.C., Ekbom, A., Brandt, L., and Ekselius, L. (2009). Excess mortality, causes of death and prognostic factors in anorexia nervosa. *British Journal of Psychiatry,* **194,** 10–17.

Papez, J. W. (1937). A proposed mechanism of emotion. *Archives of Neurology*, **38**, 725–743.

Pardo, C.A., and Eberhart, C.G. (2007). The neurobiology of autism. *Brain Pathology*, **17**, 434–447.

Park, S., Holzman, P.S., and Goldman-Rakic, P.S. (1995). Spatial working memory deficits in the relatives of schizophrenic patients. *Archives of General Psychiatry*, **52**, 821–828.

Parker, G.J.M., Luzzi, S., Alexander, D.C., Wheeler-Kingshott, C.A.M., Ciccarelli, O., and Lambon Ralph, M.A. (2005). Lateralization of ventral and dorsal auditory-language pathways in the human brain. *NeuroImage*, **24**, 656–666.

Passingham, R.E., Bengtsson, S.L., and Lau, H.C. (2010). Medial frontal cortex: From self-generated action to reflection on one's own performance. *Trends in Cognitive Sciences*, **14**, 16–21.

Patil, S.T., Zhang, L., Martenyi, F., Lowe, S.L., Jackson, K.A., Andreev, B.V., Avedisova, A.S., Bardenstein, L.M., Gurovich, I.Y., Morozova, M.A., Mosolov, S.N., Neznanov, N.G., Reznik, A.M., Smulevich, A.B., Tochilov, V.A., Johnson, B.G., Monn, J.A., and Schoepp, D.D. (2007). Activation of mGlu2/3 receptors as a new approach to treat schizophrenia: A randomized phase 2 clinical trial. *Nature Medicine*, **13**, 1102–1107.

Patterson, R.D., and Johnsrude, I.S. (2008). Functional imaging of the auditory processing applied to speech sounds. *Philosophical Transactions of the Royal Society B*, **363**, 1023–1035.

Paus, T. (2001). Primate anterior cingulate cortex: Where motor control, drive and cognition interface. *Nature Reviews Neuroscience*, **2**, 417–424.

Paus, T., Koski, L., Caramanos, Z., and Westbury, C. (1998). Regional differences in the effects of task difficulty and motor output on blood flow response in the human anterior cingulate cortex: A review of 107 PET activation studies. *NeuroReport,* **9**, R37–R47.

Pawela, C.P., Biswal, B.B., Cho, Y.R., Kao, D.S., Li, R., Jones, S.R., Schulte, M.L., Matloub, H.S., Hudetz, A.G., and Hyde, J.S. (2008). Resting-state functional connectivity of the rat brain. *Magnetic Resonance in Medicine*, **59**, 1021–1029.

Pearce, J.M.S. (2004). Richard Morton: Origins of anorexia nervosa. *European Neurology,* **52**, 191–192.

Pearce, J.M.S. (2006). Sir William Withey Gull (1816–1890). *European Neurology,* **55**, 53–56.

Pearlson, G.D., Wong, D.F., Tune, L.E., Ross, C.A., Chase, G.A., Links, J.M., Dannals, R.F., Wilson, A.A., Ravert, H.T., Wagner, H.N., and DePaulo, J.R. (1995). In vivo d2 dopamine receptor density in psychotic and nonpsychotic patients with bipolar disorder. *Archives of General Psychiatry*, **52**, 471–477.

Pelphrey, K.A., Morris, J.P., and McCarthy, G. (2005). Neural basis of eye gaze processing deficits in autism. *Brain*, **128**, 1038–1048.

Perlman, W.R., Weikert, C.S., Akil, M., and Kleinman, J.E. (2004). Postmortem investigations of the pathophysiology of schizophrenia: The role of susceptibility genes. *Journal of Psychiatry and Neuroscience*, **29**, 287–293.

Perner, J. (1991). *Understanding the Representational Mind.* Cambridge, MIT Press.

Perris, C. (1966). A study of bipolar (manic-depressive) and unipolar recurrent depressive psychoses. *Acta Psychiatrica Scandinavica*, **194**, 68–82.

Perry, R.J., Graham, A., Williams, G., Rosen, H., Erzinclioglu, S., Weiner, M., Miller, B., and Hodges, J. (2006). Patterns of frontal lobe atrophy in frontotemporal dementia: A volumetric MRI study. *Dementia and Geriatric Cognitive Disorders*, **22**, 278–287.

Perry, R.J., and Hodges, J.R. (2000). Differentiating frontal and temporal variant frontotemporal dementia from Alzheimer's disease. *Neurology*, **54**, 2277–2284.

Persico, A.M., and Bourgeron, T. (2006). Searching for ways out of the autism maze: Genetic, epigenetic and environmental clues. *Trends in Neurosciences*, **29**, 349–358.

Peters, F., Perani, D., Herholz, K., Holthoff, V., Beuthien-Baumann, B., Sorbi, S., Pupi, A., Degueldre, C., Lemaire, C., Collette, F., and Salmon, S. (2006). Orbitofrontal dysfunction related to both apathy and disinhibition in frontotemporal dementia. *Dementia and Geriatric Cognitive Disorders*, **21**, 373–379.

Petrides, M. (1996). Specialized systems for the processing of mnemonic information within the frontal cortex. *Philosophical Transactions Royal Society London B*, **351**, 1455–1462.

Petrides, M., Cadoret, G., and Mackey, S. (2005). Orofacial somatomotor responses in the macaque monkey homologue of Broca's area. *Nature*, **435**, 1235–1238.

Petrides, M., and Pandya, D.N. (1999). Dorsolateral prefrontal cortex: Cytoarchitectural analysis in the human and the macaque brain and corticocortical connection patterns. *European Journal of Neuroscience*, **11**, 1011–1036.

Petrides, M., and Pandya, D.N. (2001). Comparative cytoarchitectonic analysis of the human and the macaque ventrolateral prefrontal cortex and corticocortical connection patterns in the monkey. *European Journal of Neuroscience*, **16**, 291–310.

Pettegrew, J.R., Keshavan, M., Panchalingam, K., Strychor, S., Kaplan, D.B., Tretta, M.G., and Allen, M. (1991). Alterations in brain high-energy phosphate and membrane phospholipid metabolism in first-episode, drug naive schizophrenics: A pilot study of the dorsal prefrontal cortex by in vivo phosphorus 31 nuclear magnetic resonance spectroscopy. *Archives of General Psychiatry*, **48**, 63–568.

Phillips, M.L., Drevets, W.C., Rauch, S.L., and Lane, R. (2003a). Neurobiology of emotion perception I: The neural basis of normal emotion perception. *Biological Psychiatry*, **54**, 504–514.

Phillips, M.L., Drevets, W.C., Rauch, S.L., and Lane, R. (2003b). Neurobiology of emotion perception II: Implications for major psychiatric disorders. *Biological Psychiatry*, **54**, 515–528.

Phillips, M.L., Young, A.W., Scott, S.K., Calder, A.J., Andrew, C., Giampietro, V., Williams, S.C.R., Bullmore, E.T., Brammer, M., and Gray, J.A. (1998). Neural responses to facial and vocal expressions of fear and disgust. *Proceedings of the Royal Society London B*, **265**, 1809–1817.

Phillips, M.L., Young, A.W., Senior, C., Brammer, M., Andrew, C., Calder, A.J., Bullmore, E.T., Perrett, D.I., Rowland, D., Williams, S.C.R., Gray, J.A., and David, A.S. (1997). A specific neural substrate for perceiving facial expressions of disgust. *Nature,* **389**, 495–498.

Pierson, A., Jouvent, R., Quintin, P., Perez-Diaz, F., and Leboyer, M. (2000). Information processing deficits in relatives of manic depressive patients. *Psychological Medicine*, **30**, 545–555.

Pinker, S. (1995). Language is a human instinct. In J. Brockman (Ed.), *The Third Culture* (pp. 232–238). New York, Simon & Schuster.

Plutchik, R. (1980). *Emotion: A Psychoevolutionary Synthesis*. New York, Harper and Row.

Pobric, G., Jefferies, E., and Ralph, M.A.L. (2007). Anterior temporal lobes mediate semantic representation: Mimicking semantic dementia by using rTMS in normal participants. *Proceedings of the National Academy of Sciences of the USA*, **104**, 20137–20141.

Pollard, K.S., Salama, S.R., Lambert, N., Lambot, M-A., Coppens, S., Pedersen, J.S., Katzman, S., King, B., Onodera, C., Siepel, A., Kern, A.D., Dehay, C., Igel, H., Ares, M., Jr., Vanderhaeghen, P., and Haussler, D. (2006). An RNA gene expressed during cortical development evolved rapidly in humans. *Nature,* **443,** 167–172.

Posner, M.I. (1994). Attention: The mechanisms of consciousness. *Proceedings of the National Academy of Sciences of the USA*, **91**, 7398–7403.

Povinelli, D.J., Bering, J.M., and Giambrone, S. (2000). Toward a science of other minds: Escaping the argument by analogy. *Cognitive Science*, **24**, 509–541.

Povinelli, D.J., and Preuss, T.M. (1995). Theory of mind: Evolutionary history of a cognitive specialization. *Trends in Neurosciences*, **18**, 418–424.

Premack, D. (2007). Human and animal cognition: Continuity and discontinuity. *Proceedings of the National Academy of Sciences of the USA*, **104**, 13861–13867.

Premack, D., and Premack, A. (2003). *Original Intelligence: Unlocking the Mystery of Who We Are*. New York, McGraw-Hill.

Premack, D., and Woodruff, G. (1978). Does the chimpanzee have a theory of mind? *Behavioral and Brain Sciences*, **4**, 515–526.

Preuschoff, K., Quartz, S.R., and Bossaerts, P. (2008). Human insula activation reflects risk prediction errors as well as risk. *Journal of Neuroscience,* **28**, 2745–2752.

Preuss, T.M. (1995). Do rats have prefrontal cortex? The Rose-Woolsey-Akert program reconsidered. *Journal of Cognitive Neuroscience*, **7**, 1–24.

Preuss, T.M. (2000). What's human about the human brain? In M.S. Gazzaniga (Ed.), *The New Cognitive Neurosciences* (pp. 1219–1234). Cambridge, MIT Press.

Preuss, T.M., Cáceres, M., Oldham, M.C., and Geschwind, D.H. (2004). Human brain evolution: Insights from microarrays. *Nature Reviews Genetics*, **5**, 85–860.

Preuss, T.M., and Goldman-Rakic, P.S. (1989). Connections of the ventral granular frontal cortex of macaques with perisylvian premotor and somatosensory areas: Anatomical evidence for somatic representation in primate frontal association cortex. *Journal of Comparative Neurology*, **282**, 293–316.

Prinz, W. (1997). Perception and action planning. *European Journal of Cognitive Psychology*, **9**, 129–154.

Proctor, A.W., Qurne, M., and Francis, P.T. (1999). Neurochemical features of frontotemporal dementia. *Dementia and Geriatric Cognitive Disorders*, **10**, 8–84.

Quiroz, J.A., Singh, J., Gould, T.D., Denicoff, K.D., Zarate, C.A., and Manji, H.K. (2004). Emerging experimental therapeutics for bipolar disorder: Clues from the molecular pathophysiology. *Molecular Psychiatry*, **9**, 756–776.

Quraishi, S., and Frangou, S. (2002). Neuropsychology of bipolar disorder: A review. *Journal of Affective Disorders*, **72**, 209–226.

Rahman, S., Sahakian, B.J., Hodges, J.R., Rogers, R.D., and Robbins, T.W. (1999). Specific cognitive deficits in mild frontal variant frontotemporal dementia. *Brain*, **122**, 1469–1493.

Raichle, M.E., Fiez, J.A., Videen, T.O., MacLeod, A.-M.K., Pardo, J.V., Fox, P.T., and Petersen, S.E. (1994). Practice related changes in human brain functional anatomy during nonmotor learning. *Cerebral Cortex*, **4**, 8–26.

Raichle, M.E., and Gusnard, D.A. (2005). Intrinsic brain activity sets the stage for expression of motivated behavior. *Journal of Comparative Neurology,* **493**, 167–176.

Raichle, M.E., MacLeod, A.M., Snyder, A.Z., Powers, W.J., Gusnard, D.A., and Shulman, G.L. (2001). A default mode of brain function. *Proceedings of the National Academy of Sciences of the USA,* **98**, 676–682.

Raichle, M.E., and Snyder, A.Z. (2007). A default mode of brain function: A brief history of an evolving idea. *NeuroImage*, **37**, 1083–1090.

Raison, C.L., Capuron, L., and Miller, A.H. (2006). Cytokines sing the blues: Inflammation and the pathogenesis of depression. *Trends in Immunology*, **27**, 24–31.

Rajkowska, G. (2000). Postmortem studies in mood disorders indicate altered numbers of neurons and glial cells. *Biological Psychiatry*, **48**, 766–777.

Rakic, P. (1995). A small step for the cell, a giant leap for mankind: A hypothesis of neocortical expansion during evolution. *Trends in Neurosciences*, **18**, 383–388.

Ramnani, N., and Owen, A.M. (2004). Anterior prefrontal cortex: Insights into function from anatomy and neuroimaging. *Nature Reviews Neuroscience*, **5**, 184–194.

Rankin, K.P., Gorno-Tempini, M.L., Allison, S.C., Stanley, C.M., Glenn, S., Weiner, M.W., and Miller B.L. (2006). Structural anatomy of empathy in neurodegenerative disease. *Brain*, **129**, 2945–2956.

Rankin, K.P., Kramer, J.H., and Miller, B.L. (2005). Patterns of cognitive and emotional empathy in frontotemporal lobar degeneration. *Cognitive and Behavioural Neurology*, **18**, 28–36.

Rapoport, J.L., Addington, A.M., and Frangou, S. (2005). The neurodevelopmental model of schizophrenia: Update 2005. *Molecular Psychiatry*, **10**, 434–449.

Rapaport, J.L., Giedd, J., Kumra, S., Jacobsen, L., Smith, A., Nelson, J., and Hamburger, S. (1997). Childhood-onset schizophrenia: Progressive ventricular change during adolescence. *Archives of General Psychiatry*, **54**, 897–903.

Reiman, E.M., Lane, R.D., Ahern, G.L., Schartz, G.E., Davidson, R.J., Friston, K.J., Yun, L.-S., and Chen, K. (1997). Neuroanatomical correlates of externally and internally generated human emotion. *American Journal of Psychiatry*, **154**, 918–925.

Reith, J., Benkelfat, C., Sherwin, A., Yasuhara, Y., Kuwabara, H., Andermann, F., Bachneff, S., Cumming, P., Diksic, M., Dyve, S.E., Etienne, P., Evans, A.C., Lal, S., Shevell, M., Savard, G., Wong, D.F., Chouinard, G., and Gjedde, A. (1994). Elevated dopa decarboxylase activity in living brain of patients with psychosis. *Proceedings of the National Academy of Sciences of the USA*, **91**, 11651–11654.

Ribasés, M., Gratacòs, M., Fernández-Aranda, F., Bellodi, L., Boni, C., Anderluh, M., Cavallini, M.C., Cellini, E., Di Bella, D., Erzegovesi, S., Foulon, C., Gabrovsek, M., Gorwood, P., Hebebrand, J., Hinney, A., Holliday, J., Hu, X., Karwautz, A., Kipman, A., Komel, R., Nacmias, B., Remschmidt, H., Ricca, V., Sorbi, S., Tomori, M.,

Wagner, G., Treasure, J., Collier, D.A., and Estivill, X. (2005). Association of BDNF with restricting anorexia nervosa and minimum body mass index: A family-based association study of eight European populations. *European Journal of Human Genetics,* **13**, 428–434.

Riley, B., and Kendler, K.S. (2006). Molecular genetic studies of schizophrenia. *European Journal of Human Genetics*, **14**, 669–680.

Rilling, J.K., Barks, S.K., Parr, L.A., Preuss, T.M., Faber, T.L., Pagnoni, G., Bremner, J.D., and Votaw, J.R. (2007). A comparison of resting-state brain activity in humans and chimpanzees. *Proceedings of the National Academy of Sciences of the USA*, **104**, 17146–17151.

Rimol, L., Agartz, I., Djurovic, S., Brown, A., Roddey, J., Kahler, A., Mattingsdal, M., Athanasiu, L., Joyner, A., Schork, N., Halgren, E., Sunder, K., Melle, I., Dale, A., and Andreassen, O. (2010). Sex-dependent association of common variants of microcephaly genes with brain structure. *Proceedings of the National Academy of Science of the USA*, **107**, 384–388.

Rizzo, L., Danion, J-M., Van der Linden, M., and Grangé, D. (1996). Patients with schizophrenia remember that an event has occurred, but not when. *British Journal of Psychiatry*, **168**, 427–431.

Rizzolatti, G., and Craighero, L. (2004). The mirror-neuron system. *Annual Review of Neuroscience*, **27**, 169–192.

Roberson, E.D. (2006). Frontotemporal dementia. *Current Neurology and Neuroscience Reports*, **6**, 481–489.

Roberson, E.D., Hesse, J.H., Rose, K.D., Slama, H., Johnson, J.K., Yaffe, K., Forman, M.S., Miller, C.A., Trojanowski, J.Q., Kramer, J.H., and Miller, B.L. (2005). Frontotemporal dementia progresses to death faster than Alzheimer disease. *Neurology*, **65**, 719–725.

Robinson, L.J., Thompson, J.M., Gallagher, P., Goswami, U., Young, A.H., Ferrier, N., and Moore, P.B. (2006). A meta-analysis of cognitive deficits in euthymic patients with bipolar disorder. *Journal of Affective Disorders*, **93**, 105–115.

Robinson, T.E., and Becker, J.B. (1986). Enduring changes in brain and behaviour produced by chronic amphetamine administration: A review and evaluation of animal models of amphetamine psychosis. *Brain Research Reviews*, **11**, 157–198.

Rogers, L., and Andrew, R. (2002). *Comparative Vertebrate Lateralization*. Cambridge, UK, Cambridge University Press.

Rolls, E.T. (1999). The functions of the orbitofrontal cortex. *Neurocase*, **5**, 301–312.

Rolls, E.T. (2000). The orbitofrontal cortex and reward. *Cerebral Cortex*, **10**, 284–294.

Rommelse, N.N.J., Altink, M.E., Fliers, E.A., Martin, N.C., Buschgens, C.J.M., Hartman, C.A., Buitelaar, J.K., Faraone, S.V., Sergeant, J.A., and Oosterlaan, J. (2009). Comorbid problems in ADHD: Degree of association shared endophenotypes, and formation of distinct subtypes. Implications for a future DSM. *Journal of Abnormal Child Psychology,* **37**, 793–804.

Rosen, H.J., Allison., S.C., Schauer, G.F., Gorno-Tempini, M.L., Weiner, M.W., and Miller, B.L. (2005). Neuroanatomical correlates of behavioural disorders in dementia. *Brain*, **128**, 2612–2625.

Rosen, H.J., Gorno-Tempini, M.L., Goldman, W.P., Perry, R.J., Schuff, N., Weiner, M., Feiwell, R., Kramer, J.H., and Miller, B.L. (2002). Patterns of brain atrophy in frontotemporal dementia and semantic dementia. *Neurology*, **58**, 198–208.

Rosenthal, N.E., Sack, D.A., Gillin, J.C., Lewy, A.J., Goodwin, F.K., Davenport, Y., Mueller, P.S., Newsome, D.A., and Wehr, T.A. (1984). Seasonal affective disorder: A description of the syndrome and preliminary findings with light therapy. *Archives of General Psychiatry*, **41**, 72–80.

Ross, C.A., Margolis, R.L., Reading, S.A.J., Pletnikov, M., and Coyle, J.T. (2006). Neurobiology of schizophrenia. *Neuron*, **52**, 139–153.

Roth, R.M., Flashman, L.A., Saykin, A.J., McAllister, T.W., and Vidaver, R. (2004). Apathy in schizophrenia: Reduced frontal lobe and neuropsychological deficits. *American Journal of Psychiatry*, **161**, 157–159.

Rowe, A.D., Bullock, P.R., Polkey, C.E., and Morris, R.G. (2001). 'Theory of mind' impairments and their relationship to executive functioning following frontal lobe excisions. *Brain*, **124**, 600–616.

Rowen, L., Young, J., Birditt, B., Kaur, A., Madan, A., Philipps, D.L., Quin, S., Minx, P., Wilson, R.K., Hood, L., and Graveley, B.R. (2002). Analysis of the human neurexin genes: Alternative splicing and the generation of protein diversity, *Genomics*, **79**, 587–597.

Russell, T., and Sharma, T. (2003). Social cognition at the neural level: Investigations in autism, psychopathy and schizophrenia. In M. Brune, H. Ribbert, and W. Schiefenhövel (Eds.), *The Social Brain: Evolution and Pathology* (pp. 253–276). Chichester, West Sussex, England, John Wiley and Sons.

Sabri, O., Erkwoh, R., Schreckenberger, E.M., Cremerius, U., Schulz, G., Dickmann, C., Kaiser, E.M., Steinmeyer, E.M., Sass, H., and Buell, U. (1997). Regional cerebral blood flow and negative/positive symptoms in 24 drug-naïve schizophrenics. *Journal of Nuclear Medicine*, **38**, 181–188.

Saetre, P., Emilsson, L., Axelsson, E., Kreuger, J., Lindholm, E., and Jazin, E. (2007). Inflammation-related genes up-regulated in schizophrenia brains. *BMC Psychiatry*, **7**: 1–10.

Salisbury, D.F., Kuroki, N., Kasai, K., Shenton, M.E., and McCarley, R.W. (2007). Progressive and interrelated functional and structural evidence of post-onset brain reduction in schizophrenia. *Archives of General Psychiatry*, **64**, 521–529.

Salisbury, D.F., Shenton, M.E., Sherwood, A.R., Fischer, I.A., Yurgelun-Todd, D.A., Tohen, M., and McCarley, R.W. (1998). First-episode schizophrenic psychosis differs from first-episode affective psychosis and controls in P300 amplitude over left temporal lobe. *Archives of General Psychiatry*, **55**, 173–180.

Saltzman, C. (1998). *Portrait of Dr. Gachet*. New York, Viking.

Sanfey, A.G., Rilling, J.K., Aronson, J.A., Nystrom, L.E., and Cohen, J.D. (2003). The neural basis of economic decision-making in the ultimatum game. *Science,* **300**, 1755–1758.

Sapolsky, R.M. (2000). The possibility of neurotoxicity in the hippocampus in major depression: A primer on neuron death. *Biological Psychiatry*, **48**, 755–765.

Sargent, P.A., Kjaer, K.H., Bench, C.J., Rabiner, E.A., Messa, C., Meyer, J., Gunn, R.N., Grasby, P.M., and Cowen, P.J. (2000). Brain serotonin$_{1A}$ receptor binding measured by positron emission tomography with [^{11}C]WAY-100635. *Archives of General Psychiatry*, **57**, 174–180.

Savage-Rumbaugh, E.S. (1986). *Ape Language: From Conditioned Response to Symbol.* New York, Columbia University Press.

Schlaggar, B.L., and O'Leary, D.D.M. (1993). Patterning of the barrel field in somotosensory cortex with implications for the specification of neocortical areas. *Perspectives on Developmental Neurobiology*, **1**, 81–91.

Schmid, C.D., Melchior, B., Masek, K., Puntambekar, S.S., Danielson, P.E., Lo, D.D., Sutcliffe, J.G., and Carson, M.J. (2009). Differential gene expression LPS/IFN activated microglia and macrophages: In vitro versus in vivo. *Journal of Neurochemistry,* **109**, 117–125.

Schmitz, T.W., and Johnson, S.C. (2006). Self-appraisal decisions evoke dissociated dorsal-ventral aMPFC networks. *NeuroImage*, **30,** 1050–1058.

Schoenemann, P.T., Sheehan, M.J., and Glotzer, L.D. (2005). Prefrontal white matter volume is disproportionately larger in humans than in other primates. *Nature Neuroscience*, **8**, 242–252.

Schore, A.N. (2003). *Affect Dysregulation and Disorders of the Self*. New York, Norton.

Schretlen, D.J., Cascella, N.G., Meyer, S.M., Kingery, L.R., Testa, S.M., Munro, C.A., Pulver, A.E., Rivkin, P., Rao, V.A., Diaz-Asper, C.M., Dickerson, F.B., Yolken, R.H., and Pearlson, G.D. (2007). Neuropsychological functioning in bipolar disorder and schizophrenia. *Biological Psychiatry*, **62**, 179–186.

Schröder, J., Buchsbaum, M.S., Siegel, B.V., Geider, F.J., Lohr, J., Tang, C., Wu, J., and Potkin, S.G. (1996). Cerebral metabolic activity correlates of subsyndromes in chronic schizophrenia. *Schizophrenia Research*, **19**, 41–53.

Schroeter, M.L., Raczka, K., Neumann, J., and von Cramon, D.Y. (2008). Neural networks in frontotemporal dementia: A meta-analysis. *Neurobiology of Aging*, **29**, 418–426.

Schulkin, J. (2007). Autism and the amygdala: An endocrine hypothesis. *Brain and Cognition*, **65**, 87–99.

Schultz, W. (2001). Reward signaling by dopamine neurons. *The Neuroscientist,* **7,** 293–302.

Schultz, R.T., Gauthier, I., Klin, A., Fulbright, R.k., Anderson, A.W., Volkmar, F., Skudlarski, P., Lacadie, C., Cohen, D.J., and Gore, J.C. (2000). Abnormal ventral temporal cortical activity during face discrimination among individuals with autism and Asperger syndrome. *Archives of General Psychiatry*, **57**, 331–340.

Scott, M.M., and Deneris, E.S. (2005). Making and breaking serotonin neurons in autism. *International Journal of Developmental Neuroscience*, **23**, 277–285.

Scott, S.K., and Johnsrude, I.S. (2003). The neuroanatomical and functional organization of speech perception. *Trends in Neurosciences*, **26**, 100–107.

Scott, S.K., and Wise, R.J.S. (2004). The functional neuroanatomy of prelexical processing in speech perception. *Cognition*, **92**, 13–45.

Sebat, J., Lakshmi, B., Malhotra, D., Troge, J., Lese-Martin, C., Walsh, T., Yamrom, B., Yoon, S., Krasnitz, A., Kendall, J., Leotta, A., Pai, D., Zhang, R., Lee, Y.-H., Hicks, J., Spence, S.J., Lee, A.T., Puura, K., Lehtimäki, T., Ledbetter, D., Gregersen, P.K., Bregman, J., Sutcliffe, J.S., Jobanputra, V., Chung, W., Warburton, D., King, M.-C., Skuse, D., Geschwind, D.H., Gilliam, T.C., Ye, K., and Wigler, M. (2007). Strong association of de novo copy number mutations with autism. *Science*, **316**, 445–449.

Seeley, W.W. (2008). Selective functional, regional, and neuronal vulnerability in frontotemporal demential. *Current Opinion in Neurology,* **21,** 701–707.

Seeley, W.W., Carlin, D.A., Allman, J.M., Macedo, M.N., Bush, C., Miller, B.L., and DeArmond, S.J. (2006). Early frontotemporal dementia targets neurons unique to apes and humans. *Annals of Neurology*, **60**, 660–667.

Seeley, W.W., Crawford, R., Rascovsky, K., Kramer, J.H., Weiner, M., Miller, B.L., and Gorno-Tempini, M.L. (2008). Frontal paralimbic network atrophy in very mild behavioral variant frontotemporal dementia. *Archives of Neurology*, **65**, 249–255.

Seeley, W.W., Crawford, R.K., Zhou, J., Miller, B.L., and Greicius, M.D. (2009). Neurodegenerative diseases target large-scale human brain networks. *Neuron*, **62**, 42–52.

Seeley, W.W., Menon, V., Schatzberg, A.F., Keller, J., Glover, G.H., Kenna, H., Reiss, A.L., and Greicius, M.D. (2007). Dissociable intrinsic connectivity networks for salience processing and executive control. *Journal of Neuroscience*, **27**, 2349–2356.

Seeman, P. (1987). Dopamine receptors and the dopamine hypothesis of schizophrenia. *Synapse*, **1**, 133–152.

Selemon, L.D., Rajkowska, G., and Goldman-Rakic, P.S. (1995). Abnormally high neuronal density in the schizophrenia cortex. A morphometric analysis of prefrontal area 9 and occipital area 17. *Archives of General Psychiatry*, **52**, 805–818.

Selemon, L.D., Rajkowska, G., and Goldman-Rakic, P.S. (1998). Elevated neuronal density in prefrontal area 46 in brains from schizophrenia patients: Application of a three-dimensional, stereologic counting method. *Journal of Comprehensive Neurology*, **392**, 402–412.

Semendeferi, K., Armstrong, E., Schleicher, A., Zilles, K., and Van Hoesen, G.W. (2001). Prefrontal cortex in humans and apes: A comparative study of area 10. *American Journal of Physical Anthropology*, **114**, 224–241.

Senju, A., Tojo, Y., Yaguchi, K., and Hasegawa, T. (2005). Deviant gaze processing in children with autism: An ERP study. *Neuropsychologia*, **43**, 1297–1306.

Servan-Schreiber, D., Carter, C.S., Bruno, R.M., and Cohen, J.D. (1998). Dopamine and the mechanisms of cognition: Part II. D-amphetamine effects in human subjects performing a selective attention task. *Biological Psychiatry*, **43**, 723–729.

Servan-Schreiber, D., Cohen, J., and Steingard, S. (1996). Schizophrenic deficits in the processing of context: A test of a theoretical model. *Archives of General Psychiatry*, **53**, 1105–1112.

Seltzer, M.M., Shattuck, P., Abbeduto, L., and Greenberg, J.S. (2004). Trajectory of development in adolescents and adults with autism. *Mental Retardation and Developmental Disabilities Research Reviews*, **10**, 234–247.

Senft, S.L., and Woolsey, T.A. (1991). Growth of thalamic afferents into mouse barrel cortex. *Cerebral Cortex,* **1**, 308–335.

Serretti, A., and Mandelli, L. (2008). The genetics of bipolar disorder: Genome 'hot regions', genes, new potential candidates and future directions. *Molecular Psychiatry*, **13**, 742–771.

Sexton, C.E., Mackay, C.E., and Ebmeier, K.P. (2009). A systematic review of diffusion tensor imaging studies in affective disorders. *Biological Psychiatry*, **66**, 814–823.

Shagass, C. (1975). EEG and evoked potentials in the psychoses. In D.X. Freedman (Ed.), *Biology of the Major Psychoses* (pp. 101–127). New York, Raven Press.

Shannon, R.V., Zeng, F.G., Kamath, V., Wygonski, J., and Ekelid, M. (1995). Speech recognition with primarily temporal cues. *Science*, **270**, 303–304.

Shapleske, J., Rossell, S.L., Woodruff, P.W.R., and David, A.S. (1999). The planum temporale: A systematic, quantitative review of its structural, functional and clinical significance. *Brain Research Reviews*, **29**, 26–49.

Sharma, T., Lancaster, E., Sigmundsson, T., Lewis, S., Takei, N., Gurling, H., Barta, P., Pearlson, G., and Murray, R.M. (1999). Lack of normal pattern of cerebral asymmetry in familial schizophrenic patients and their relatives: The Maudsley Family Study. *Schizophrenia Research,* **40**, 111–120.

Sharp, S.I., McQuillin, A., and Gurling, H.M.D. (2009). Genetics of attention-deficit hyperactivity disorder (ADHD). *Neuropharmacology,* **57**, 590–600.

Shaw, P., Lalonde, F., Lepage, C., Rabin, C., Eckstrand, K., Sharp, W., Greenstein, D., Evans, A., Giedd, J.N., and Rapoport, J. (2009). Development of cortical asymmetry in typically developing children and its disruption in attention-deficit/hyperactivity disorder. *Archives of General Psychiatry,* **66**, 888–896.

Sheline, Y.I. (2003). Neuroimaging studies of mood disorder effects on the brain. *Biological Psychiatry*, **54**, 338–352.

Shelton, R.C., and Weinberger, D.R. (1986). X-ray computerized tomography studies in schizophrenia: a review and synthesis. In S.R. Steinhauer, J. H. Gruzelier, and J. Zubin (Eds.), *Handbook of Schizophrenia, Volume 1: The Neurology of Schizophrenia* (pp. 207–250). Amsterdam, Elsevier.

Shenton, M.E., Dickey, C.C., Frumin, M., and McCarley, R.W. (2001). A review of MRI findings in schizophrenia. *Schizophrenia Research*, **49**, 1–52.

Shepard, P.D., Holcomb, H.H., and Gold, J.M. (2006). The presence of absence: Habenular regulation of dopamine neurons and the encoding of negative outcomes. *Schizophrenia Bulletin,* **32**, 417–421.

Shergill, S.S., Kanaan, R.A., Chitnis, X.A., O'Daly, O., Jones, D.K., Frangou, S., Williams, S.C.R., and Howard, R.J. (2007). A diffusion tensor imaging study of fasciculi in schizophrenia. *American Journal of Psychiatry*, **164**, 467–473.

Sherman, S.M. (2001). Thalamic relay functions. *Progress in Brain Research*, **134**, 51–69.

Sherwood, C.C., Stimpson, C.D., Raghanti, M.A., Wildman, D.E., Uddin, M., Grossman, L.I., Goodman, M., Redmond, J.C., Bonar, C.J., Erwin, J.M., and Hof, P.R. (2006). Evolution of increased glia-neuron ratios in the human frontal cortex. *Proceedings of the National Academy of Sciences of the USA*, **103**, 13606–13611.

Shin, L.M., Dougherty, D.D., Orr, S.P., Pitman, R.K., Lasko, M., Macklin, M.L., Alpert, N.M., Fischman, A.J., and Rauch, S.L. (2000). Activation of anterior paralimbic structures during guilt-related script-driven imagery. *Biological Psychiatry*, **48**, 43–50.

Shiori, T., Kato, T., Inubuski, T., Murashita, J., and Takahashi, S. (1994). Correlations of phosphomonoesterase measured by phosphorus-31 magnetic resonance spectroscopy in the frontal lobes and negative symptoms in schizophrenia. *Psychiatry Research: Neuroimaging*, **55**, 223–235.

Shiah, I.-S., and Yatham, L.N. (2000). Serotonin in mania and in the mechanism of action of mood stabilizers: A review of clinical studies. *Bipolar Disorders*, **2**, 77–92.

Shorter, E. (1997). *A History of Psychiatry.* Toronto, John Wiley and Sons.

Sigman, M., Spence, S.J., and Wang, A.T. (2006). Autism from developmental and neuropsychological perspectives. *Annual Review of Clinical Psychology*, 2006, **2**, 327–355.

Sigmundsson, T., Suckling, J., Maier, M., Williams, S.C.R., Bullmore, E.T., Greenwood, K.E., Fukuda, R., Ron, M.A., and Toone, B.K. (2001). Structural abnormalities in frontal, temporal, and limbic regions and interconnecting white matter tracts in schizophrenic patients with prominent negative symptoms. *American Journal of Psychiatry*, **158**, 234–243.

Silbersweig, D.A., Stern, E., Frith, C., Cahill, C., Holmes, A., Gootoonk, S., Seaward, J., McKenna, P., Chua, S.E., Schnorr, L., Jones, T., and Frackowiak, R.S.J. (1995). A functional neuroanatomy of hallucinations in schizophrenia. *Nature*, **378**, 176–179.

Silver, H., Feldman, P., Bilker, W., and Gur, R.C. (2003). Working memory deficit as a core neuropsychological dysfunction in schizophrenia. *American Journal of Psychiatry*, **160**, 1809–1816.

Simms, M.L., Kemper, T.L., Timbie, C.M., Bauman, M.L., and Blatt, G.J. (2009). The anterior cingulate cortex in autism: Heterogeneity of qualitative and quantitative cytoarchitectonic features suggest possible subgroups. *Acta Neuropathologica,* **118**, 673–684.

Singer, T., Kiebel, S.J., Winston, J.S., Dolan, R.J., and Frith, C.D. (2004b). Brain responses to the acquired moral status of faces. *Neuron*, **41**, 653–662.

Singer, T., Seymour, B., O'Doherty, J., Kaube, H., Dolan, R.J., and Frith, C.D. (2004a). Empathy for pain involves the affective but not sensory components of pain. *Science,* **303**, 1157–1162.

Rizzolatti, G., and Sinigalia, C. (2008). *Mirrors in the Brain.* New York, Oxford.

Small. D.M., Zatorre, R.J., Dagher, A., Evans, A., and Jones-Gotman, M. (2001). Changes in brain activity related to eating chocolate: From pleasure to aversion. *Brain*, **124**, 1720–1733.

Smith, C.A., and Lazarus, R.S. (1990). Emotion and adaptation. In L.A. Pervin (Ed.), *Handbook of Personality: Theory and Research* (pp. 609–637). New York, Guilford.

Smith, C.U.M. (1982). Evolution and the problem of the mind: Part II. John Hughlings Jackson. *Journal of the History of Biology*, **15**, 241–262.

Soares, J.C. (2003). Contributions from brain imaging to the elucidation of pathophysiology of bipolar disorder. *International Journal of Neuropsychopharmacology*, **6**, 171–180.

Soares, J.C., and Innis, R.B. (1999). Neurochemical brain imaging investigations of schizophrenia. *Biological Psychiatry*, **46**, 600–615.

Sommer, I.E.C, Ramsey, N.F., Mandl, R.C.W., van Oel, C.J., and Kahn, R.S. (2004). Language activation in monozygotic twins discordant for schizophrenia. *British Journal of Psychiatry*, **184**, 128–135.

Southgate, V., and Hamilton, A.F.deC. (2008). Unbroken mirrors: Challenging a theory of autism. *Trends in Cognitive Sciences*, **12**, 225–229.

Spence, S.A., Brooks, D.J., Hirsch, S.R., Liddle, P.F., Meehan, J., and Grasby, P.M. (1997). A PET study of voluntary movement in schizophrenic patients experiencing passivity phenomena (delusions of alien control). *Brain*, **120**, 1997–2011.

Spence, S.A., Farrow, T.F.D., Herford, A.E., Wilkinson, I.D., Zheng, Y., and Woodruff, P.W.R. (2001). Behavioural and functional anatomical correlates of deception in humans. *NeuroReport,* **12**, 2849–2853.

Spence, S.A., Liddle, P.F., Stefan, M.D., Hellewell, J.S.E., Sharma, T., Friston, K.J., Hirsch, S.R., Frith, C.D., Murray, R.M., Deakin, J.F.W., and Grasby, P.M. (2000). Functional anatomy of verbal fluency in people with schizophrenia and those at genetic risk: Focal dysfunction and distributed disconnectivity reappraised. *British Journal of Psychiatry*, 176, 52–63.

Spencer, K.M., Nestor, P.G., Niznikiewicz, M.A., Klump, M.C., Frumin, M., Shenton, M.E., and McCarley, R.W. (2004). Neural synchrony indexes disordered perception and cognition in schizophrenia. *Proceedings of the National Academy of Sciences of the USA*, **101**, 17288–17293.

Sporn, A.L., Greenstein, D.K., Gogtay, N., Jeffries, N.O., Lenane, M., Gochman, P., Clasen, L.S., Blumenthal, J., Giedd, J.N., and Rapaport, J.L. (2003). Progressive brain volume loss during adolescence in childhood-onset schizophrenia. *American Journal of Psychiatry*, **160**, 2181–2189.

Spreng, R.N., Mar, R.A., and Kim, A.S.N. (2009). The common neural basis of autobiographical memory, prospection, navigation, theory of mind and the default mode: A quantitative meta-analysis. *Journal of Cognitive Neuroscience*, **21**, 489–510.

Sprong, M., Schothorst, P., Vos, E., Hox, J., and Van Engeland, H. (2007). Theory of mind in schizophrenia. *British Journal of Psychiatry*, **191**, 5–13.

Squire, L. (1992). Memory and the hippocampus: A synthesis of findings with rats, monkeys and humans. *Psychological Review,* **99**, 195–231.

Sridharan, D., Levitin, D.J., and Menon, V. (2008). A critical role for the right fronto-insular cortex in switching between central-executive and default-mode networks. *Proceedings of the National Academy of Sciences of the USA*, **105**, 12569–12574.

Stanley, J.A., Williamson, P.C., Drost, D.J., Carr, T., Rylett, J., Malla, A., and Thompson, R.T. (1995). In vivo prefrontal 31P magnetic resonance spectroscopy in schizophrenic patients. *Archives of General Psychiatry*, **52**, 399–406.

Stanley, J.A., Williamson, P.C., Drost, D.J., Rylett, J., Carr, T., Malla, A., and Thompson, R.J. (1996). An in vivo proton magnetic resonance spectroscopy study of schizophrenic patients. *Schizophrenia Bulletin*, **22**, 597–609.

Steele, J.D., and Lawrie, S.M. (2004). Segregation of cognitive and emotional function in the prefrontal cortex: A stereotactic meta-analysis. *NeuroImage*, **21**, 868–875.

Stefanis, N., Frangou, S., Yakeley, J., Sharma, T., O'Connell, P., Morgan, K., Sigmudsson, T., Taylor, M., and Murray, R. (1999). Hippocampal volume reduction in schizophrenia: effects of genetic risk and pregnancy and birth complications. *Biological Psychiatry*, **46**, 697–702.

Stefansson, H., Sigurdsson, E., Steinthorsdottir, V., Bjornsdottir, S., Sigmundsson, T., Ghosh, S., Brynjolfsson, J., Gunnarsdottir, S., Ivarsson, O., Chou, T.T., Hjaltason, O., Birgisdottir, B., Jonsson, H., Gudnadottir, V.G., Gudmundsdottir, E., Bjornsson, A., Ingvarsson, B., Ingason, A., Sigfusson, S., Hardardottir, H., Harvey, R.P., Lai, D., Zhou, M., Brunner, D., Mutel, V., Gonzalo, A., Lemke, G., Sainz, J., Johannesson, G., Andresson, T., Gudbjartsson, D., Manolescu, A., Frigge, M.L., Gurney, M.E., Kong, A., Gulcher, J.R., Petursson, H., and Stefansson, K. (2002). *Neuroregulin 1* and susceptibility to schizophrenia. *American Journal of Human Genetics*, **71**, 877–892.

Steinvorth, S., Corkin, S., and Halgren, E. (2006). Ecphory of autobiographical memories: An fMRI study of recent and remote memory retrieval. *NeuroImage*, **30**, 285–298.

Stevens, J.R. (1973). An anatomy of schizophrenia? *Archives of General Psychiatry*, **29**, 177–189.

Stevens, J.R. (1982). Neuropathology of schizophrenia. *Archives of General Psychiatry*, **39**, 1131–1139.

Still, G.F. (2006). Some abnormal psychical conditions in children. Excerpts from three lectures. *Journal of Attention Disorders*, **10**, 126–136.

Stoll, A.L., Renshaw, P.F., Yurgelun-Todd, D.A., and Cohen, B. (2000). Neuroimaging in bipolar disorder: What have we learned? *Biological Psychiatry*, **48**, 505–517.

Strakowski, S.M., DelBello, M.P., and Adler, C.M. (2005). The functional neuroanatomy of bipolar disorder: A review of neuroimaging findings. *Molecular Psychiatry*, **10**, 105–116.

Strakowski, S.M., DelBello, M.P., Zimmerman, M.E., Getz, G.E., Mills, N.P., Ret J., Shear, P., and Adler, C.M. (2002). Ventricular and periventricular structural volumes in first- versus multiple-episode bipolar disorder. *American Journal of Psychiatry*, **159**, 1841–1847.

Straub, R.E., Jiang, Y., MacLean, C.J., Ma, Y., Webb, B.T., Myakishev, M.V., Harris-Kerr, C., Wormley, B., Sadek, H., Kadambi, N., Cesare, A.J., Gibberman, A., Wang, X., O'Neill, F.A., Walsh, D., and Kendler, K.S. (2002). Genetic variation in the 6p22.3 gene *DTNBP1*, the human ortholog of the mouse dysbindin gene, is associated with schizophrenia. *American Journal of Human Genetics*, **71**, 337–348.

Stuss, D.T., Gallup, G.G., and Alexander, M.P. (2001). The frontal lobes are necessary for 'theory of mind.' *Brain*, **124**, 279–286.

Stuss, D., and Levine, B. (2002). Adult clinical neuropsychology: Lessons from studies of the frontal lobes. *Annual Review of Psychology*, **53**, 401–433.

Suddath, R.L., Christison, G.W., Torrey, E.F., Casanova, M.F., and Weinberger, D.R. (1990). Anatomical abnormalities in the brains of monozygotic twins discordant for schizophrenia. *New England Journal of Medicine*, **322**, 789–794.

Suddendorf, T., and Busby, J. (2003). Mental time travel in animals? *Trends in Cognitive Sciences*, **9**, 391–396.

Suddendorf, T., and Whiten, A. (2001). Mental evolution and development: Evidence for secondary representation in children, great apes, and other animals. *Psychological Bulletin*, **127**, 629–650.

Südhof, T.C. (2008). Neuroligins and neurexins link synaptic function to cognitive disease. *Nature*, **455**, 903–911.

Sullivan, P.F., Kendler, K.S., and Neale, M.C. (2003). Schizophrenia as a complex trait: Evidence from a meta-analysis of twin studies. *Archives of General Psychiatry,* **60**, 1187–1192.

Swash, M. (2005). John Hughlings Jackson (1835–1911). *Journal of Neurology*, **252**, 745–746.

Swerdlow, N.R., and Geyer, M.A. (1998). Using an animal model of deficient sensorimotor gating to study the pathophysiology and new treatments of schizophrenia. *Schizophrenia Bulletin*, **24**, 285–301.

Swerdlow, N.R., and Koop, G.F. (1987). Dopamine, schizophrenia, mania, and depression: Toward a unified hypothesis of cortico-striato-pallido-thalamic function. *Behavioural and Brain Sciences*, **10**, 197–245.

Swerdlow, N.R., Martinez, Z.A., Hanlon, F.M., Platten, A., Farid, M., Auerbach, P., Braff, D.L., and Geyer, M. (2000). Toward understanding the biology of a complex phenotype: Rat strain and substrain differences in sensorimotor gating: Disruptive effects of dopamine agonists. *Journal of Neuroscience*, **20**, 4325–4336.

Szatmari, P., Bartolucci, G., and Bremner R. (1989). Asperger's syndrome and autism: Comparison of early history and outcome. *Developmental Medicine and Child Neurology*, **31**, 709–720.

Szebenyi, G., Bollati, F., Bisbal, M., Sheridan, S., Faas, L., Wray, R., Haferkamp, S., Nguyen, S., Caceres, A., and Brady, S.T. (2005). Activity-driven dendritic remodeling requires microtubule-associated protein1A. *Current Biology*, **15**, 1820–1826.

Taber, M.T., and Fibiger, H.C. (1995). Electrical stimulation of the prefrontal cortex increases dopamine release in the nucleus accumbens of the rat: Modulation by metabotropic glutamate receptors. *Journal of Neuroscience*, **15**, 3896–3904.

Takahashi, T., Wood, S.J., Yung, A.R., Soulsby, B., McGorry, P.D., Susuki, M., Kawasaki, Y., Phillips, L.J., Velakoulis, D., and Pantelis, C. (2009). Progressive gray matter reduction of superior temporal gyrus during transition to psychosis. *Archives of General Psychiatry*, **66**, 366–376.

Tamminga, C.A., Thaker, G.K., Buchanen, R., Kirkpatrick, B., Alphs, L.D., Chase, T.N., and Carpenter, W.T. (1992). Limbic system abnormalities identified in schizophrenia using positron emission tomography with fluorodeoxyglucose and neocortical alterations with deficit syndrome. *Archives of General Psychiatry*, **49**, 522–530.

Tantam, D. (1988). Asperger's syndrome. *Journal of Child Psychology and Psychiatry*, **29**, 245–255.

Tek, C., Gold, J., Blaxton, T., Wilk, C., McMahon, R.P., and Buchanan, R.W. (2002). Visual perceptual and working memory impairments in schizophrenia. *Archives of General Psychiatry,* **59,** 146–153.

Tenn, C.C., Fletcher, P.J., and Kapur, S. (2003). Amphetamine-sensitized animals show a sensorimotor gating and neurochemical abnormality similar to that of schizophrenia. *Schizophrenia Research*, **64**, 103–114.

Teramitsu, I., Kudo, L.C., London, S.E., Geschwind, D.H., and White, S.A. (2004). Parallel FoxP1 and FoxP2 expression in songbird and human brain predicts functional interaction. *Journal of Neuroscience*, **24**, 3152–3163.

Théberge, J., Al-Semaan, Y., Williamson, P.C., Menon, R.S., Neufeld, R.W.J., Schaefer, B., Densmore, M., and Drost, D.J. (2003). Glutamate and glutamine in the anterior cingulate and thalamus of medicated patients with chronic schizophrenia and healthy comparison subjects measured with 4.0-T proton MRS. *American Journal of Psychiatry*, **160**, 2231–2233.

Théberge, J., Bartha, R., Drost, D.J., Menon, R.S., Malla, A., Takhar, J., Neufeld, R.W.J., Rogers, J., Pavlosky, W., Schaefer, B., Densmore, M., Al-Semaan, Y., and Williamson, P.C. (2002). Glutamate and glutamine measured with 4.0 T proton MRS in never-treated patients with schizophrenia and healthy volunteers. *American Journal of Psychiatry*, **159**, 1944–1946.

Théberge, J., Williamson, K., Aoyama, N., Drost, D., Manchanda, R., Malla, A., Northcott, S., Menon, R.S., Neufeld, R.W.J., Rajakumar, N., Pavlosky W., Densmore, M., Schaefer, B., and Williamson, P.C. (2007). Longitudinal gray matter and glutamatergic metabolite losses in first episode schizophrenia. *British Journal of Psychiatry*, **191**, 325–334.

Thomas, D.M., Francescutti-Verbeem, D.M., and Kuhn, D.M. (2006). Gene expression profile of activated microglia under conditions associated with dopamine neuronal damage. *The FASEB Journal*, **20**, 515–517

Thompson, P.M., Vidal, C., Giedd, J.N., Gochman, P., Blumenthal, J., Nicolson, R., Toga, A.W., and Rapaport, J.L. (2001). Mapping adolescent brain change reveals dynamic wave of accelerated gray matter loss in very early-onset schizophrenia. *Proceedings of the National Academy of Sciences of the USA*, **98**, 11650–11655.

Tobias, P.V. (1987). The brain of *Homo habilis*: A new level of organization in cerebral evolution. *Journal of Human Evolution*, **16**, 741–761.

Tohen, M., Zarate, C.A., Hennen, J., Khalsa, H.-M.K., Strakowski, S.M., Gebre-Medhin, P., Salvatore, P., and Baldessarini, R.J. (2003). The McLean-Harvard first-episode mania study: Prediction of recovery and first recurrence. *American Journal of Psychiatry*, **160**, 2099–2107.

Tomasello, M., Carpenter, M., Call, J., Behne, T., and Moll, H. (2005). Understanding and sharing intentions: The origins of cultural cognition. *Behavioral and Brain Sciences*, **28**, 675–735.

Tononi, G., and Edelman, G.M. (1998a). Consciousness and complexity. *Science*, **282**, 1846–1851.

Tononi, G., and Edelman, G.M. (1998b). Consciousness and the integration of information in the brain. *Advances in Neurology*, **77**, 245–279.

Torres, I.J., Boudreau, V.G., and Yatham, L.N. (2007). Neuropsychological functioning in euthymic bipolar disorder: A meta-analysis. *Acta Psychiatrica Scandinavica*, **434**, 17–26.

Toru, M., Watanabe, S., Shibuya, H., Nishikawa, T., Noda, K., Mitsushio, H., Ichikawa, H., Kurumaji, A., Takashima, M., Mataga, N., and Ogawa, A. (1988). Neurotransmitters, receptors and neuropeptides in post-mortem brains of schizophrenic patients. *Acta Psychiatrica Scandinavica*, **78**, 121–137.

Tosato, S., Dazzan, P., and Collier, D. (2005). Association between the neuroregulin 1 gene and schizophrenia: A systematic review. *Schizophrenia Bulletin*, **31**, 613–617.

Tsai, G., Passani, L.A., Slusher, B.S., Carter, R., Baer, L., Kleinman, J.E., and Coyle, J.T. (1995). Abnormal excitatory neurotransmitter metabolism in schizophrenic brains. *Archives of General Psychiatry*, **52**, 829–836.

Tsuang, M.T., Woolson, R.F., and Fleming, J.A. (1979). Long-term outcome of the major psychoses I. Schizophrenia and affective disorders compared with psychiatrically symptom-free surgical conditions. *Archives of General Psychiatry*, **36**, 1295–1301.

Tyler, L.K., and Marslen-Wilson, W. (2008). Fronto-temporal brain systems supporting spoken language comprehension. *Philosophical Transactions of the Royal Society B*, **363**, 1037–1054.

Uddin, M., Wildman, D.E., Liu, G., Xu, W., Johnson, R.M., Hof, P.R., Kapatos, G., Grossman, L.J., and Goodman, M. (2004). Sister grouping of chimpanzees and humans as revealed by genome-wide phylogenetic analysis of brain gene expression profiles. *Proceedings of the National Academy of Sciences of the USA*, **101**, 2957–2962.

Ullrich, B., Ushkaryov, Y.A., and Südhof, T.C. (1995). Cartography of neurexins: More than 1000 isoforms generated by alternative splicing and expressed in distinct subsets of neurons. *Neuron,* **14,** 497–507.

Ullsperger, M., and von Cramon, D.Y. (2003). Error monitoring using external feedback: Specific roles of the habenular complex, the reward system, and the cingulate motor area revealed by functional magnetic resonance imaging. *Journal of Neuroscience,* **23**, 4308–4314.

Umbricht, D., Schmid, L., Koller, R., Vollenweider, F.X., Hell, D., and Javitt, D.C. (2000). Ketamine-induced deficits in auditory and visual context-dependent processing in healthy volunteers: Implications for models of cognitive deficits in schizophrenia. *Archives of General Psychiatry*, **57**, 1139–1147.

Valicenti-McDermott, M.D., McVicar, K., Cohen, H.J., Wershil, B.K., and Shinnar, S. (2008). Gastrointestinal symptoms in children with autism spectrum disorder and language regression. *Pediatric Neurology,* **39**, 392–398.

Vallender, E.J., Mekel-Bobrov, N., and Lahn, B.T. (2008). Genetics of human brain evolution. *Trends in Neurosciences*, **31**, 637–644.

Van der Does, A.J.M., and Van den Bosch, R.J. (1992). What determines Wisconsin Card Sorting performance in schizophrenia? *Clinical Psychological Reviews*, **12**, 567–583.

Van der Loos, H., and Woolsey, T.A. (1973). Somatosensory cortex: Structural alterations following early injury to sense organs. *Science,* **179,** 395–398.

Vanderschuren, L.J., Schmidt, E.D., De Varies, T.J., Van Moorsel, A.P., Tilders, F.J.H., and Schoffelmeer, A.N.M. (1999). A single exposure to amphetamine is sufficient to induce long-term behavioural, neuroendocrine, and sensitization in rats. *Journal of Neuroscience*, **19**, 9579–9586.

van der Stelt, O., Belger, A., and Lieberman, J.A. (2004). Macroscopic fast neuronal oscillations and synchrony in schizophrenia. *Proceedings of the National Academy of Sciences of the USA*, **101**, 17567–17568.

Vanhollebeke, B., Nielsen, M.J., Watanabe, Y., Truc, P., Vanhamme, L., Nakajima, K., Moestrup, S.K., and Pays, E. (2007). Distinct roles of haptoglobin-related protein and apolipoprotein L-I in trypanolysis by human serum. *Proceedings of the National Academy of Sciences of the USA*, **104**, 4118–4123.

Vargas, D.L., Nascimbene, C., Krishnan, C., Zimmerman, A.W., and Pardo, C.A. (2005). Neuroglial activation and neuroinflammation in the brain of patients with autism. *Annals of Neurology,* **57**, 67–81.

Varma, A.R., Adams, W., Lloyd, J.J., Carson, K.J., Snowden, J.S., Testa, H.J., Jackson, A., and Neary, D. (2002). Diagnostic patterns of regional atrophy on MRI and regional cerebral blood flow change on SPECT in young onset patients with Alzheimer's disease, frontotemporal dementia and vascular dementia. *Acta Neurologica Scandinavica*, **105**, 261–269.

Varrone, A., Pappatà, S., Caracò, C., Soricelli, A., Milan, G., Quarantelli, M., Alfano, B., Postiglione, A., and Salvatore, M. (2002). Voxel-based comparison of rCBF SPECT images in frontotemporal dementia and Alzheimer's disease highlights the involvement of different cortical networks. *European Journal of Nuclear Medicine*, **29**, 1447–1454.

Velakoulis, D., Walterfang, M., Mocellin, R., Pantelis, C., and McLean, C. (2009). Frontotemporal dementia presenting as schizophrenia-like psychosis in young people: Clinicopathological series and review of cases. *British Journal of Psychiatry*, **194**, 298–305.

Versace, A., Almeida, J.R.C., Hassel, S., Walsh, N.D., Novelli, M., Klein, C.R., Kupfer, D.J., and Phillips, M.L. (2008). Elevated left and reduced right orbitomedial prefrontal fractional anisotropy in adults with bipolar disorder revealed by tract-based spatial statistics. *Archives of General Psychiatry*, **65**, 1041–1052.

Vidal, C.N., Nicolson, R., DeVito, T.J., Hayashi, K.M., Geaga, J.A., Drost, D.J., Williamson, P.C., Rajakumar, R., Sui, Y., Dutton, R.A., Toga, A.W., and Thompson, P.M. (2006). Mapping corpus callosum deficits in autism: An index of aberrant cortical connectivity. *Biological Psychiatry*, **60**, 218–225.

Vidal, C.N., Rapoport, J.L., Hayashi, K.M., Geaga, J.A., Sui, Y., McLemore, L.E., Alaghband, Y., Gochman, P., Blumenthal, J., Gogtay, N., Nicolson, R., Toga, A.W., and Thompson, P.M. (2006). Dynamically spreading frontal and cingulate deficits mapped in adolescents with schizophrenia. *Archives of General Psychiatry*, **63**, 25–34.

Videbech, P. (2000). PET measurements of brain glucose metabolism and blood flow in major depressive disorder: A critical review. *Acta Psychiatrica Scandinavica*, **101**, 11–20.

Vita, A., De Peri L., Silenzi, C., and Dieci, M. (2006). Brain morphology in first-episode schizophrenia: A meta-analysis of quantitative magnetic resonance imaging studies. *Schizophrenia Research*, **82**, 75–88.

Vogt, B.A. (2009a). Regions and subregions of the cingulate cortex. In B.A. Vogt (Ed.), *Cingulate Neurobiology and Disease* (pp. 3–30). New York, Oxford University Press.

Vogt, B.A. (2009b). Architecture, neurocytology and comparative organization of monkey and human cingulate cortices. In B.A. Vogt (Ed.), *Cingulate Neurobiology and Disease* (pp. 65–93). New York, Oxford University Press.

Vogt, B.A., and Laureys, S. (2005). Posterior cingulate, precuneal and retrospenial cortices: Cytology and components of the neural network correlates of consciousness. *Progress in Brain Research*, **150**, 205–217.

Vogt, B.A., and Vogt, L.J. (2009). μ-Opioid receptors, placebo map, descending systems, and cingulate-mediated control of vocalization. In B.A. Vogt (Ed.), *Cingulate Neurobiology and Disease* (pp. 339–364). New York, Oxford University Press.

Volk, D.W., Austin, M.C., Pierri, J.N., Sampson, A.R., and Lewis, D.A. (2000). Decreased glutamic acid decarboxylase$_{67}$ messenger RNA expression in a subset of prefrontal cortical R-aminobutyric acid neurons in subjects with schizophrenia. *Archives of General Psychiatry*, **57**, 237–245.

Volkow, N.D., Wang, G-J., Fowler, J.S., and Ding, Y-S. (2005). Imaging the effects of methylphenidate on brain dopamine: New model on its therapeutic actions for attention-deficit/hyperactivity disorder. *Biological Psychiatry,* **57**, 1410–1415.

Volkow, N.D., Wang, G-J., Kollins, S.H., Fowler, J.S., Wigal, T.L., Newcorn, J.H., Telang, F., Fowler, J.S., Zhu, W., Logan, J., Ma, Y., Pradham, K., Wong, C., and Swanson, J.M. (2005). Evaluating dopamine reward pathway in ADHD: Clinical implications. *Journal of the American Medical Association*, **302**, 1084–1091.

Volz, H-P., Gaser, C., and Sauer, H. (2000a). Supporting evidence for the model of cognitive dysmetria in schizophrenia- a structural magnetic resonance imaging study using deformation-based morphometry. *Schizophrenia Research*, **46**, 45–56.

Volz, H-P., Riehemann, S., Maurer, I., Smesney, S., Sommer, M., Rzanny, R., Hostein, W., Czekalla, J., and Sauer, H. (2000b). Reduced phosphodiesters and high-energy phosphates in the frontal lobe of schizophrenic patients: A ^{31}P chemical shift spectroscopic imaging study. *Biological Psychiatry*, **47**, 954–961.

Volz, H-P., Rzanny, R., May, S., Hegervald, H., Preufler, B., Hajek, M., Kaiser, W.A., and Sauer, H. (1997). ^{31}P magnetic resonance spectroscopy in the dorsolateral prefrontal cortex of schizophrenics with a volume selective technique: Preliminary findings. *Biological Psychiatry*, **41**, 644–648.

Volz, H.P., Rzanny, R., Riehemann, S., May, S., Hegewald, H., Preussler, B., Hubner, G., Kaiser, W.A., and Sauer, H. (1998a). ^{31}P magnetic resonance spectroscopy in the frontal lobe of major depressed patients. *European Archives of Psychiatry and Clinical Neuroscience*, **248**, 289–295.

Volz, H-P., Rzanny, R., Rossger, G., Hubner, G., Kreitschmann-Andermahr, I., Kaiser, W.A., and Sauer, H. (1998b). ^{31}P Phosphorous magnetic resonance spectroscopy of the dorsolateral prefrontal region in schizophrenics: A study including 50 patients and 36 controls. *Biological Psychiatry*, **44**, 399–404.

Voorn, P., Vanderschuren, L.J.M.J., Groenewegen, H.J., Robbins, T., and Pennartz, C.M.A. (2004). Putting a spin on the dorsal-ventral divide of the striatum. *Trends in Neurosciences*, **27**, 468–474.

Walker, E., and Lewine, R.J. (1990). Prediction of adult-onset schizophrenia from childhood home movies of the patients. *American Journal of Psychiatry*, **147**, 1052–1056.

Wallace, S., Coleman, M., Pascalis, O., and Bailey, A. (2006). A study of impaired judgement of eye-gaze direction and related face-processing deficits in autism spectrum disorders. *Perception*, **35**, 1651–1664.

Walsh, T., McClelland, J.M., McCarthy, S.E., Addington, A.M., Pierce, S.B., Cooper, G.M., Nord, A.S., Kusenda, M., Malhotra, D., Bhandari, A., Stray, S.M., Rippey, C.F., Roccanova, P., Makarov, V., Lakshmi B., Findling, R.L., Sikich, L., Stromberg, T., Merriman, B., Gogtay, N., Butler, P., Eckstrand, K., Noory, L., Gochman, P., Long, R., Chen, Z., Davis, S., Baker, C., Eichler, E.E., Meltzer, P.S., Nelson, S.F., Singleton, A.B., Lee, M.K., Rapoport, J.L., King, M.-C., and Sebat, J. (2008). Rare structural variants disrupt multiple genes in neurodevelopmental pathways in schizophrenia. *Science*, **320**, 539–543.

Wang, F., Kalmar, J.H., He Y., Jackowski, M., Chepenik, L.G., Edmiston, E.E., Tie, K., Gong, G., Shah, M.P., Jones, M., Uderman, J., Constable, R.T., and Blumberg, H.P. (2009). Functional and structural connectivity between the perigenual anterior cingulate and amygdala in bipolar disorder. *Biological Psychiatry*, **66**, 516–521.

Wang, F., Sun, Z., Cui, L., Du, X., Wang, X., Zhang, H., Cong, Z., Hong, N., and Zhang, D. (2004). Anterior cingulum abnormalities in male patients with schizophrenia determined through diffusion tensor imaging. *American Journal of Psychiatry*, **161**, 573–575.

Wang, Y., Cui, J., Chan, R.C.K., Deng, Y., Shi, H. Hong, X., Li, Z., Yu, X., Gong, Q., and Shum, D. (2009). Meta-analysis of prospective memory in schizophrenia: Nature, extent, and correlates. *Schizophrenia Research*, **114**, 64–70.

Ward, K.E., Friedman, L., Wise, A., and Schulz, S.C. (1996). Meta-analysis of brain and cranial size in schizophrenia. *Schizophrenia Research*, **22**, 197–213.

Wassef, A., Baker, J., and Kochan, L.D. (2003). GABA and schizophrenia: A review of basic science and clinical studies. *Journal of Clinical Psychopharmacology*, **23**, 601–640.

Waters, F.A.V., Maybery, M.T., Badcock, J.C., and Michie, P.T. (2004). Context memory and binding in schizophrenia. *Schizophrenia Research*, **68**, 119–125.

Waterworth, D.M., Bassett, A.S., and Brzustowicz, L.M. (2002). Recent advances in the genetics of schizophrenia. *Cellular and Molecular Life Sciences*, **59**, 331–348.

Watson, K.K., Jones, T.K., and Allman, J.M. (2006). Dendritic architecture of the Von Economo neurons. *Neuroscience*, **141**, 1107–1112.

Watson, K.K., Matthew, B.J., and Allman, J.A. (2007). Brain activation during sight gags and language-dependent humor. *Cerebral Cortex,* **17**, 314–324.

Wehr, T.A. (1992). Improvement of depression and triggering of mania by sleep deprivation. *Journal of the American Medical Association*, **267**, 548–551.

Weinberger, D.R. (1987). Implications of normal brain development for the pathogenesis of schizophrenia. *Archives of General Psychiatry*, **44**, 660–669.

Weinberger, D.R., Berman, K.F., and Zec, R.F. (1986). Physiological dysfunction of dorsolateral cortex in schizophrenia: I. Regional cerebral blood flow (rCBF) evidence. *Archives of General Psychiatry*, **43**, 114–124.

Wentz, E., Gillberg, I.C., Anckarsäter, H., Gillberg, C., and Råstam, M. (2009). Adolescent-onset anorexia nervosa: 18-year outcome. *British Journal of Psychiatry,* **194,** 168–174.

Whitty, P., Clarke, M., McTigue, O., Browne, S., Gervin, G., Kamali, M., Lane, A., Kinsella, A. Waddington, J., Larkin, C., and O'Callaghan, E. (2006). Diagnostic specificity and predictors of neurological soft signs in schizophrenia, bipolar disorder and other psychoses over the first 4 years of illness. *Schizophrenia Research*, **86**, 110–117.

Wible, C.G., Anderson, J., Shenton, M.E., Kricun, A., Hirayasu, Y., Tanaka, S., Levitt, J.J., O'Donnell, B.F., Kikinis, R., Jolesz, F.A., and McCarley, R.W. (2001). Prefrontal cortex, negative symptoms, and schizophrenia: An MRI study. *Psychiatry Research: Neuroimaging*, **108**, 65–78.

Williams, D.L., Goldstein, G., and Minshew, N.J. (2006a). Neuropsychological functioning in children with autism: Further evidence for disordered complex information-processing. *Child Neuropsychology*, **12**, 279–298.

Williams, J.B.W., Gibbon, M., First, M.B., Spitzer, R.L., Davies, M., Borus, J., Howes, M.J., Kane, J., Pope, H.G., Rounsaville, B., and Wittchen, H.-U. (1977). The Structured Clinical Interview for DSM-III-R(SCID)II. Multisite test-retest reliability. *Archives of General Psychiatry,* **4**, 1229–1235.

Williams, J.G., Higgins, J.P.T., and Brayne, C.E.G. (2006b). Systematic review of prevalence studies of autism spectrum disorders. *Archives of Disease in Childhood*, **91**, 8–15.

Williams, N.A., Close, J.P., Giouzeli, M., and Crow, T.J. (2006c). Accelerated evolution of *Protocadherin11X/Y*: A candidate gene-pair for cerebral asymmetry and language. *American Journal of Medical Genetics Part B (Neuropsychiatric Genetics)*, **141B**, 623–633.

Williamson, P. (2006). *Mind, Brain, and Schizophrenia.* New York, Oxford University Press.

Williamson, P. (2007). Are anticorrelated networks relevant to schizophrenia? *Schizophrenia Bulletin*, **33**, 994–1003.

Williamson, P., Drost, D., Stanley, J., Carr, T., Morrison, S., and Merskey, H. (1991). Localized phosphorus 31 nuclear magnetic resonance spectroscopy in chronic schizophrenic patients and normal controls. *Archives of General Psychiatry*, **48**, 578.

Wilson, T.W., Rojas, D.C., Reite, M.L., Teale, P.D., and Rogers, S.J. (2007). Children and adolescents with autism exhibit reduced MEG steady-state gamma responses. *Biological Psychiatry*, **62**, 192–197.

Wing, L. (1991). The relationship between Asperger's syndrome and Kanner's autism. In U. Frith (Ed.), *Autism and Asperger Syndrome.* Cambridge, U.K., Cambridge University Press.

Winokur, G., and Clayton, P. (1967). Family history studies I: Two types of affective disorders separated according to genetic and clinical factors. In J. Wortis (Ed.), *Recent Advances in Biological Psychiatry* (pp. 35–50), volume 9. New York, Plenum.

Winokur, J., Cryell, W., Endicott, J., and Akiskal, H. (1993). Further distinctions between manic-depressive illness (bipolar disorder) and primary depressive disorder. *American Journal of Psychiatry*, **150**, 1176–1186.

Wise, R.J.S. (2003). Language systems in normal and aphasic human subjects: Functional imaging studies and inferences from animal studies. *British Medical Bulletin*, **65**, 95–119.

Wise, S.P., Murray, E.A., and Gerfen, C.R. (1996). The frontal cortex-basal ganglia system in primates. *Critical Reviews in Neurobiology*, **10**, 317–356.

Wolkin, A. Sanfilipo, M., Wolf, A.P., Angrist, B., Brodie, J.D., and Rotrosen, J. (1992). Negative symptoms and hypofrontality in chronic schizophrenia. *Archives of General Psychiatry*, **49**, 959–965.

Wood, J.N., and Grafman, J. (2003). Human prefrontal cortex: Processing and representational perspectives. *Nature Reviews Neuroscience*, **4**,139–147.

Wood, S.J., Pantelis, C., Velakoulis, D., Yücel, M., Fornito, A., and McGorry, P.D. (2008). Progressive changes in the development toward schizophrenia: Studies in subjects at increased symptomatic risk. *Schizophrenia Bulletin*, **34**, 322–329.

Wood, S.J., Velakoulis, D., Smith, D.J., Bond, D., Stuart, G.W., McGorry, P.D., Brewer, W.J., Bridle, N., Eritaia, J., Desmond, P., Singh, B., Copolov, D., and Pantelis, C. (2001). A longitudinal study of hippocampal volume in first episode psychosis and chronic schizophrenia. *Schizophrenia Research*, **52**, 37–46.

Woodruff, P.W.R., Wright, I.C., Bullmore, E.T., Brammer, M., Howard, R.J., Williams, S.C.R., Shapleske, J., Rossell, S., David, A.S., McGuire, P.K., and Murray, R.M. (1997). Auditory hallucinations and the temporal cortical response to speech in schizophrenia: A functional magnetic resonance imaging study. *American Journal of Psychiatry*, **154**, 1676–1682.

Woods, B.T. (1998). Is schizophrenia a progressive neurodevelopmental disorder? Toward a unitary pathogenetic mechanism. *American Journal of Psychiatry*, **155**, 1661–1670.

Woods, B.T., and Yurgelin-Todd, D. (1991). Brain volume loss in schizophrenia: When does it occur and is it progressive? *Schizophrenia Research*, **5**, 202–204.

Woods, B.T., Yurgelin-Todd, D., Goldstein, J., Seidman, L.J., and Tsuang, M.T. (1996). MRI brain abnormalities in schizophrenia: One process or more? *Biological Psychiatry*, **40**, 585–596.

Woods, C.G., Bond, J., and Wolfgang, E. (2005). Autosomal recessive primary microcephaly (MCPH): A review of clinical, molecular, and evolutionary findings. *American Journal of Human Genetics*, **76**, 717–728.

Woodward, J., and Allman, J. (2007). Moral intuition: Its neural substrates and normative significance. *Journal of Physiology-Paris,* **101**, 179–202.

Woolley, J.D., Gorno-Tempini, M.-L., Seeley, W.W., Rankin, K., Lee, S.S., Matthews, B.R., and Miller, B.L. (2007). Binge eating is associated with right orbitofrontal-insular-striatal atrophy in frontotemporal dementia. *Neurology*, **69**, 1424–1433.

Wright, A.A. (1998). Auditory list memory in rhesus monkeys. *Psychological Science*, **9**, 91–98.

Wright, I.C., Rabe-Hesketh, S., Woodruff, P.W.R., David, A.S., Murray, R.M., and Bullmore, E.T. (2000). Meta-analysis of regional brain volumes in schizophrenia. *American Journal of Psychiatry*, **157**, 16–25.

Wu, J.C., and Bunney, W.E. (1990). The biological basis of an antidepressant response to sleep deprivation and relapse: Review and hypothesis. *American Journal of Psychiatry*, **147**, 14–21.

Yacubian, J., de Castro, C.C., Ometto, M., Barbosa, E., de Camargo, C.P., Tavares, H., Cerri, G.G., and Gattaz, W.F. (2002). 31 P-spectroscopy of frontal lobe in schizophrenia: Alterations in phospholipids and high-energy phosphate metabolism. *Schizophrenia Research*, **58**, 117–122.

Yang, M.S., and Gill, M. (2007). A review of gene linkage, association and expression studies in autism and an assessment of convergent evidence. *International Journal of Developmental Neurosience*, **25**, 69–85.

Yang, Y., and Schmitt, H.P. (2001). Frontotemporal dementia: Evidence for impairment of ascending serotoninergic but not noradrenergic innervation. Immunocytochemical and quantitative study using a graph method. *Acta Neuropathologica*, **101**, 256–270.

Yatham, L.N., Liddle, P.F., Shiah, I.-S., Lam, R.W., Ngan, E., Scarrow, G., Imperial, M., Stoessl, J., Sossi, V., and Ruth, J. (2002). PET study of [^{18}F]6-fluoro-L-dopa uptake in neuroleptic- and mood-stabilizer-naïve first-episode nonpsychotic mania: Effects of treatment with divalproex sodium. *American Journal of Psychiatry*, **159**, 768–774.

Yeap, S., Kelly, S.P., Sehatpour, P., Magno, E., Garavan, H., Thakore, J.H., and Foxe, J.J. (2008). Visual sensory processing deficits in schizophrenia and their relationship to disease state. *European Archives of Psychiatry and Clinical Neuroscience,* **258,** 305–316.

Yildiz, A., Demopoulis, C.M., Moore, C.M., Renshaw, P.F., and Sachs, G.S. (2001). Effect of lithium on phosphoinositide metabolism in human brain: A proton decoupled 31P nuclear magnetic resonance spectroscopy study. *Biological Psychiatry*, **50**, 3–7.

Yildiz-Yesiloglu, A., and Ankerst, D.P. (2006a). Review of ^{1}H magnetic resonance spectroscopy findings in major depressive disorder: A meta-analysis. *Psychiatry Research; Neuroimaging*, **147**, 1–25.

Yildiz-Yesiloglu, A., and Ankerst, D.P. (2006b). Neurochemical alterations of the brain in bipolar disorder and their implications for pathophysiology: A systematic review of the in vivo proton magnetic resonance spectroscopy findings. *Progress in Neuro-Psychopharmacology and Biological Psychiatry*, **30**, 969–995.

Young, K.A., Manaye, K.F., Liang, C, Hicks, P.B., and German, D.C. (2000) Reduced number of mediodorsal and anterior thalamic neurons in schizophrenia. *Biological Psychiatry*, **47**, 944–953.

Young, L.T., Warsh, J.J., Kish, S.J., Shannak, K., and Hornykeiwicz, O. (1994). Reduced brain 5-HT and elevated NE turnover and metabolites in bipolar affective disorder. *Biological Psychiatry*, **35**, 121–127.

Yukie, M., and Shibata, H. (2009). Temporocingulate interactions in the monkey. In B.A. Vogt (Ed.), *Cingulate Neurobiology and Disease* (pp. 145–162). New York, Oxford University Press.

Yurgelun-Todd, D.A., Gruber, S.A., Kanayama, G., Killgore, W.D.S., Baird, A.A., and Young, A.D. (2000). fMRI during affect discrimination in bipolar affective disorder. *Bipolar Disorders*, **2**, 237–248.

Yurgelun-Todd, D.A., Renshaw, P.F., Gruber, S.A., Ed, M., Waternaux, C., and Cohen, B.M. (1996). Proton magnetic resonance spectroscopy of the temporal lobes in schizophrenics and normal controls. *Schizophrenia Research*, **19**, 55–59.

Zahn, R., Moll, J., Krueger, F., Huey, E.D., Garrido, G., and Grafman, J. (2007). Social concepts are represented in the superior anterior temporal cortex. *Proceedings of the National Academy of Sciences of the USA*, **104**, 6430–6435.

Zakzanis, K.K., and Hansen, K.T. (1998). Dopamine D_2 densities and the schizophrenic brain. *Schizophrenia Research*, **32**, 201–206.

Zakzanis, K.K., Poulin, P., Hansen, K.T., and Jolic, D. (2000). Searching the schizophrenic brain for temporal lobe deficits: A systematic review and meta-analysis. *Psychological Medicine*, **30**, 491–504.

Zatorre, R.J., and Gandour, J.T. (2008). Neural specializations for speech and pitch: Moving beyond dichotomies. *Philosophical Transactions of the Royal Society B*, **363**, 1087–1104.

Zhou, Y., Liang, M., Tian, L., Wang, K., Hao, Y., Liu, H., Liu, Z., and Jiang, T. (2007). Functional disintegration in paranoid schizophrenia using resting-state fMRI. *Schizophrenia Research*, **97**, 194–205.

Zhou, Y., Shu, N., Liu, Y., Song, M., Hao, Y., Liu, H., Yu, C., Liu, Z., and Jiang, T. (2008). Altered resting-state functional connectivity and anatomical connectivity of hippocampus in schizophrenia. *Schizophrenia Research*, **100**, 120–132.

Zilbovicius, M., Meresse, I., Chabane, N., Brunelle, F., Samson, Y., and Boddaert, N. (2006). Autism, the superior temporal sulcus and social perception. *Trends in Neurosciences*, **29**, 359–366.

Zipursky, R.B., Lambe, E.K., Kapur, S., and Mikulis, D.J. (1998). Cerebral gray matter volume deficits in first episode psychosis. *Archives of General Psychiatry*, **55**, 540–546.

Zipursky, R.B., Lim, K.O., Sullivan, E.V., Brown, B.W., and Pfefferbaum, A. (1992). Widespread cerebral gray matter volume deficits in schizophrenia. *Archives of General Psychiatry*, **49**, 195–205.

Zucker, N.L., Losh, M., Bulik, C.M., LaBar, K.S., Piven, J., and Pelphrey, K.A. (2007). Anorexia nervosa and autism spectrum disorders: Guided investigation of social cognitive endophenotypes. *Psychological Bulletin,* **133,** 976–1006.

Index

Note: Page numbers followed by "*f*" denote figures.